Neurochemical Correlates of Cerebral Ischemia

Advances in Neurochemistry

SERIES EDITORS

B. W. Agranoff, *University of Michigan, Ann Arbor*
M. H. Aprison, *Indiana University School of Medicine, Indianapolis*

ADVISORY EDITORS

J. Axelrod	F. Margolis	P. Morell	J. S. O'Brien
F. Fonnum	B. S. McEwen	W. T. Norton	E. Roberts

A Continuation Order Plan is available for this series. A continuation order will bring delivery of each new volume immediately upon publication. Volumes are billed only upon actual shipment. For further information please contact the publisher.

Neurochemical Correlates of Cerebral Ischemia

Edited by

Nicolas G. Bazan
Louisiana State University Medical Center
New Orleans, Louisiana

Pierre Braquet
Institut Henri Beaufour
Paris, France

and

Myron D. Ginsberg
University of Miami School of Medicine
Miami, Florida

PLENUM PRESS • NEW YORK AND LONDON

Library of Congress Cataloging-in-Publication Data

Neurochemical correlates of cerebral ischemia / edited by Nicolas G.
  Bazan, Pierre Braquet, and Myron D. Ginsbery.
       p.   cm. -- (Advances in neurochemistry ; v. 7)
    Includes bibliographical references and index.
    ISBN 0-306-43944-1
    1. Cerebral ischemia--Pathophysiology. 2. Neurochemistry.
  I. Bazán, Nicolás G. II. Braquet, P. (Pierre) III. Ginsberg, Myron
  D. IV. Series.
    [DNLM: 1. Brain Damage, Chronic--metabolism. 2. Cerebral
  Ischemia--metabolism. 3. Cerebral Ischemia--physiopathology.
  4. Neurochemistry.   W1 AD684E v.7 / /WL 355 N4943]
  QP356.3.H37 vol. 7
  [RC388.5]
  599'.0188 s--dc20
  [616.8'1]
  DNLM/DLC
  for Library of Congress   92-9177
                                                                CIP

ISBN 0-306-43944-1

© 1992 Plenum Press, New York
A Division of Plenum Publishing Corporation
233 Spring Street, New York, N.Y. 10013

Printed in the United States of America

CONTRIBUTORS

TAKAO ASANO • *Department of Neurosurgery, Saitama Medical Center, Saitama Medical School, Saitama, Japan*

A. BAETHMANN • *Institute for Surgical Research, Klinikum Grosshadern, Ludwig Maximilians University, 8000 München 70, and Institute of Neurosurgical Pathophysiology, University of Mainz, 6500 Mainz, Germany*

ROHIT BAKSHI • *Departments of Neurology and Neurosurgery, University of California, San Francisco, California*

NICOLAS G. BAZAN • *LSU Eye Center and Neuroscience Center, LSU Medical Center School of Medicine, New Orleans, Louisiana*

PIERRE BRAQUET • *Institut Henri Beaufour, 92350 Le Plessis Robinson, Paris, France*

PAK H. CHAN • *CNS Injury and Edema Research Center, Department of Neurology, School of Medicine, University of California, San Francisco, California*

THELMA CHAN • *CNS Injury and Edema Research Center, Department of Neurology, School of Medicine, University of California, San Francisco, California*

CHU KUANG CHEN • *Departments of Pediatrics and Neurology, Neuroscience Program, University of Michigan, Ann Arbor, Michigan*

SYLVIA CHEN • *CNS Injury and Edema Research Center, Department of Neurology, School of Medicine, University of California, San Francisco, California*

LILLIAN CHU • *CNS Injury and Edema Research Center, Department of Neurology, School of Medicine, University of California, San Francisco, California*

RHOBERT W. EVANS • *Department of Anesthesiology and Critical Care Medicine, University of Pittsburgh, School of Medicine, Pittsburgh, Pennsylvania*

ALAN I. FADEN • *Departments of Neurology and Neurosurgery, University of California, San Francisco, California*

AKHLAQ A. FAROOQUI • *Department of Medical Biochemistry, The Ohio State University, Columbus, Ohio*

TAHIRA FAROOQUI • *Division of Pharmacology, College of Pharmacy, The Ohio State University, Columbus, Ohio*

STEPHEN K. FISHER • *Department of Pharmacology, University of Michigan, Ann Arbor, Michigan*

MYRON D. GINSBERG • *Cerebral Vascular Disease Research Center, Department of Neurology, University of Miami School of Medicine, Miami, Florida*

STEVEN H. GRAHAM • *Departments of Neurology and Neurosurgery, University of California, San Francisco, California*

GEORGE A. GREGORY • *CNS Injury and Edema Research Center, Department of Neurology, School of Medicine, University of California, San Francisco, California*

J. A. HELPERN • *Center for Stroke Research, Department of Neurology, Henry Ford Hospital and Health Science Center, Detroit, Michigan, and Department of Physics, Oakland University, Rochester, Michigan*

YUTAKA HIRASHIMA • *Department of Medical Biochemistry, The Ohio State University, Columbus, Ohio*

LLOYD A. HORROCKS • *Department of Medical Biochemistry, The Ohio State University, Columbus, Ohio*

K.-A. HOSSMANN • *Department of Experimental Neurology, Max Planck Institute for Neurological Research, D-5000 Cologne 41, Germany*

SHIGEKI IMAIZUMI • *CNS Injury and Edema Research Center, Department of Neurology, School of Medicine, University of California, San Francisco, California*

MICHAEL V. JOHNSTON • *Departments of Pediatrics and Neurology, Johns Hopkins University and Kennedy Institute, Baltimore, Maryland*

JUDITH A. KELLEHER • *CNS Injury and Edema Research Center, Department of Neurology, School of Medicine, University of California, San Francisco, California*

O. KEMPSKI • *Institute for Surgical Research, Klinikum Grosshadern, Ludwig Maximilians University, 8000 München 70, and Institute of Neurosurgical Pathophysiology, University of Mainz, 6500 Mainz, Germany*

PATRICK M. KOCHANEK • *Department of Anesthesiology and Critical Care Medicine, University of Pittsburgh, School of Medicine, Pittsburgh, Pennsylvania*

KYUYA KOGURE • *Department of Neurology, Institute of Brain Diseases, 1-1 Seiryo-Machi, Aoba-Ku, Sendai, Japan*

JOSEPH C. LAMANNA • *Departments of Neurology and Physiology/ Biophysics, Case Western Reserve University School of Medicine and University Hospitals of Cleveland, Cleveland, Ohio*

MATTHIAS LEMKE • *Departments of Neurology and Neurosurgery, University of California, San Francisco, California*

STEVEN R. LEVINE • *Center for Stroke Research, Department of Neurology, Henry Ford Hospital and Health Science Center, Detroit, Michigan*

W. DAVID LUST • *Laboratory of Experimental Neurosurgery, Department of Neurosurgery, Case Western Reserve University School of Medicine and University Hospitals of Cleveland, Cleveland, Ohio*

G. B. MARTIN • *Department of Emergency Medicine, Henry Ford Hospital and Health Science Center, Detroit, Michigan*

BRIAN MELDRUM • *Department of Neurology, Institute of Psychiatry, London, United Kingdom*

SHINICHI NAKANO • *Department of Neurology, Institute of Brain Diseases, 1-1 Seiryo-Machi, Aoba-Ku, Sendai, Japan*

EDWIN M. NEMOTO • *Department of Anesthesiology and Critical Care Medicine, University of Pittsburgh, School of Medicine, Pittsburgh, Pennsylvania*

W. PASCHEN • *Department of Experimental Neurology, Max Planck Institute for Neurological Research, D-5000 Cologne 41, Germany*

ROBERT A. RATCHESON • *Laboratory of Experimental Neurosurgery, Department of Neurosurgery, Case Western Reserve University School of Medicine and University Hospitals of Cleveland, Cleveland, Ohio*

WARREN R. SELMAN • *Laboratory of Experimental Neurosurgery, Department of Neurosurgery, Case Western Reserve University School of Medicine and University Hospitals of Cleveland, Cleveland, Ohio*

TAKAO SHIMIZU • *Department of Biochemistry, Faculty of Medicine, University of Tokyo, Tokyo, Japan*

FAYE S. SILVERSTEIN • *Departments of Pediatrics and Neurology, Neuroscience Program, University of Michigan, Ann Arbor, Michigan*

DANIEL STATMAN • *Departments of Pediatrics and Neurology, Neuroscience Program, University of Michigan, Ann Arbor, Michigan*

GRACE Y. SUN • *Biochemistry Department, University of Missouri, Columbia, Missouri*

TAKASHI WATANABE • *Division of Neurosurgery, Institute of Neurological Sciences, Tottori University of Medicine, Yonago, Japan*

PHILLIP WEINSTEIN • *Departments of Neurology and Neurosurgery, University of California, San Francisco, California*

K. M. A. WELCH • *Center for Stroke Research, Department of Neurology, Henry Ford Hospital and Health Science Center, Detroit, Michigan*

FRANK A. WELSH • *Division of Neurosurgery, University of Pennsylvania, Philadelphia, Pennsylvania*

DAVID F. WILSON • *Department of Biochemistry and Biophysics, Medical School, University of Pennsylvania, Philadelphia, Pennsylvania*

SABRINA YUM • *Departments of Neurology and Neurosurgery, University of California, San Francisco, California*

PREFACE

This volume summarizes current knowledge on neurochemical correlates of cerebral ischemia, emphasizing their relevance to function and their pathophysiological significance.

The study of neurochemical correlates of cerebral ischemia and trauma provides a strong foundation for the definition of mechanisms of damage, the identification of possible therapeutic targets, and the assessment of new drugs. The pathophysiological roles of oxygen radicals, protein and polyamine metabolism, biologically active lipids, metabolic alterations, excitatory amino acid neurotransmitters, cell signaling, second messengers, inositol lipids, pyruvate dehydrogenase, and other neurochemical events are described.

We thank the authors for their efforts in contributing updates of their work for inclusion in this volume. Although we have a central focus throughout this book and, therefore, unity, we did not want to impose restrictions on the contributors. The outcome is well balanced, partially overlapping in some cases, and in many instances includes discussion of the clinical relevance of the neurochemical correlates described as well as future research directions. This book is not the proceedings of a meeting but reflects the achievement of our goal to generate a source of current ideas on the subject.

The Editors

CONTENTS

CHAPTER 3

ROLE OF PYRUVATE DEHYDROGENASE IN ISCHEMIC INJURY

FRANK A. WELSH

CHAPTER 4

DISTURBANCES OF PROTEIN AND POLYAMINE METABOLISM AFTER REVERSIBLE CEREBRAL ISCHEMIA

K.-A. HOSSMANN AND W. PASCHEN

CHAPTER 5

OXYGEN DEPENDENCE OF NEURONAL METABOLISM

DAVID F. WILSON

CHAPTER 6

DYSMETABOLISM IN LIPID BRAIN ISCHEMIA

KYUYA KOGURE AND SHINICHI NAKANO

CHAPTER 7

INVOLVEMENT OF CALCIUM, LIPOLYTIC ENZYMES, AND FREE FATTY ACIDS IN ISCHEMIC BRAIN TRAUMA

AKHLAQ A. FAROOQUI, YUTAKA HIRASHIMA, TAHIRA FAROOQUI, AND LLOYD A. HORROCKS

CHAPTER 8

ARACHIDONIC ACID LIPOXYGENASE PRODUCTS PARTICIPATE IN THE PATHOGENESIS OF DELAYED CEREBRAL ISCHEMIA

TAKASHI WATANABE, TAKAO ASANO, AND TAKAO SHIMIZU

CHAPTER 9

BIOCHEMICAL CHANGES AND SECONDARY TISSUE INJURY AFTER
BRAIN AND SPINAL CORD ISCHEMIA/REPERFUSION

ALAN I. FADEN, PHILLIP WEINSTEIN, ROHIT BAKSHI, SABRINA YUM,
MATTHIAS LEMKE, AND STEVEN H. GRAHAM

CHAPTER 10

FREE FATTY ACID LIBERATION IN THE PATHOGENESIS AND THERAPY
OF ISCHEMIC BRAIN DAMAGE

EDWIN M. NEMOTO, RHOBERT W. EVANS, AND PATRICK M. KOCHANEK

CHAPTER 11

CEREBRAL ISCHEMIA AND POLYPHOSPHOINOSITIDE METABOLISM

GRACE Y. SUN

CHAPTER 12

PROTECTION AGAINST ISCHEMIC BRAIN DAMAGE BY EXCITATORY AMINO ACID ANTAGONISTS

BRIAN MELDRUM

CHAPTER 13

ACUTE ALTERATIONS IN PHOSPHOINOSITIDE TURNOVER

FAYE S. SILVERSTEIN, CHU KUANG CHEN, STEPHEN K. FISHER, DANIEL STATMAN, AND MICHAEL V. JOHNSTON

CHAPTER 14

NEW INSIGHTS INTO THE ROLE OF OXYGEN RADICALS IN CEREBRAL ISCHEMIA

PAK H. CHAN, SYLVIA CHEN, SHIGEKI IMAIZUMI, LILLIAN CHU, JUDITH A. KELLEHER, GEORGE A. GREGORY, AND THELMA CHAN

CHAPTER 15

BIOCHEMICAL FACTORS AND MECHANISMS OF SECONDARY BRAIN DAMAGE IN CEREBRAL ISCHEMIA AND TRAUMA

A. BAETHMANN AND O. KEMPSKI

CHAPTER 16

MODULATORS OF NEURAL CELL SIGNALING AND TRIGGERING OF GENE EXPRESSION FOLLOWING CEREBRAL ISCHEMIA

NICOLAS G. BAZAN

CHAPTER 17

CELLULAR AND METABOLIC SIGNIFICANCE OF CELLULAR ACID-BASE SHIFTS IN HUMAN STROKE

K. M. A. WELCH, STEVEN R. LEVINE, G. B. MARTIN, AND J. A. HELPERN

Neurochemical Correlates of Cerebral Ischemia

INTRODUCTION
Current Biochemical and Molecular Approaches to the Study of Cerebral Ischemia

MYRON D. GINSBERG, PIERRE BRAQUET, and NICOLAS G. BAZAN

1. INTRODUCTION

Cerebral ischemia—the most prevalent form of clinical stroke—is a medical problem of the first magnitude. Despite rather convincing evidence of declining

MYRON D. GINSBERG • *Cerebral Vascular Disease Research Center, Department of Neurology, University of Miami School of Medicine, Miami, Florida.* *PIERRE BRAQUET* • *Institut Henri Beaufour, 92350 Le Plessis Robinson, Paris, France.* *NICOLAS G. BAZAN* • *LSU Eye Center and Neuroscience Center, LSU Medical Center School of Medicine, New Orleans, Louisiana.*

Neurochemical Correlates of Cerebral Ischemia, Volume 7 of *Advances in Neurochemistry*, edited by Nicolas G. Bazan, Pierre Braquet, and Myron D. Ginsberg. Plenum Press, New York, 1992.

incidence of and mortality from stroke over the past decades (Scheinberg, 1988), it remains the third leading cause of death in the United States, as well as the major source of chronic disability, whose cost is reckoned in billions of dollars per annum and whose emotional impact is devastating (Hachinski and Norris, 1985). Traditional therapeutic approaches, largely supportive and directed at systemic factors, have tended to create a nihilistic attitude toward the potential for effective therapy of this disorder. This attitude is now changing as a result of impressive scientific advances, often carried out at a very basic level, that are shedding light on basic stroke pathomechanisms and are suggesting promising therapeutic approaches, some of which are now beginning to enter the clinical arena.

The problem of ischemic brain injury may be introduced by considering the high and incessant metabolic demand of the brain, its absolute dependence upon glucose provision, and its consequent susceptibility to functional, electrical, bioenergetic, and ionic failure as cerebral perfusion declines below critical threshold levels (Astrup *et al.*, 1977; Heiss and Rosner, 1983; Sokoloff, 1976). The attempts of ischemic tissue to continue its metabolic activity in the face of restricted oxygen supply are inevitably short-lived (Baron, 1985). In Chapter 5 of this volume, D. F. Wilson carefully considers the manner in which neuronal metabolism critically depends upon oxygen provision to tissue.

Current biochemical and molecular approaches to brain ischemia necessitate the rigorous use of controlled experimental animal preparations (Garcia, 1984; Molinari, 1988; Molinari and Laurent, 1976). The particular utility of rodent ischemia models has been recently reviewed (Ginsberg and Busto, 1989). When one surveys current work being carried out in in vivo ischemia models as well as in simpler neuronal-slice or cell culture systems, certain areas emerge as pivotal foci of research interest. Many of these factors are reviewed in Chapter 9 of this volume by A. I. Faden *et al.*, who underscore the multifactorial nature of secondary factors in ischemic injury and emphasize the likelihood that effective pharmacotherapy will probably necessitate the use of combinations of effective agents. In Chapter 2 of this volume, W. D. Lust *et al.* provide a broad review of the metabolic correlates of focal cerebral ischemia, emphasizing the factors that influence deterioration of the "perifocal" region. In Chapter 15 of this volume, A. Baethmann *et al.* discuss potential factors mediating secondary damage in the settings of head injury and ischemia; they propose three guidelines for assessing the importance of these mediators: (1) that such substances be shown to be induced by cerebral damage; (2) that they be formed and released in proportion to insult severity; and (3) that specific inhibition of their release or function lead to reduced damage. To epitomize, comprehending ischemic brain injury is, of necessity, a polyglot endeavor requiring a broad purview and a menu of complementary experimental approaches. In the paragraphs below, attention is directed to the most salient of these areas.

2. ROLE OF CALCIUM ION AND ENZYME ACTIVATION IN ISCHEMIA

Ionized calcium functions widely as a cellular messenger and intracellular regulator (Carafoli, 1987). Although cellular calcium dyshomeostasis has been postulated to be critical in producing cellular injury in general (Cheung *et al.*, 1986) and ischemic brain injury in particular (Hass, 1981), both experimental-animal and clinical efforts directed at blocking voltage-sensitive calcium channels have met with only mixed therapeutic success in averting the consequences of brain ischemia (Ginsberg, 1989). It is probable that calcium enters neurons during ischemia not only through voltage-dependent ion channels but also through agonist-dependent and even nonspecific ion channels as cellular bioenergetics deteriorate. In addition, calcium is probably released as well from intracellular storage sites during ischemia. From these considerations, one would suspect that blockade of voltage-dependent calcium channels alone might not necessarily confer cerebroprotection. In experimental studies, when calcium channel blockers exhibit effectiveness, this is typically most impressive with pre-ischemic adminis-tration, and patterns of tissue rescue at times are suggestive of a hemodynamic mechanism (Ginsberg, 1989). We have recently described a dramatic protective effect of a novel phenylalklyamine calcium channel blocker in experimental ischemia (Nakayama *et al.*, 1988), but the mechanism of its protective effect may involve its associated serotonin S_2-antagonist property; this remains to be clari-fied, and studies are in progress.

The deleterious sequelae of ischemia-induced increases in intracellular cyto-solic calcium are thought to be mediated via activation of phospholipases. In Chapter 7 of this volume, A. A. Farooqui *et al.* emphasize that phospholipase activation is a complex and multifactorial process involving several different enzyme systems; there may be differential activation of two distinct types of phospholipase A_2 in ongoing ischemia. In Chapter 11, G. Y. Sun considers in detail the area of polyphosphoinositide metabolism and its relationship to intra-cellular signal transduction; she also discusses possible mechanisms triggering polyphosphoinositide breakdown in ischemia. In Chapter 10, E. M. Nemoto *et al.* analyze how phospholipid hydrolysis and free fatty acid accumulation contribute to ischemic brain injury.

In Chapter 3, F. A. Welsh considers another important enzyme, pyruvate dehydrogenase, located in mitochondria and activated during ischemia but inhib-ited during postischemic recirculation. He proposes the "working hypothesis" that activation of calcium-dependent protein kinases leads to the phosphorylation of many proteins, including pyruvate dehydrogenase, during recirculation; the re-sulting inhibition of this enzyme causes a decreased generation of NADH reducing equivalents needed for oxidative phosphorylation. In Chapter 4, K.-A. Hossmann and W. Paschen provide a general review of the subject of protein metabolism in ischemia and the emerging area of selective gene expression; these authors also consider the relevance of polyamine metabolism to ischemic cell death.

3. NEUROTRANSMITTER MEDIATION OF ISCHEMIC BRAIN INJURY

It has become firmly established that excitotoxic mechanisms play a pivotal role in at least some forms of hypoxic/ischemic neuronal injury (Meldrum, 1989; Rothman and Olney, 1986, 1987), which are directly relevant to the human setting of brain injury following cardiac arrest (Petito *et al.*, 1987), and probably to focal ischemic stroke. It is quite probable, however, that multiple neurotransmitter/ neuromodulatory systems participate in mediating neuronal damage. Strong evidence has been adduced for the participatory role of the dopaminergic system in injury to striatal neurons (Globus *et al.*, 1987, 1988a, b). Importantly, these studies have raised the possibility that dopamine and glutamate act in concert to damage vulnerable neurons (Globus *et al.*, 1988b). Combined treatment with a dopamine D-1 agonist and an *N*-methyl-D-aspartate (NMDA) receptor blocker has been shown to protect against ischemic injury—an effect not observed with either agent alone (Globus *et al.*, 1988c). Antagonists of the NMDA receptor have themselves met with mixed success in achieving cerebroprotection (Shearman, 1989). In Chapter 12 of this volume, B. Meldrum reviews the issue of cerebral protection afforded by excitatory amino acid antagonists. In general, this is an area of extraordinary clinical interest which will continue to be extensively explored. In Chapter 13, F. S. Silverstein *et al.* discuss the intriguing ability of the excitatory neurotransmitter agonist quisqualate to stimulate the turnover of inositol phospholipids in tissues obtained from hypoxic-ischemic brain—the cerebral insult thus serving to augment the responsiveness of neural tissue to this agonist.

4. PLASMA GLUCOSE LEVEL AND THE ROLE OF BRAIN ACIDOSIS

Studies over the past decade have unequivocally established the injurious role of elevated plasma glucose levels in the setting of brain ischemia (Ginsberg *et al.*, 1980; Myers and Yamaguchi, 1977; Nedergaard, 1987; Pulsinelli *et al.*, 1982; Welsh *et al.*, 1980). Recent evidence of compartmentalization of hydrogen ion buffering within glial cells during ischemia (Kraig *et al.*, 1985, 1986) suggests that tissue necrosis may be triggered by the exhaustion of glial buffering capacity. The deleterious effect of glucose appears to be present only in regions potentially susceptible to collateral perfusion but not in zones of end-arterial supply (Prado *et al.*, 1988). Translating these findings to the clinical setting is difficult, however, owing in part to the confounding facts that diabetics generally tend to fare worse after a stroke and that stress-induced hyperglycemia may occur secondarily following acute stroke and complicate the interpretation of the significance of elevated plasma glucose levels. Nonetheless, this area of concern remains therapeutically significant, deserving of further clinical exploration. In Chapter 17 of this volume, K. M. A. Welch *et al.* discuss the ability of ^{31}P magnetic resonance spectroscopy to provide measurements of regional intracellular pH in humans. Their data underscore the variability of brain pH and energetics in acute clinical stroke and direct attention to the puzzling tissue alkalosis that is observed following the initial acidosis of early stroke. Preliminary findings from this group support the notion that high plasma glucose levels contribute to brain acidosis and poor outcome. Additionally, their pilot data in patients studied during after cardiac arrest serve to emphasize the potential value of this type of clinical application of the technique.

5. IMPORTANCE OF BRAIN TEMPERATURE IN ISCHEMIC INJURY

Although it has long been appreciated that major reductions of whole-body temperature protect against cerebral ischemic injury (Rosomoff, 1957), recent studies from our laboratory have convincingly shown that a mild degree of selective brain hypothermia may also confer significant cerebroprotection (Busto *et al.*, 1989a, b; Ginsberg *et al.*, 1989). These promising results strongly encourage the need for both neurochemical investigations of the factors mediating this protective effect and further experimental and, eventually, clinical studies in the setting of cardiac arrest and stroke.

6. OXYGEN RADICALS AND LIPID-DERIVED MEDIATORS OF ISCHEMIC INJURY

In an era in which clot-specific thrombolytic therapy for early acute ischemic stroke is undergoing active clinical exploration (Levy *et al.*, 1989; Zivin, 1989), one must reconsider whether cerebral reperfusion itself contributes to brain injury and, if so, whether this injury is mediated via oxygen radical mechanisms. Although oxygen radicals are often proposed as a mechanism of ischemic brain injury (Siesjö, 1981), the unequivocal demonstration that they play an important role in mediating parenchymal brain damage in ischemia has proven extremely elusive. Nonetheless, convincing evidence of oxygen radical generation has been obtained from studies on the pial surface (Wei and Kontos, 1987), suggesting that these radicals have a blood vessel origin; topical free-radical scavengers effect reversal of vascular abnormalities observed following complete ischemia (Kontos, 1989). In Chapter 14 of this volume, P. H. Chan *et al.* emphasize some of the newer important aspects of oxygen radical involvement in brain injury and emphasize how arachidonic acid, whose metabolism involves the generation of oxygen radicals, can have several pathological effects on cellular systems, including the intercalation of arachidonate into lipid membranes; its action as an intracellular messenger, leading to calcium mobilization and activation of protein kinases; and its role in inhibiting glutamate uptake. These authors address the important issue of superoxide dismutase as a therapeutic agent and discuss the measures that must be taken to enhance its accessibility to brain cells. In Chapter 8 of this volume, T. Watanabe *et al.* implicate the activation of lipoxygenase pathways as possibly relevant to the pathogenesis of cerebral vasospasm in subarachnoid hemorrhage.

7. CONCLUDING OBSERVATIONS

The study of cerebral ischemia is now well positioned to benefit from the explosion of insights provided by recent developments in cellular and molecular neuroscience. The development of novel therapeutic strategies for ischemic stroke must of necessity rely upon rigorous basic-science approaches, directed at understanding (1) the mechanism of brain-parenchymal injury, (2) cerebrovascular responses, and (3) the biochemical and molecular mechanisms underlying synaptic plasticity and recovery of function in stroke (Feeney and Sutton, 1987).

ACKNOWLEDGMENTS

Dr. Ginsberg is the recipient of a Jacob Javits Neuroscience Investigator Award and receives support from U.S. Public Health Service grants NS-05820 and NS-22603. He is indebted to Helen Valkowitz for preparing the typescript.

REFERENCES

Astrup, J., Symon, L., Branston, N. M., and Lassen, N. A., 1977, Cortical evoked potential and extracellular K^+ and H^+ at critical levels of brain ischemia, *Stroke* **8**:51–57.

Baron, J. C, 1985, Positron tomography in cerebral ischemia. A review, *Neuroradiology* **27**:509–516.

Busto, R., Dietrich, W. D., Globus, M. Y.-T., Valdes, I., Scheinberg, P., and Ginsberg, M. D, 1987, Small differences in intraischemic brain temperature critically determine the extent of ischemic neuronal injury, *J. Cereb. Blood Flow Metab.* **7**:729–738.

Busto, R., Dietrich, W. D., Globus, M. Y.-T., and Ginsberg, M. D, 1989*a*, Postischemic moderate hypothermia inhibits CA1 hippocampal ischemic neuronal injury, *Neurosci. Lett.* **101**:299–304.

Busto, R., Dietrich, W. D., Globus, M. Y.-T., and Ginsberg, M. D, 1989*b*, The importance of brain temperature in cerebral ischemic injury, *Stroke* **20**:1113–1114.

Busto, R., Globus, M. Y.-T., Dietrich, W. D., Martinez, E., Valdes, I., and Ginsberg, M. D, 1989c, Effect of mild hypothermia on ischemia-induced release of neurotransmitters and free fatty acids in rat brain, *Stroke* **20**:904–910.

Carafoli, E, 1987, Intracellular calcium homeostasis, *Annu. Rev. Biochem.* **56**:395–433.

Cheung, J. Y., Bonventre, J. V., Malis, C. D., and Leaf, A, 1986, Calcium and ischemic injury, *N. Engl. J. Med.* **314**:1670–1676.

Feeney, D. M., and Sutton, R. L, 1987, Pharmacotherapy for recovery of function after brain injury, *Crit. Rev. Neurobiol.* **3**:135–197.

Garcia, J. H, 1984, Experimental ischemic stroke: A review, *Stroke* **15**:5–14.

Ginsberg, M. D, 1989, Efficacy of calcium channel blockers in brain ischemia—a critical assessment, *in*, "Pharmacology of Cerebral Ischemia 1988—Proceedings of the Second International Symposium on Pharmacology of Cerebral Ischemia" (J. Krieglstein, ed.), pp. 65–73, Wissenschaftliche Verlagsgesellschaft mbH, Stuttgart, Germany.

Ginsberg, M. D., and Busto, R, 1989, Progress review: Rodent models of cerebral ischemia, *Stroke* **20**: 1627–1642.

Ginsberg, M. D., Busto, R., Castella, Y., Valdes, I., and Loor, J, 1989, The protective effect of moderate intra-ischemic brain hypothermia is associated with improved postischemic glucose utilization and blood flow, *J. Cereb. Blood Flow Metab.* **9**(Suppl. 1):S380.

Ginsberg, M. D., Welsh, F. A., and Budd, W. W, 1980, Deleterious effect of glucose pretreatment on recovery from diffuse cerebral ischemia in the cat. I. Local cerebral blood flow and glucose utilization, *Stroke* **11**:347–354.

Globus, M. Y.-T., Busto, R., Dietrich, W. D., Martinez, E., Valdes, I., and Ginsberg, M. D, 1988a, Effect of ischemia on the in vivo release of striatal dopamine, glutamate, and gamma-aminobutyric acid studied by intracerebral microdialysis, *J. Neurochem.* **51**:1455–1464.

Globus, M. Y.-T., Busto, R., Dietrich, W. D., Martinez, E., Valdes, I., and Ginsberg, M. D, 1988b, Intra-ischemic extracellular release of dopamine and glutamate is associated with striatal vulnerability to ischemia, *Neurosci. Lett.* **91**:36–40.

Globus, M. Y.-T., Dietrich, W. D., Busto, R., Valdes, I., and Ginsberg, M. D, 1988c, The combined treatment with a dopamine D-1 antagonist (SCH-23390) and NMDA receptor blocker (MK-801) dramatically protects against ischemia-induced hippocampal damage, *J. Cereb. Blood Flow Metab.* **8**(Suppl. 1):S5.

Globus, M. Y.-T., Ginsberg, M. D., Dietrich, W. D., Busto, R., and Scheinberg, P, 1987, Substantia nigra lesion protects against ischemic damage in the striatum, *Neurosci. Lett.* **80**:251–256.

Hachinski, V., and Norris, J. W, 1985, "The Acute Stroke," FA Davis, Philadelphia.

Hass, W. K, 1981, Beyond cerebral blood flow, metabolism, and ischemic thresholds: An examination of the role of calcium in the initiation of cerebral infarction, *in* "Cerebral Vascular Disease 3. Proceedings of the 10th International Salzburg Conference" (J. S. Meyer, H. Lechner, M. Reivich, E. O. Ott, and A. Aranibar, eds.), pp. 3–17, Excerpta Medica, Amsterdam.

Heiss, W.-D., and Rosner, G, 1983, Functional recovery of cortical neurons as related to degree and duration of ischemia, *Ann. Neurol.* **14**:294–301.

Kontos, H. A, 1989, Oxygen radicals in cerebral ischemia, *in* "Cerebrovascular Diseases. Sixteenth Research (Princeton) Conference" (M. D. Ginsberg and W. D. Dietrich, eds.), pp. 365–371, Raven Press, New York.

Kraig, R. P., Pulsinelli, W. A., and Plum, F, 1985, Hydrogen ion buffering during complete brain ischemia, *Brain Res.* **342**:281–290.

Kraig, R. P., Pulsinelli, W. A., and Plum, F, 1986, Carbonic acid buffer changes during complete brain ischemia, *Am. J. Physiol.* **250**:R348–R357.

Levy, D. E., Brott, T., Haley, E. C., Barsan, W. G., Olinger, C. P., Reed, R. L., and Marler, J. R, 1989, A safety study of tissue plasminogen activator (rt-PA) in the hyperacute phase of ischemic stroke, *in* "Cerebrovascular Diseases. Sixteenth Research (Princeton) Conference" (M. D. Ginsberg and W. D. Dietrich, eds.), pp. 21–27, Raven Press, New York.

Meldrum, B, 1989, Excitotoxicity in ischemia: An overview, *in* "Cerebrovascular Diseases. Sixteenth Research (Princeton) Conference" (M. D. Ginsberg and W. D. Dietrich, eds.), pp. 47–60, Raven Press, New York.

Molinari, G. F, 1988, Editorial. Why model strokes? *Stroke* **19:**1195–1197.

Molinari, G. F., and Laurent, J. P., 1976, A classification of experimental models of brain ischemia, *Stroke* **7:**14–17.

Myers, R. E., and Yamaguchi, S, 1977, Nervous system effects of cardiac arrest in monkeys. Preservation of vision, *Arch. Neurol.* **34:**65–74.

Nakayama, H., Ginsberg, M. D., and Dietrich, W. D, 1988, (S)-emopamil, a novel calcium channel blocker and serotonin S_2 antagonist, markedly reduces infarct size following middle cerebral artery occlusion in the rat, *Neurology* **38:**1667–1673.

Nedergaard, M, 1987, Transient focal ischemia in hyperglycemic rats is associated with increased cerebral infarction, *Brain Res.* **408:**79–85.

Petito, C. K., Feldmann, E., Pulsinelli, W. A., and Plum, F, 1987, Delayed hippocampal damage in humans following cardiorespiratory arrest, *Neurology* **37:**1281–1286.

Prado, R., Ginsberg, M. D., Dietrich, W. D., Watson, B. D., and Busto, R, 1988, Hyperglycemia increases infarct size in collaterally perfused but not end-arterial vascular territories, *J. Cereb. Blood Flow Metab.* **8:**186–192.

Pulsinelli, W. A., Waldman, S., Rawlinson, D., and Plum, F, 1982, Moderate hyperglycemia augments ischemic brain damage: A neuropathologic study in the rat, *Neurology* **32:**1239–1246.

Rosomoff, H. L, 1957, Hypothermia and cerebral vascular lesions. II. Experimental interruption followed by inductions of hypothermia, *Arch. Neurol. Psychiatry* **78:**454–464.

Rothman, S. M., and Olney, J. W, 1986, Glutamate and the pathophysiology of hypoxic-ischemic brain damage, *Ann. Neurol.* **19:**105–111.

Rothman, S. M., and Olney, J. W, 1987, Excitotoxicity and the NMDA receptor, *Trends Neurosci.* **10:**299–302.

Scheinberg, P, 1988, Controversies in the management of cerebral vascular disease, *Neurology* **38:**1609–1616.

Shearman, G. T, 1989, Effect of the NMDA antagonist MK-801 in animal models of focal and global cerebral ischemia, *in* "Cerebrovascular Diseases. Sixteenth Research (Princeton) Conference" (M. D. Ginsberg and W. D. Dietrich, eds.), pp. 73–77, Raven Press, New York.

Siesjö, B. K, 1981, Cell damage in the brain: A speculative synthesis, *J. Cereb. Blood Flow Metab.* **1:**155–185.

Sokoloff, L, 1976, Circulation and energy metabolism of the brain, *in* "Basic Neurochemistry" (G. J. Siegel, R. W. Albers, R. Katzman, and B. W. Agranoff, eds.), pp. 388–413, Little, Brown and Co, Boston.

Wei, E. P., and Kontos, H. A, 1987, Oxygen radicals in cerebral ischemia, *Physiologist* **30:**122.

Welsh, F. A., Ginsberg, M. D., Rieder, W., and Budd, W. W, 1980, Deleterious effect of glucose pretreatment on recovery from diffuse cerebral ischemia in the cat. II. Regional metabolite levels, *Stroke* **11:**355–363.

Zivin, J. A, 1989, A perspective on the future of thrombolytic stroke therapy, *in* "Cerebrovascular Diseases. Sixteenth Research (Princeton) Conference" (M. D. Ginsberg and W. D. Dietrich, eds.), pp. 33–37, Raven Press, New York.

CHAPTER 2

METABOLIC CORRELATES OF FOCAL ISCHEMIA

WARREN R. SELMAN, JOSEPH C. LAMANNA, ROBERT A. RATCHESON, and W. DAVID LUST

1. INTRODUCTION

1.1. Definition of Focal Ischemia

Stroke in humans is a syndrome consisting of the abrupt onset of a focal neurological deficit. The etiology of stroke is varied, but the majority of strokes are due to brain infarction from arterial occlusion (Walker *et al.*, 1981; Robins and Baum, 1981). The rest are attributed to infarction, intracerebral hemorrhage, and subarachnoid hemorrhage. Experimental focal ischemia produced by intracranial vessel occlusion closely resembles the clinical manifestations of cerebral ischemia presenting as stroke. The presence of different perfusion zones following vessel

WARREN R. SELMAN, ROBERT A. RATCHESON, and W. DAVID LUST • *Laboratory of Experimental Neurosurgery, Department of Neurosurgery, Case Western Reserve University School of Medicine and University Hospitals of Cleveland, Cleveland, Ohio.* *JOSEPH C. LAMANNA* • *Departments of Neurology and Physiology/Biophysics, Case Western Reserve University School of Medicine and University Hospitals of Cleveland, Cleveland, Ohio.*

Neurochemical Correlates of Cerebral Ischemia, Volume 7 of *Advances in Neurochemistry*, edited by Nicolas G. Bazan, Pierre Braquet, and Myron D. Ginsberg. Plenum Press, New York, 1992.

occlusion is responsible for the unique characteristics of focal, as opposed to global, ischemia. The variability of the collateral circulation and of tissue perfusion renders the experimental investigation of focal ischemia inherently more difficult than the investigation of global ischemia. The complexity of focal stroke is further compounded by an incomplete understanding of the control mechanisms regulating blood flow of the brain under normal and pathological conditions. Our working hypothesis is that the normal coupling mechanisms among function, blood flow, and metabolism are perturbed during and after ischemia and, furthermore, that the pathophysiologies in the focal and perifocal regions are distinct. For this reason, the results discussed in this chapter are prefaced by an overview of the physiology of energy metabolism and blood flow in the brain. The chapter will then briefly review the clinical significance of stroke in an attempt to underscore the importance of, and the problems with, focal ischemia models; finally, the biochemical correlates to brain injury following irreversible focal ischemia will be described in some detail.

2. BLOOD-FLOW–METABOLISM–FUNCTION COUPLING

2.1. General Considerations

It is well known that the brain is dependent, on a moment-to-moment basis, on the delivery of glucose and oxygen for its energy supply. Brain work (utilization of energy) is exactly balanced by oxidative metabolism (energy production) as long as there are sufficient supplies of substrates (mainly glucose) and oxygen and continual removal of reduced metabolic end products. Although the dependence of the brain on oxygen and glucose is easily acknowledged; and while the coupled nature of the relationships among function, metabolism, and supply is usually recognized, the coupling mechanisms responsible for the fine control of this system are not very well understood (Siesjö, 1978, 1984).

Fundamentally, it is most logical that the entire coupled system is driven by the work function, i.e., energy demand. Energy demand in the brain is anisotropic, varying both spatially and temporally. The interrelationship among energy demand, energy production, and substrate supply/end product removal can be fully understood only by using experimental paradigms which control or measure spatial heterogeneity and also allow reasonable temporal resolution. Figure 1 presents the probable interrelationships (solid arrows) between each of the variables in diagram form. Neuronal activity directly stimulates metabolism, and increased metabolism directly results in increased blood flow. Less well understood are hypothetical mechanisms (dashed arrows) whereby neuronal activity, independent of metabolic requirements, could directly control blood flow through activation of vasomotor neurons at any level within the cerebrovasculature. Additionally, there is some evidence that primary changes in blood flow could lead

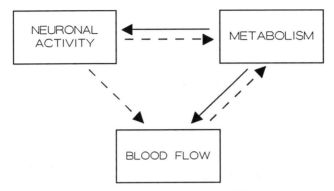

FIGURE 1. Interrelationship of neuronal activity, metabolism, and blood flow in the central nervous system. The solid arrows represent known control mechanisms, whereas the dashed arrows indicate putative physiological regulatory interactions that may also be invoked under pathological conditions within the brain.

to changes in metabolism, independent of neuronal activity, based on suggested control of metabolism by substrate or oxygen limitation. It is possible but unlikely that blood flow changes per se directly affect neuronal firing, independent of metabolism. This would be indicative of the presence of a nonmetabolically based neuronal blood flow sensor circuit. It is an implausible mechanism because blood flow is not a critical variable; the critical variables are delivery of glucose and delivery of oxygen, which are more likely candidates for neuronal sensor circuits. Glucose delivery and oxygen delivery are determined by capillary surface area and permeability, as well as by blood concentration and flow rate. As will be seen, the distinction between blood flow and delivery has important implications for understanding the compensatory mechanisms triggered in response to pathological challenges to the brain.

It must be remembered that unique conditions exist in the brain which affect the relationship between energy demand, energy metabolism, and substrate and oxygen delivery, such as high surface-area-to-cell-volume ratios; cell processes that are at a significant distance from the cell body and its nucleus; strict requirements for stable and well-controlled excitable membrane ion distributions; a more or less continuous global level of synaptic activity, with extreme heterogeneity locally; and enclosure in a rigid container which limits the changes in volume of the various compartments.

2.2. Brain Work

Brain work is difficult to quantify. In tissues such as muscle, where mechanical work is done along with generation of heat, thermodynamic work can be measured and converted directly to quantitative energy usage terms. There is no easy analogy to this in brain tissue because the specialized function of the brain is information processing, for which we have no solid thermodynamic theoretical foundation. Therefore, it is more troublesome to describe brain work, yet full comprehension of brain physiology and pathology ultimately depends explicitly on an accurate definition of this term.

2.2.1. Categories of Work

There are two main categories of energy utilization in the brain: the homeostatic energy consumption that maintains cell integrity, and the work done in carrying out the specialized functions of the brain.

2.2.1.1. Homeostatic As in most other cells and tissues of the body, most of the homeostatic work in the brain is biosynthetic work, for example, metabolic pathways involving polysaccharides, lipids, proteins, and nucleic acids. Homeostatic energy requirements may be responsible for as much as half of the normal energy production by the resting brain.

2.2.1.2. Specialized The specialized function of the brain is the reception, transmission, and storage of information as performed by neurons. Glial and endothelial cells have specialized functions which maintain the external and internal milieux that allow the neurons to perform their function. The specialized, active work done by brain tissue amounts primarily to osmotic work, including both axonal transport and ion transport, the latter of which is presumed to be the most costly energetically. The ion transport system that is responsible for the majority of brain energy consumption is, not surprisingly, (Na^+, K^+)-ATPase. Compartmental distributions of other ions, especially calcium, hydrogen, and bicarbonate ions, ultimately depend for regulation on metabolism, either directly through ATP-utilizing pumps or indirectly through the energy available in the sodium gradient. In addition to the control of ion gradients, a certain energy cost is associated with transmitter synthesis and reuptake and with protein phosphorylation reactions.

2.3. Brain Energy Metabolism

The first leg in the diagram of Figure 1 is the couple between neuronal activity and metabolism. The components of this couple are shown schematically in Figure 2. The initiating event is the efflux of K^+ accompanying neuronal activation (Lothman *et al.*, 1975). ATP is used by (Na^+, K^+)-ATPase to restore the potassium gradient and hence the membrane potential. ADP produced in this reaction relieves the rate limitation on the respiratory chain enzymes, promoting oxygen and substrate consumption for rephosphorylation as brain mitochondria to make a transition from state 4 to state 3 (Rosenthal and LaManna, 1975). As a result of these metabolic reactions, the cell uses the energy available from the oxidation of

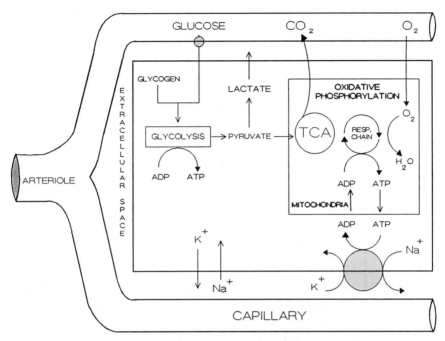

FIGURE 2. Schematic of energy homeostasis in the brain. The solid rectangle represents the intracellular compartment composed of both glia and neurons which are served by the capillaries. The two major compartments within the cell are the cytoplasm and the mitochondrion. See the text for a discussion of the dynamic processes which couple metabolism, blood flow, and function.

substrate-reducing equivalents which are provided by glucose with water as the end product. In removing the reducing equivalents from glucose, carbon dioxide is produced. Therefore, for the cells to function, the energy-dissipative reactions must be balanced by continuous input of glucose and oxygen, continuous removal of carbon dioxide, and osmotic control of cell water.

The relationship between ATP utilization and brain function should be understood within the framework of its dynamic range (Erecinska and Silver, 1989). Suppression of much of the synaptic activity by inducing barbiturate coma to the point of electroencephalographic (EEG) silence results in a 50% reduction of oxygen consumption. Similar reductions have been produced by blockage of the (Na^+, K^+)-ATPase in slices and in vivo. On the other hand, brain metabolism can be increased at least 2.5 times during the intense neuronal activity induced by generalized seizure activity. Thus, basal oxygen consumption is about twice the minimum for homeostatic needs and can be increased manyfold in response to increased neuronal activity.

The consequence of an interrupted delivery of glucose is energy failure due to lack of reducing equivalents. Some tissue reserve of glucosyl units is available for short times through the tissue glycogen content, but this is not large. For example, at a normal rate of glucose consumption on the order of 0.5 μmol/g (wet wt) per min, the available glucosyl units from glycogen, about 3 μmol/g (wet wt), would be able to provide 10 minutes of substrate for oxidative metabolism. Alternative substrate sources of reducing equivalents can be used, and ketone bodies, if available, could support oxidative metabolic requirements in the face of insufficient glucose supply (Hawkins *et al.*, 1986).

Acute extreme changes in glucose availability alter neuronal function, energy metabolism, and blood flow, demonstrating some degree of rebalance in the system in attempt at compensation (see, e.g., Bryan *et al.*, 1986; Duckrow and Bryan, 1987; Duckrow *et al.*, 1987; Hollinger and Bryan, 1987).

Complete lack of oxygen quickly results in energy failure of the tissue through a full reductive stop in mitochondrial chain component redox states (Kreisman *et al.*, 1981*b*). In the presence of continued glycolytic substrate availability, ATP will continue to be generated anaerobically at about 5% of the efficiency (glucose used for ATP produced) of the oxidative reactions and with concomitant production of lactate, which results in an acid and osmotic load (Rapoport *et al.*, 1986). Hypoxia and hyperoxia are also environmental conditions which must be compensated for to maintain efficient functional capacity (LaManna *et al.*, 1984, 1987).

It is certain that heterogeneous metabolic compartments exist in brain tissue. The first level for considering heterogeneity would be categories based on the cell types: neurons, glia, and endothelial cells (without regard for the cell subtypes within each category, which may also have significantly different energy requirements). Neurons are a likely site of oxidative metabolism. The influx of Na^+ ions during activation should be a strong stimulus to (Na^+, K^+)-ATPase. Mitochondria and other enzyme systems are present in high concentration. It must be remembered that there may be a different metabolic component in the dendritic region than in the soma or axon. The relative contribution of glial cells to energy metabolism is unclear. Recent suggestions indicate that the glial cell might be the site of anaerobic-like energy production through glycolysis (Fox *et al.*, 1988). There is some evidence that glycolytic lactate production can occur in the presence of oxygen, but the link to the glial cell has never been definitively made.

Capillary endothelial cells represent a very small volume, and their contribution to brain metabolism will be greatly overshadowed by that of their neighbor glial and neuronal cells. Nevertheless, their metabolic activity must be important to their own function since they contain significant numbers of mitochondria and must do work in their blood-brain barrier functional capacity. Their primary source of energy may be fatty acids; their glucose consumption in the presence of fatty acids is very low (Goldstein and Betz, 1983).

The existence of heterogeneity between cellular types and also within the intracellular milieu has the potential to greatly affect the tissue response to focal ischemia, which adds a third level of regional heterogeneity. As just one example, heterogeneity in intracellular pH in focal ischemia (LaManna *et al.*, 1986) could result in extreme variations in tissue glycolytic rates (Hochachka and Mommsen, 1983).

2.4. Brain Perfusion

2.4.1. General Considerations

The delivery of glucose and oxygen and the removal of carbon dioxide (and, at times, other end products of metabolism such as lactate and adenosine) are dependent on the tissue blood supply. The brain has some unusual conditions which affect the mechanisms that control the blood supply. For example, the brain must be isolated from the systemic arterial blood pressure. This is due to at least two reasons. (1) Overall blood volume cannot be allowed to change much because the brain is in a rigid container of more or less fixed volume, filled by brain cellular volume (80 to 85%), extracellular fluid (10 to 15%), and intravascular blood (2 to 5%). Changes in the volume of any of these compartments must be compensated for by changes in the others. (2) Significant rises in capillary pressure would have significant structural consequences for the tight junctions on cerebral capillaries. The majority of the isolation mechanisms occur through neurogenic and myogenic control down through the level of the larger arterioles. Neural control at this level originates primarily from the peripheral sympathetic ganglia acting through vasoconstrictor alpha-adrenergic receptors.

2.4.2. Intrinsic Control of Small Vessels

At the level of the capillary, the control mechanisms must be somewhat more complex. There are two primary variables which affect the delivery of substrate and oxygen: flow rate and blood volume. Blood volume is an indicator of capillary surface area, and in this regard, endothelial cell permeability to a given substance must be considered. These variables are usually referred to by the general term "permeability × surface area product" or simply PS. If there were no physiological changes in surface area, the blood flow term would be sufficient to describe delivery. However, changes in surface area (also reflected in changes in capillary blood volume) are likely to occur, and so the more simplistic view of cerebral blood flow is too limited.

2.4.2.1. Stewart-Hamilton Central Volume Principle The connection between flow and volume is most easily understood by the central-volume principle in which the capillary mean transit time (MTT) is the capillary blood volume (CBV) divided by the tissue blood flow (CBF):

$$MTT = CBV/CBF$$

Changes in both blood flow and blood volume occur during compensatory responses to pathological challenges (Shockley and LaManna, 1988). Another way of considering this relationship is that mean transit time is related to the red cell velocity and the capillary path length. The data show that there is a distribution of flow rates in the capillary bed. Since entrance pressure must be about the same, the main variable must be the path length or capillary length. The arterial network of the cerebral cortex, at the level of the terminal vascular bed, appears to consist of four to six levels of branching between the pial arteriole and the capillaries with characteristic "dichotomous" or "stirrup" branches (Motti *et al.*, 1986). This arrangement produces a rather wide distribution of possible capillary path lengths; a range of 18 to 277 μm has been reported for the interbranch segment length in a series of 100 samples (Motti *et al.*, 1986).

2.4.2.2. *Capillary Recruitment* The mechanism most discussed for changes in blood volume is capillary recruitment (Weiss, 1988). Although still controversial as a phenomenon in brain tissue, capillary recruitment is well known in other vascular beds such as skeletal muscle. Most of the physiological evidence favors capillary recruitment, but most anatomical studies fail to demonstrate "empty" capillaries. One difficulty in determining the role of capillary recruitment is in the definition of terms. The argument has primarily centered around what is meant by "open" or "closed" capillaries. If one takes the view that some capillaries are completely closed and thus not perfused with blood except when recruited, then one is hard pressed to explain the anatomical data that cannot identify more than a small percentage of capillaries that do not contain blood. However, if one takes the view that there is a continuum of red blood cell flow rates and a distribution of capillary mean transit times in the brain, then there will be some proportion of vessels which contain blood (and thus, are anatomically "open") but which have extremely long transit times. Physiologically these act as if "closed." Mechanisms which could act to control capillary perfusion at the microvessel level (below the level of vascular smooth muscle) include contraction of endothelial cells and changes in cell volume of pericytes, glia, or endothelial cells which surround microvessels.

These issues remain to be determined experimentally. The issue is important because of the theoretical distinctions between mechanisms that increase blood flow through increased flow rate and those that increase blood flow by increased blood volume. For example, the delivery of oxygen, which is highly diffusible, can be increased by an increased flow rate without necessarily increasing capillary blood volume. Although the acute compensatory response to hypoxia is an increase in the capillary mean transit time as a result of both blood volume and blood flow increases (LaManna *et al.*, 1984; Shockley and LaManna, 1988), the chronic adaptation involves only an increased flow rate (augmented by increased hematocrit) with a return to normal of the capillary blood volume (LaManna *et al.*, 1989). Equivalent reasoning can be applied to the acute and chronic compensatory responses to hyperglycemia (Kikano *et al.*, 1989; Harik and LaManna, 1988). In this situation, blood flow increases only in the acute response, the chronic response apparently involving changes in capillary permeability.

2.5. Coupling Factors

There must, then, be signals for increased tissue blood perfusion during increased tissue work. It has become clear that these signals do not involve a hypoxic drive mechanism as found in other organs such as in skeletal muscle. In physiologically well-controlled preparations, mitochondrial metabolism and tissue oxygen tension always increase with tissue activation, whether the tissue is activated by direct electrical stimulation, spreading depression, or even seizures (LaManna *et al.*, 1987; Kreisman *et al.*, 1981a). Potential signals for increased perfusion include extracellular potassium ion release, adenosine, carbon dioxide, or even protons. It is also quite possible that the signal is of direct neuronal origin. These possibilities are the subject of intensive current investigation (Collins, 1987; Siesjö, 1984).

The importance of the factors discussed in this section is especially amplified when focal ischemia is considered. The complicating effects of the relationships between the physiological variables and their control mechanisms will become apparent when the data from the focal ischemia model are presented below. First, however, we would like to present a description of focal ischemia in its clinical aspects, since the choice of experimental model must consider clinical relevance.

3. FOCAL ISCHEMIA IN HUMANS

3.1. Morbidity and Mortality

Epidemiological evidence demonstrates that both the frequency and severity of cerebrovascular disease have diminished in the past 20 years (Wolf *et al.*, 1986). The major impact in the reduction of stroke morbidity and mortality has come from better recognition and control of risk factors such as systemic hypertension. Nevertheless, little progress has been made in improving the treatment of strokes; this leaves stroke as the third leading cause of death and the major cause of chronic disability in the United States (Wolf *et al.*, 1986; Goldberg and Kurland, 1962; Kannel and Wolf, 1983). The need to develop effective therapeutic strategies to ameliorate the devastating consequences of stroke remains urgent.

3.2. Etiology

Considerable controversy exists regarding the etiology of focal ischemia. Two mechanisms may coexist or operate independently: thrombosis and embolism. The outcome of either embolic or thrombotic stroke may be modified by the consequences of reperfusion. Embolic material may fragment or dislodge, and a thrombosis may recanalize, resulting in restoration of blood flow to the tissue. This reperfusion can result in increased damage due to conversion of a so-called bland or nonhemorrhagic infarction to a hemorrhagic infarction.

3.3. Dependence of Brain Function on Blood Flow

Integrated neurological, neurophysiological, and neuropathological studies in focal ischemia have demonstrated a correlation between regional cerebral blood flow and brain function (Rossen *et al.*, 1943). Correlation of clinical symptoms and cerebral blood flow studies suggests that flows between 20 and 25 ml/100 g per min are borderline for normal synaptic transmission (Symon *et al.*, 1974; Boysen *et al.*, 1974; Sundt *et al.*, 1974). Experimental investigations have further defined this relationship. A threshold relationship between electrical activity and blood flow changes after middle cerebral artery occlusion has been demonstrated in primates (Branston *et al.*, 1974). Massive potassium efflux occurs at a blood flow substantially lower than that for electrical failure (Astrup *et al.*, 1977). The concept of an "ischemic penumbra" has been used to define the regions of the brain with blood flow between the thresholds for electrical and membrane failure. The lower threshold was presumed to be that for infarction, whereas the higher represented a condition more consistent with reversible injury. The duration of ischemia is a critical factor in the equation and is known to affect these thresholds; i.e., the more profound the ischemia, the shorter time the tissue can survive before infarction (Jones *et al.*, 1981; Rosner and Heiss, 1983).

3.4. Paralysis Versus Infarction

The ultimate fate of the perifocal region, however, is a matter of controversy. Strong *et al.* (1983*a, b*) demonstrated a reduction of electrocortical activity after 2 hours of middle cerebral artery occlusion in the cat without evidence of membrane damage, only to note evidence of incomplete infarction in the marginal gyrus on pathological examination. Lassen and Vorstrup (1984) suggested that the cells in the ischemic penumbra may exist in a dangerous state in which irreversible cell damage can occur. Crockard *et al.* (1987) suggested that the loss of electrical activity at the higher flow threshold corresponds to the onset of energy failure and that potassium efflux is associated with loss of glial rather than neuronal function.

Thus, the role of the perifocal region in the evolution of ischemic damage is unresolved.

4. EXPERIMENTAL MODELS OF FOCAL ISCHEMIA

4.1. General Considerations

An experimental model of focal ischemia requires an animal model in which (1) the vascular occlusion results in predictable changes in blood flow, (2) the parenchymal lesion closely resembles the pathological changes observed in human stroke, (3) the method of ischemia production is compatible with reperfusion, (4) a multidisciplinary approach with investigative techniques of appropriate regional resolution can be used to study the different pathological processes which contribute to ischemic injury, and (5) adequate numbers of animals are available to ensure statistical significance at a reasonable cost. The behavior, motor and sensory integration, amount of neocortex, and function and architecture of the cerebral vasculature are important factors in determining the adequacy of experimental models (Moossy, 1979).

Previously reported physiological and clinical observations would suggest that the model of single-artery occlusion in subhuman primates is the closest to an ideal model of ischemic stroke (Symon *et al.*, 1974). Although much information can be gained from these animals, ethical considerations, expense, and the difficulty in obtaining large enough numbers for therapeutic trials dictate that other models be used.

Rodent models are inexpensive to obtain and maintain, and large numbers can be used for concurrent biochemical, metabolic, and pathological studies requiring statistical analyses. The laboratory rat is one of the most thoroughly studied animals with respect to physiology and metabolism. Although other species have been used for certain rapidly occurring biochemical events associated with ischemia, no other models are as feasible as rodents. The cerebral circulation and distribution of infarction in rats are similar to those in humans (Yamori *et al.*, 1976; Rieke *et al.*, 1981). This model permits a correlation among metabolic function, regional cerebral blood flow analysis, edema formation, physiological function, and pathological outcome to provide possible routes for improving therapeutic intervention. Such analyses are not possible in models in which there is only one end point.

4.2. Middle Cerebral Artery Occlusion

The goal of any model of focal ischemia is to produce consistent zones of altered perfusion. Although a variety of arterial occlusions have been used, middle cerebral artery (MCA) occlusion has provided a more consistent region of focal ischemia than has cervical carotid manipulation.

4.2.1. Anatomy

A prime anatomical consideration in MCA occlusion is the site of occlusion in relation to the lenticulostriate perforators and more distal branches. The lenticulostriate arteries are considered to be at least functional, if not anatomical, end arteries. Thus occlusion at or proximal to their origin should effectively preclude collateral perfusion of the structures involved and may lead to a different pattern of infarction from that which occurs if occlusion is distal to the origin of the lenticulostriate perforators. Finally, segmental occlusion which occurs with endovascular embolic occlusion, or extravascular occlusion along a given length of the vessel, may restrict collateral flow through lenticulostriate arteries more than a single-point extravascular occlusion would, and thus the pattern of infarction may be affected not only by the site, but also by the type of occlusion.

4.2.2. Location and Method of Occlusion

Alteration of brain circulation by arterial occlusion was reported as early as 1836, when Cooper ligated the carotid and vertebral arteries in dogs (Cooper, 1836). Flourens (1847) subsequently described the effect of embolic occlusion. The various methods of occlusion that have been used can be broadly grouped into intravascular or extravascular and permanent or temporary. These methods are summarized in Table 1 for the permanent-occlusion models and Table 2 for the reversible-occlusion models.

Although endovascular techniques with emboli most closely resemble the pathogenesis of clinical ischemia, there is more variability in the site of occlusion. Furthermore, with autologous clot, the time of occlusion before reperfusion is difficult to control. Removable intravascular obstruction can overcome some of these variables, but the exact site of occlusion remains difficult to predict.

Extravascular techniques have included coagulation, ligature or clip placement, and the use of inflatable cuffs. Although these techniques permit precise knowledge of the site of occlusion, there is concern about the effects of the intracranial surgery needed to perform the occlusion. Furthermore, the reliability of reperfusion after prolonged occlusion is not always readily established.

4.2.3. Species and Strain Differences

MCA occlusion has been reported in various species ranging from mice to subhuman primates. It has been suggested that smaller vertebrate animals react differently from subhuman primates to middle cerebral artery occlusion, but

TABLE 1. Permanent Occlusion Models

Location of occlusion[a]	Method of occlusion; strain[a]	Comments[a]	References
Proximal to RB	Coagulation; SD	Developed proximal-occlusion model and documented blood flow alterations	Tamura et al. (1981); Tyson et al. (1984)
Proximal to RB	Coagulation; SD	Length and location of occlusion important correlate to pathology and neurologic deficit	Bederson et al. (1986)
Proximal to RB	Coagulation; SD	Quantitation of stroke volume	Osborne et al. (1987)
Proximal to LSB	Coagulation; SD, W, F, SHR	Quantitation of stroke volume, cortical infarction, most consistent in SHR	Duverger and Mac-Kenzie (1988)
Proximal to LSB	Coagulation; W	Autoradiographic determination of blood flow, glucose, metabolism, pH	Sako et al. (1985); Nedergaard et al. (1986)
Proximal to RB	Coagulation; SD	Metabolic assays on basis of anatomical regions	Nowicki et al. (1988)
Proximal to RB	Coagulation; SD	Metabolic assays on basis of perfusion patterns	Selman et al. (1987)
Distal to RF	Coagulation; W	Small cortical infarct and no infarct in young rats	Robinson (1981); Coyle (1982)
Distal	Coagulation of selective branches; SD	Cortical infarct in selected territories	Rubino and Young (1988)
Distal (?)	Embolus secondary to homologous clot; W	Territories outside MCA distribution may be affected	Kudo et al. (1982)
Distal (?)	Nonocclusive photo-coagulation CCA; ?	Emboli pathophysiology similar to man	Futrell et al. (1989)

[a]Abbreviations: W, Wistar; F, Fisher; SD, Sprague-Dawley; SHR, spontaneously hypertensive; RB, rhinal branch; LSB, lenticulostriate branch; RF, rhinal fissure; CCA, common carotid artery.

differences in the location and method of occlusion make such comparisons difficult at best.

Among rat models of focal ischemia, strain variation in susceptibility to vessel occlusion has been well documented. Initial studies demonstrated that the Fisher 344 strain was the most susceptible to cerebral infarction with carotid occlusion in the neck (Payan and Conard, 1977). Recent studies confined to MCA occlusion demonstrate that the least variability with respect to volume of infarction

TABLE 2. Reversible Occlusion Models

Location of occlusion[a]	Method of occlusion; strain[a]	Comments[a]	References
Proximal to RB	Snare; SD	Temporary ischemia, direct reperfusion, determination of ischemic edema	Shigeno *et al.* (1985)
Proximal to LSB	Endovascular occlusion ICA, ACA, and MCA; SD	Temporary occlusion of MCA without craniotomy	Zea Longa *et al.* (1989)
Distal to RB	Photocoagulation of CCA with acute recanalization; SD	Occlusion without violating dura; direct reperfusion	Nakayama *et al.* (1988)
Distal RB	Coagulation of distal MCA plus snare ligation of CCS; W, F, SHR	Quantitation stroke volume, SHR more consistent cortex infarct, easier to access to MCA, but reperfusion only through collaterals	Brint *et al.* (1988)

[a]Abbreviations: W, Wistar; F, Fisher; SD, Sprague-Dawley; SHR, spontaneously hypertensive; RB, rhinal branch; LSB, lenticulostriate branch; ICA, internal carotid artery; ACA, anterior cerebral artery; CCA, common carotid artery.

may be obtained with spontaneously hypertensive rats (Brint *et al.*, 1988; Duverger and MacKenzie, 1988).

5. METABOLIC CORRELATES OF FOCAL ISCHEMIA

5.1. Rationale for Measuring Energy and Glucose-Related Metabolites in Focal Ischemia

The hydrolysis of ATP provides a major portion of the energy required for brain function, and glucose is normally the sole metabolic substrate for the production of ATP (see above). It is not surprising, then, that the viability of brain tissue following an insult can be evaluated by the measurement of the endogenous concentrations of glucose and energy-related metabolites. Although the concentrations of these metabolites provide some insights into the energy status of the tissue, the results, alone, measure neither evolving brain damage nor the functional state of the tissue. First, the depletion of the high-energy phosphates and of glucosyl reserves cannot be equated with irreversible brain damage. The depletion of energy stores occurs within 2 minutes of ischemia, a time that does not elicit irreversible brain damage. It is likely that brain injury arises from energy depletion only when a time threshold is exceeded. Second, a normal metabolite profile is permissive to, but does not guarantee the existence of, cell function. Ostensibly viable tissue can be paralyzed for a number of reasons, and this loss of function is quite distinct from that resulting from tissue infarction. Nevertheless, the results from the measurement of energy-related metabolites can be useful in understanding the pathophysiology of ischemia.

Experience has shown, however, that there are problems in applying these methods to the investigation of focal ischemia. One of the major drawbacks to focal models of ischemia has been the variability in the dimensions of the affected regions following a single-vessel occlusion, and the sampling of tissue according to anatomical landmarks has proven to be unreliable (Ratcheson and Ferrendelli, 1980; Welsh, 1984). Several studies have measured metabolites in various brain regions following focal ischemia, and the results are flawed by the apparent heterogeneity of the blood flow to the tissues sampled (Ratcheson and Ferrendelli, 1980; Selman et al., 1987; Nowicki et al., 1988). It is necessary, therefore, to measure brain perfusion in conjunction with performing metabolic studies of focal ischemia. Certain limitations ascribed to focal models of ischemia may be negated by the promising results from studies on spontaneously hypertensive rats, but by being more reproducible, the SHR model of focal stroke may well be less relevant to the human condition (Brint et al., 1988; Grabowski et al., 1988).

5.2. Experimental Protocol

Sprague-Dawley rats weighing 250 to 300 g were prepared and the MCA occluded as described previously (Tamura et al., 1981; Selman et al., 1987). The rats were reanesthetized, and the brains were frozen in situ at 20 min, 6 hr and 24 hr after the occlusion of the MCA (Ponten et al., 1973). The brains were removed at $-20°C$ and sectioned at a thickness of 20 μm, and selected sections were either lyophilized or stained with hematoxylin and eosin and with thionin. The tissue was dissected and the metabolites measured as described by Lowry and Passonneau (1972) and Lust et al. (1981). Three samples of contralateral cortex from each brain were assayed routinely and then averaged to give the value shown for cortical area no. 1. The sites for the remaining samples were dissected from the ipsilateral cortex and are presented in Figure 3. Statistical differences ($P < 0.05$) were determined by analysis of variance (ANOVA) with Duncan's method performed for individual comparisons.

5.3. Localization of Focal and Perifocal Sites by Using Neutral Red

To minimize the problems created by sampling tissue on the basis of anatomical landmarks, 2 ml of a 2% solution of the weak base chromophore neutral red (NR) was slowly infused into rats approximately 30 minutes prior to in situ fixation of the brain. The advantages of this approach to the investigation of

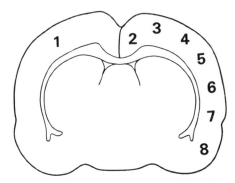

FIGURE 3. Schematic of coronal section of rat brain indicating dissection sites for metabolite analyses. The animals were prepared and the tissues processes as described in the text. Three samples were taken from the contralateral cortex of lyophilized sections, and the metabolites were analyzed. The values for the metabolites from area 1 represent the mean of three samples from the contralateral cortex. Since the magnitude of the perifocal region varied both with time after occlusion and between animals, this region cannot be assigned a set of numbers for all times and every rat. Nevertheless, the cingulate cortex was routinely found in areas 2 and 3 and the ischemic cortex in areas 7 and 8. The perifocal region at the earlier period of ischemia was found in areas 4 through 6 depending on the animal and was nonexistent at 1 day of ischemia. Therefore, the focal region extended from area 4 to area 8 at 1 day after irreversible focal ischemia.

focal ischemia are many, but perhaps most important is the ability to visualize the areas of altered perfusion during both sectioning and dissection (Figure 4). In this study, the rats in each time group were selected on the basis of the perfusion patterns, with the animals not exhibiting a reduction of perfusion in the ipsilateral cortex being discarded. The metabolites were measured in small pieces of tissue weighing approximately 1 µg. This approach thus reduces, but does not eliminate, the problems associated with the variability in the size and shape of the focal and perifocal regions among the experimental animals. Future studies will correlate the metabolite concentrations in discrete pieces of tissue either with the intensity of the NR in the same region determined by color film histophotometry or with the intracellular pH of the tissue determined by the ratio of the charged and uncharged forms of NR (LaManna, 1987; LaManna *et al.*, 1986).

5.4. Maturation of Focal and Perifocal Regions Determined by NR Intensity

The NR profiles were examined in representative photographs taken from rat brains during sectioning, and the areas were measured for the focal region (i.e., absence of NR staining), perifocal region (i.e., presence of patchy staining with NR) and cingulate cortex, a region of the ipsilateral cortex apparently served by

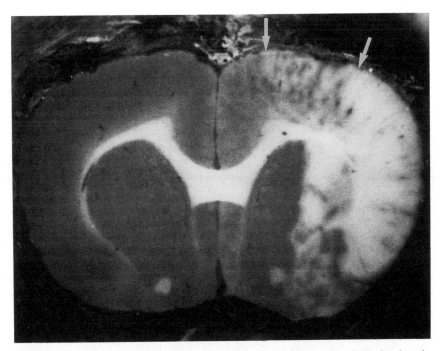

FIGURE 4. Photograph of rat brain 1 hr following MCA occlusion. NR was injected 30 min prior to in situ fixation as described in the text. Focal areas are devoid of NR, whereas those in the perifocal region are intermediately stained (the arrows designate the medial and lateral borders of this region) and the remaining regions have a homogeneous staining pattern. Note that NR uptake into white matter is much lower than the uptake into gray matter. Brains from animals which did not exhibit this characteristic type of NR distribution were not included in this study. Generally, the dorsolateral striatum was also affected, but the perifocal region was small or nonexistent.

the anterior cerebral artery. The medial and lateral boundaries of the perifocal region are indicated by the arrows in Figure 4. It is evident that in a 1-day period following the occlusion of the MCA, the perifocal region decreases concomitant with a large increase in infarct size from about 38 to 72% of the total ipsilateral cortex (Figure 5). The major changes occur between 6 and 24 hr of occlusion, coinciding temporally with the development of demonstrable tissue damage.

5.5. Time Course of High-Energy Phosphate Changes Following Focal Ischemia

The high-energy phosphate (HEP) concentrations (i.e., sum of ATP + P-creatine) in the various cortical areas were measured at 20 min, 6 hr, and 1 day

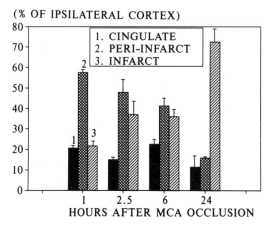

(% OF IPSILATERAL CORTEX)

FIGURE 5. Relative areas of cingulate cortex (solid bars), perifocal cortex (cross-hatched bars), and focal ischemic cortex (slashed bars) at various times after MCA occlusion. The total area of the cortex ipsilateral to the occlusion was determined, and the relative size of each region was measured at 1, 2.5, 6, and 24 hr after occlusion. The results are presented as the mean of four determinations ± 1 SEM for each time period.

following occlusion of the MCA of the rat (Figure 6). Although the pattern of HEP depression was similar at both 20 min and 6 hr of occlusion, there was a marked change by 1 day of occlusion. At 20 min and 6 hr of occlusion, the levels of HEP gradually decreased, moving laterally and ventrally from the midline of the cortex. This transition in energy reserves from normally perfused tissue to that for ischemic tissue was more abrupt by 1 day of occlusion, as indicated by the depletion of HEP in areas 5 and 6. We conclude from these results that the fall in the energy status of the ischemic tissue, like that for global ischemia, is relatively rapid, occurring within 20 min of occlusion, and, as the perfusion to the perifocal region decreases over 24 hr, so does the concentration of HEP. The elevation of HEP levels above those for control in an area medial to the affected regions indicates that the metabolism within this tissue is affected by the metabolic stress

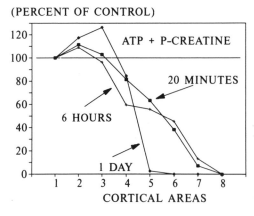

(PERCENT OF CONTROL)

FIGURE 6. Regional distribution of HEP at various stages of irreversible focal ischemia. The animals were prepared, the tissue processed, and metabolites analyzed as described in the text. The results are expressed as the percent HEP in the contralateral cortex (i.e., area 1). The cortical areas correspond to those shown in Figure 3.

in adjacent areas. In its simplest terms, this may be a form of metabolic diaschisis resulting from the loss of input from the ischemic region.

The changes observed in these studies are far more dramatic than those reported by others (Nowicki *et al.*, 1988; Germano *et al.*, 1987). When the metabolites were determined by the tissue analysis, the largest decrease in either striatum or parietal cortex was approximately 50% at 1 and 2 days after the occlusion of MCA in Fisher-344 rats. In the study with phosphate-magnetic resonance spectroscopy (MRS), absolute values were not reported but the ratio of ATP to total P_i was depressed by only 25%. The explanations for these relatively small changes in ATP were similar in both studies, having to do with the contamination of the ischemic tissue samples by adjacent tissues which apparently had near normal metabolism. This, once again, reemphasizes the importance of resolving the problem of heterogeneity in focal ischemia models, either by using an indicator to specify the level of perfusion to the tissue or by using a more consistent model such as that purported for SHR rats (Brint *et al.*, 1988).

5.6. Time Course of Changes in Glucose and Glycogen

The glucose concentrations decreased in the ischemic region by 20 min of occlusion and essentially remained constant up to 6 hr (Figure 7). The loss of this important substrate to the ischemic region is similar to that reported for global

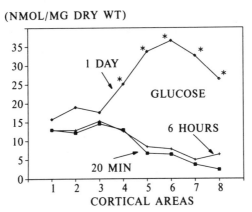

FIGURE 7. Glucose concentration in the cerebral cortex at various times after MCA occlusion. The results are expressed in nanomoles per milligram (dry wt), and each value represents the mean from four or more determinations. Significant differences ($P < 0.05$) between values at the different times of occlusion in a given area were determined by ANOVA and Duncan's method for individual comparisons and are indicated by asterisks. The differences between the values for the contralateral and the ipsilateral cortex were generally significant, but are not indicated.

ischemia (Siesjö, 1978). There was, however, a large accumulation of glucose in infarcted tissue by 1 day after occlusion, a finding similar to that described by Nowicki *et al.* (1988). Since this region is devoid of HEP and the tissue perfusion remains low, the elevation of glucose probably cannot be attributed to a reversal of the insult. It is more likely that this phenomenon is due to an inability of infarcted tissue to consume glucose in conjunction with either greater diffusion of glucose from the existing blood supply or to a restoration of some reflow in this area. In either case, both histology and metabolism indicate that the tissue is irreversibly damaged at 1 day after occlusion, with little likelihood of recovery.

Glycogen is the principle reserve of glucosyl units in the brain and is thought to reside primarily in the glia (Klatzo *et al.*, 1970). The pattern of changes in glycogen concentration with time after occlusion differ markedly from those observed for glucose. Although the glycogen levels are low in the ischemic areas, they appear to increase with time in the medial portion of the ipsilateral cortex (Figure 8). Since it is well known that glycogen increases to levels significantly greater than those for control during reflow following transient global ischemia and the magnitude of the change is greater after longer periods of ischemia (Mrsulja *et al.*, 1976; Siesjö, 1978; Arai *et al.*, 1986), this effect may be simply the response of injured tissue to an ischemic insult. Alternatively, the glycogen accumulation may represent metabolic diaschisis in areas adjacent to the ischemic focus, regions which also exhibited an elevation in HEP.

5.7. Penumbra: Viability of Concept Exceeds That for the Region

The results for perfusion, histology, and metabolism in the rat model of focal ischemia indicate that the evolution of brain damage in the focal region differs markedly from that in the perifocal region and that the critical variable may be that

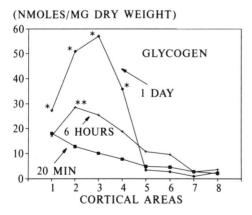

FIGURE 8. Glycogen levels in cortical areas at various times after MCA occlusion in the rat. For details, see the legend to Figure 7.

of time. The stringent definition of the penumbra has severely limited its application in stroke research, since it is difficult to simultaneously and discretely confirm (1) low extracellular potassium, (2) low blood flow, and (3) electrical quiescence in a relatively small region of the rat cortex. In this regard, a comprehensive review of focal cerebral ischemia shies away from the use of the word "penumbra" and refers to the area of marginal ischemia as the "peri-infarct zone" (Nedergaard et al., 1986). The concept of such a region encompassing the ischemic region may, nevertheless, be useful in designing experiments to minimize brain damage following focal ischemia. The metabolite profile at 1 day following MCA occlusion indicates that the tissue in the perifocal region is indistinguishable from that in the focal region. Since the onset of the pathophysiology in this region is relatively slow compared with that in the ischemic core, there is apparently a time frame for intervention, but this has disappeared by 1 day of irreversible focal ischemia.

5.8. Metabolic Correlates of the Perifocal Region

The metabolite profile in 46 pieces of tissue dissected from within the perifocal region of the brain shown in Figure 4, harvested at 1 hr after permanent irreversible ischemia was determined. Since the changes in the levels of ATP, P-creatine, and lactate were independent of sampling site (i.e., depth of cortex or medial to lateral location), the relationship of lactate concentration to ATP concentration in the same tissue was examined (Figure 9). The horizontal and vertical lines represent ±2 standard deviations of the mean for control lactate and ATP, respectively. Any value above the upper horizontal line and to the left of the vertical line is outside the 95% confidence level for the control values. Approximately 70% of the samples in the normal range for ATP exhibited an elevated lactate concentration, suggesting that an energy imbalance occurred in the perifocal region, but that it was not sufficient at 1 hr of occlusion to compromise the HEP status of the tissue. A similar finding of elevated lactate with only intermediate decreases in HEP has been reported by Busto and Ginsberg (1985) in a rat model of graded transient ischemia. These changes were observed in the dorsolateral cortex, a region exhibiting marginal, not total, ischemia.

The elevation of the lactate concentration in the perifocal region suggests an increased intracellular acidification which might explain, in part, the subsequent deterioration of this tissue. To evaluate this possibility, the levels of lactate were plotted against the P-creatine/ATP ratio from the same tissue. According to the creatine kinase equilibrium, intracellular acidification should lead to a decrease in this ratio (Veech, 1980). As shown in Figure 10, the ratio fell outside 2 SD of the control value in only 30% of the tissues examined, suggesting that the protons generated by excess lactate formation were buffered either metabolically or physically and/or removed by extrusion.

The heterogeneous patterns observed in the perifocal region might just as

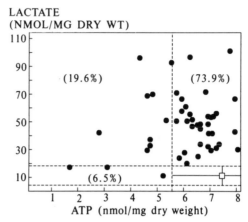

LACTATE
(NMOL/MG DRY WT)

FIGURE 9. Relationship of lactate to ATP in the perifocal region 1 hr after MCA occlusion in the rat. The perifocal region from the rat brain shown in Figure 4 was dissected into 46 discrete pieces of tissue and analyzed for ATP, P-creatine, and lactate. The dashed lines represent 2 SD from the mean determined in a minimum of six tissues from the contralateral cortex. The numbers in parentheses represent the percentages of the total tissues that had either (1) ATP within 2 SD of the mean for the control and lactate outside 2 SD of the mean for the control (73.9%), (2) lactate and ATP values outside 2 SD of their respective means (19.6%), and (3) lactate within 2 SD and ATP outside 2 SD (6.5%).

easily be explained by different responses present in different metabolic compartments.

6. SPECULATION ON THE PATHOPHYSIOLOGY OF BRAIN DAMAGE AFTER FOCAL ISCHEMIA

The metabolic fate of the ischemic focus is similar in most respects to the changes found following global ischemia. The changes in energy-related and glucose-related metabolites are evident within 20 min, and the depletion of energy stores is essentially complete. Despite the similarities, it is apparent that the ischemic core can influence the surrounding tissue, which is in direct contrast with the conditions encountered with the global models of ischemia. Because the ultimate goal of focal ischemia research is to establish an effective means of treatment, it is important to identify the factors which influence the apparent deterioration of the perifocal region with time. There are a number of possible explanations for the eventual infarction of the perifocal region, but the most plausible is that the perifocal region cannot be sustained by the collateral blood flow, thus leading to an ever-increasing level of energy imbalance in this tissue.

The discussion concerning capillary path length and capillary mean transit

P-CREATINE/ATP RATIO

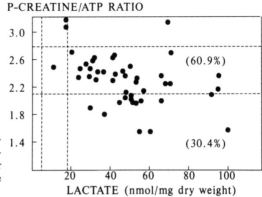

FIGURE 10. Relationship of the P-creatine/ATP ratio to the levels of lactate in the perifocal region 1 hr after MCA occlusion. For details, see the legend to Figure 9.

times might be relevant with respect to the perifocal region. Since the pathway from the collateral circulation to the regions served by the MCA would be longer, it is possible that the ability to supply nutrients and remove waste would be less efficient. Although this would not be sufficient to cause an immediate collapse of energy metabolism, the initially small, but ever-increasing, imbalance between energy production and consumption would ultimately lead to metabolic failure. This is supported by the elevation of lactate concentration in tissue which has normal or near-normal HEP at 1 hr after occlusion.

Other factors besides blood flow may influence the energy balance in the perifocal region. The loss of electrical activity in the perifocal region would tend to reduce the energy demands of the tissue by as much as 50% (Astrup, 1982) and, by doing so, actually protect against energy imbalance. This conservation of energy may be offset by an increase in energy demands elicited by spreading depression, which has been described in focal ischemia outside the territory subserved by the MCA (Nedergaard et al., 1986). The activation of the (Na^+, K^+)-ATPase during spreading depression may transiently disrupt the more precarious energy balance within the tissue owing to the decrease in blood flow. Each event would increase the deficiency in energy production, and this would be reflected by an increase in lactate production. If the buffering capacity of the tissue fails, the increased acidification would put the tissue at further risk.

Another factor to be considered in the deterioration of the perifocal region is edema. A recent report Olsson et al. (1989) demonstrated a marked decrease in the specific gravity of the cortex at 2, 6, and 24 hr after MCA occlusion, but the edema formation was evident only in spontaneously hypertensive rats and not in normotensive rats. The reason for the absence of edema in the normotensive Wistar rats may once again be related to the variable response in these animals (Brint et al., 1988). In preliminary experiments in our laboratory, an increase in the water content of both the focal and perifocal regions of the brain is evident by proton magnetic resonance imaging (MRI) in the normotensive rat, but the effect usually occurs only after 6 hr of MCA occlusion. The use of proton MRI should help to determine whether the time-dependent loss of perfusion to the perifocal region, as was indicated by NR intensity, is associated with edema formation.

In summary, a key to the slow deterioration of the perifocal region appears to be the reduction of blood flow, which in turn triggers metabolic events within the tissue. Signals from the tissue (e.g., CO_2, H^+) which might normally increase blood flow only further compromise the blood flow to the perifocal region. Alternatively, the asymmetry between energy production and consumption within the tissue increases with longer periods of MCA occlusion, eventually leading to energy failure. If both systems are operational, they would act synergistically to hasten the deterioration of the perifocal region. Further studies will attempt to dampen both of these processes in the hope of reducing the brain injury in the perifocal region.

7. THERAPEUTIC APPROACHES AGAINST FOCAL ISCHEMIA

7.1. Attributes of Focal Ischemia Impacting on Therapy

The evolution of ischemic damage in the penumbra is a vital consideration with regard to the treatment of stroke, since tissue in the penumbral region should be amenable to postischemic therapeutic intervention. Focal ischemic lesions appear to develop or mature over time (Garcia, 1984; Weinstein *et al.*, 1986). Thus, each treatment must be considered in light of its ability to offer protection at a given time after an ischemic event. There may be different "therapeutic windows" for different treatments. Recirculation may be considered the most direct form of therapy, although one in which special consideration must be given to the deleterious effects which may impact on the metabolic apparatus. Furthermore, the gross pathological damage which can occur if reperfusion is instituted too late after an ischemic event, including aggravated brain edema, hemorrhagic infarction, and brain herniation, has been well documented (Schuier and Hossmann, 1980; Dietrich *et al.*, 1987*a, b*; Hornig *et al.*, 1986).

7.2. Some Examples of Treatment Modalities

7.2.1. Hemodilution

Recirculation may not always be an immediate therapeutic option. Alternative forms of therapy will still be required in these instances. Hemodilution has been proposed as a method for the treatment of focal ischemia, although the results of such trials have been inconsistent (Grotta, 1987). It has been postulated that a decrease in hematocrit and viscosity improves microcirculatory perfusion (Kee and Wood, 1984). The effect of such perfusion changes on metabolism in marginally perfused regions must be further defined. Since hemodilution may aggravate edema and compromise the oxygen delivery to the tissue, it is important to assess both positive and negative effects of this therapy on cerebral metabolism and pathological outcome. In this manner, it may be possible to optimize the parameters of such therapy and modify the therapy to minimize any deleterious effects. Even if hemodilution alone is not protective, it may be possible to improve the delivery of other therapeutic agents by this treatment, and thus the potential for synergistic protection exists.

7.2.2. Calcium Channel Blockers

Although alterations in oxidative metabolism may underlie neuronal damage, marked increases in intracellular cytoplasmic calcium ion concentration occur in the course of ischemia and may be crucial in irreversible cell injury (Siesjö, 1981; Raichle, 1983). Calcium channel blockers have been evaluated in a variety of experimental models of ischemia. There have been conflicting results on the response to different agents (Mohamed *et al.*, 1985; Gotoh *et al.*, 1986; Germano *et al.*, 1987; Kobayashi *et al.*, 1988). It is unresolved whether the potential benefit is related to a direct effect on cellular metabolism (Siesjö, 1981; Raichle, 1983) or on an augmentation of cerebral blood flow (Harris *et al.*, 1982). Newer calcium channel blockers, which also possess serotonin antagonist properties, are protective (Bielenberg *et al.*, 1987). The possibility of combining calcium channel blockers with more potent and specific serotonin antagonists which act on different receptors (Glennon, 1986) appears to be a promising form of therapy. Whether such synergism affects blood flow and/or provides metabolic protection requires further investigation.

8. CONCLUSIONS

Our conclusions concerning the metabolic correlates of focal ischemia can be characterized by the single expression of heterogeneity. This heterogeneity plays out on several levels, each of which contributes to the overall complexity of the system. We have identified a number of levels of heterogeneity in the phenomenon of focal ischemia:

1. The first level of heterogeneity is regional heterogeneity. This distinguishes focal ischemia from generalized stroke. The gross regional partitions are the focal and perifocal regions, as well as nearby and distant regions supplied by intact vasculature.

2. The second level of heterogeneity is histological heterogeneity. This level comprises the differential metabolic responses of neuronal glial and endothelial cells (and their subtypes).
3. The third level of heterogeneity is cytological heterogeneity. This level is concerned with intracellular metabolic and functional compartments and pools.
4. The fourth level of heterogeneity is physiological heterogeneity. This level is exemplified by the diversity expressed in cerebrovascular variables, especially at the level of the capillary and the mechanisms which control its function.
5. The fifth level of heterogeneity is neuropathological heterogeneity. This level is most easily illustrated by the variability in sensitivity of cells within the regions affected by focal ischemia, i.e., a "selective vulnerability."
6. The sixth level might be considered therapeutic heterogeneity. At this level we suggest that the treatment of choice in focal ischemia depends on more than one modality and also depends directly on the determination of other variables such as the time after the ischemic event and whether reperfusion has occurred.

It is clear that a full appreciation of these levels of heterogeneity is required to understand the pathophysiology of focal ischemia and to devise rational strategies for therapy. It is also clear that the design of animal models of focal ischemia must consider heterogeneity to be a critical component.

REFERENCES

Arai, H., Passonneau, J. V., and Lust, W. D., 1986, Energy metabolism in delayed neuronal death of the CA1 neurons of the hippocampus following ischemia, *Metabol. Brain Dis.* **1**:263–278.

Astrup, J., 1982, Energy-requiring cell functions in the ischemic brain, *J. Neurosurg.* **56**:481–497.

Astrup, J., Symon, L., Branston, M., and Lassen, N. A., 1977, Cortical evoked potential and extracellular K^+ and H^+ at critical levels of brain ischemia, *Stroke* **8**:51–57.

Bederson, J. B., Pitts, L. H., Tsuji, M., Nishimura, M. C., Davis, R. L., and Bartkowski, H., 1986, Rat middle cerebral artery occlusion: Evaluation of the model and development of a neurologic examination, *Stroke* **17**:472–476.

Bielenberg, G. W., Haubruck, H., and Krieglstein, J., 1987, Effects of calcium entry blocker emopamil on postischemic energy metabolism of the isolated perfused rat brain, *J. Cereb. Blood Flow Metab.* **7**:489–496.

Boysen, G., Engell, H. C., Pistolese, G. R., Fiorani, P., Agnoli, A., and Lassen, N. A., 1974, On the critical lower level of cerebral blood flow in man with particular reference to carotid surgery, *Circulation* **49**:1023–1025.

Branston, N. M., Symon, L., Crockard, H. A., and Pasztor, E., 1974, Relationship between the cortical evoked potential and local cortical blood flow following acute middle cerebral artery occlusion in the baboon, *Exp. Neurol.* **45**:195–208.

Brint, S., Jacewicz, M., Kiessling, M., Tanabe, J., and Pulsinelli, W., 1988, Focal brain ischemia in the rat: Methods for reproducible neocortical infarction using tandem occlusion of the distal middle cerebral and ipsilateral common carotid arteries, *J. Cereb. Blood Flow Metab.* **8**:474–485.

Bryan, R. M., Keefer, K. A., and MacNeill, C., 1986, Regional cerebral glucose utilization during insulin-induced hypoglycemia in unanesthetized rats, *J. Neurochem.* **46**:1904–1911.

Busto, R., and Ginsberg, M. D., 1985, Graded focal cerebral ischemia in the rat by unilateral carotid artery occlusion and elevated intracranial pressure: Hemodynamic and biochemical characterization, *Stroke* **16**:446–476

Collins, R. C., 1987, Physiology-metabolism-blood flow couples in brain, *in* "Cerebrovascular Diseases" (W. J. Powers and R. E.Raichle, eds.), pp. 149–162, Raven Press, New York.

Cooper, A., 1836, Some experiments and observations on tying the carotid and vertebral arteries, *Guys Hosp. Rep.* **1**:458–475.

Coyle, P., 1982, Middle cerebral artery occlusion in the young rat, *Stroke* **13**:855–859.

Crockard, H. A., Gadian, D. G., Frackowiak, R. S. J., Proctor, E., Allen, K., Williams, S. R., and Ross Russell, R. W., 1987, Acute cerebral ischaemia: Concurrent changes in cerebral blood flow, energy metabolites, pH, and lactate measured with hydrogen clearance and ^{31}P and ^{1}H nuclear magnetic resonance spectroscopy. II. Changes during ischaemia, *J. Cereb. Blood Flow Metab.* **7**:394–402.

Dietrich, W. D., Busto, R., Watson, B. D., Scheinberg, P., and Ginsberg, M. D., 1987*a*, Photochemically induced cerebral infarction. II. Edema and blood brain barrier disruption, *Acta Neuropathol. (Berl)* **72**:326–334.

Dietrich, W. D., Busto, R., Yoshida, S., and Ginsberg, M. D., 1987*b*, Histopathological and hemodynamic consequences of complete versus incomplete ischemia in the rat, *J. Cereb. Blood Flow Metab.* **7**:300–308.

Duckrow, R. B., and Bryan, R. M., 1987, Regional cerebral glucose utilization during hyperglycemia, *J. Neurochem.* **48**:989–993.

Duckrow, R. B., Beard, D. C., and Brennan, R. W., 1987, Regional cerebral blood flow decreases during chronic and acute hyperglycemia, *Stroke* **18**:52–58.

Duverger, D., and MacKenzie, E. T., 1988, The quantification of cerebral infarction following focal ischemia in the rat: Influence of strain, arterial pressure, blood glucose concentration, and age, *J. Cereb. Blood Flow Metab.* **8**:449–461.

Erecinska, M., and Silver, I. A., 1989, ATP and brain function, *J. Cereb. Blood Flow Metab.* **9**:2–19.

Flourens, J. P. M., 1847, Note touchant l'action de divers substances injectees dans les arteres, *C. R. Acad. Sci.* **24**:905–908.

Fox, P. T., Raichle, M. E., Mintun, M. A., and Dence, C., 1988, Nonoxidative glucose consumption during focal physiologic neural activity, *Science* **241**:462–464.

Futrell, C., Millikan, C., Watson, B. D., Dietrich, W. D., and Ginsberg, M. D., 1988, Embolic stroke from a carotid arterial source in the rat: pathology and clinical implications, *Neurology 38*(Suppl. 1):1050–1056.

Garcia, J. H., 1984, Experimental ischemic stroke. A review, *Stroke* **15**:5–14.

Germano, I. M., Bartkowski, H. M., Cassel, M. E., and Pitts, L. H., 1987, The therapeutic value of nimodipine in experimental focal cerebral ischemia, *J. Neurosurg.* **67**:81–87.

Glennon, R. A., 1986, Central serotonin agonists and antagonists, *Neurotransmissions* **2**:1–3.

Goldberg, I. D., and Kurland, L. T., 1962, Mortality in 33 countries from disease of the nervous system, *World Neurol.* **3**:444–465.

Goldstein, G. W., and Betz, A. L., 1983, Recent advances in understanding brain capillary function, *Ann. Neurol.* **14**:389–395.

Gotoh, O., Mohamed, A. A., McCulloch, J., Graham, D. I., Harper, A. M., and Teasdale, G. M., 1986, Nimodipine and the haemodynamic and histopathological consequences of middle cerebral artery occlusion in the rat, *J. Cereb. Blood Flow Metab.* **6**:321–331.

Grabowski, M., Nordborg, C., Brundin, P., and Johansson, B. B., 1988, Middle cerebral artery occlusion in the hypertensive and normotensive rat: A study of histopathology and behavior, *J. Hypertension* **6:**405–411.

Grotta, J. C., 1987, Current status of hemodilution in acute cerebral ischemia, *Stroke* **18:**689–690.

Harik, S. I., and LaManna, J. C., 1988, Vascular perfusion and blood-brain glucose transport in acute and chronic hyperglycemia, *J. Neurochem.* **51:**1924–1929.

Harris, R. J., Branston, N. M., Symon, L., Bayhan, M., and Watson, A., 1982, The effects of a calcium antagonist, nimodipine, upon physiological responses of the cerebral vasculature and its possible influence upon focal cerebral ischaemia, *Stroke* **13:**759–766.

Hawkins, R. A., Mans, A. W., and Davis, D. W., 1986, Regional ketone body utilization by rat brain in starvation and diabetes, *Am. J. Physiol.* **250:**E169–E178.

Hochachka, P. W., and Mommsen, T. P., 1983, Protons and anaerobiosis, *Science* **219:**1391–1397.

Hollinger, B. R., and Bryan, R. M., 1987, β-Receptor-mediated increase in cerebral blood flow during hypoglycemia, *Am. J. Physiol.* **253:**H949–H955.

Hornig, C. R., Dorndorf, W., and Agnoli, A. L., 1986, Hemorrhagic cerebral infarction—a prospective study, *Stroke* **17:**179–184.

Jones, T., Morawetz, R. B., Crowell, M., Marcoux, F. W., Fitzgibbon, S. J., DeGirolami, U., and Ojemann, R. G., 1981, Thresholds of focal cerebral ischemia in awake monkeys, *J. Neurosurg.* **54:**773–782.

Kannel, W. B., and Wolf, P. A., 1983, Epidemiology of cerebrovascular disease, *in* "Cerebral Arterial Disease" (R. W. R. Russell, ed.), pp. 1–23, Churchill Livingstone, Edinburgh.

Kee, D. B., Jr., and Wood, J. H., 1984, Rheology of the cerebral circulation, *Neurosurgery* **15:**125–131.

Kikano, G. E., LaManna, J. C., and Harik, S. I., 1989, Brain perfusion in acute and chronic hyperglycemia, *Stroke* **20(8):**1027–1031.

Klatzo, I., Farkas-Bargeton, E., Guth, L., Miguel, J., and Olsson, Y., 1970, Some morphological and biochemical aspects of abnormal glycogen accumulation in the glia, *in* "Sixth International Congress of Neuropathology," pp. 351–365, Masson et Cie, Paris.

Kobayashi, S., Obana, W., Andrews, B. T., Nishimura, M. C., and Pitts, L. H., 1988, Lack of effect of nimodipine in experimental regional cerebral ischemia, *Stroke* **19:**147 (abstract).

Kreisman, N. R., LaManna, J. C., Rosenthal, M., and Sick, T. J., 1981a, Oxidative metabolic responses with recurrent seizures in rat cerebral cortex: Role of systemic factors, *Brain Res.* **218:**175–188.

Kreisman, N. R., Sick, T. J., LaManna, J. C., and Rosenthal, M., 1981b, Local tissue oxygen tension-cytochrome a,a$_3$ redox relationship in rat cerebral cortex in vivo, *Brain Res.* **218:**161–174.

Kudo, M., Aoyama, A., Ichimori, S., and Fukunaga, N., 1982, An animal model of cerebral infarction. Homologous blood clot emboli in rats, *Stroke* **13:**505–508.

LaManna, J. C., 1987, Intracellular pH determination by absorption spectrophotometry of neutral red, *Metab. Brain Dis.* **2:**167–182.

LaManna, J. C., Light, A. I., Peretsman, S. J., and Rosenthal, M., 1984, Oxygen insufficiency during hypoxic hypoxia in rat brain cortex, *Brain Res.* **293:**313–318.

LaManna, J. C., McCracken, K. A., Whittingham, T. S., and Lust, W. D., 1986, Determination of intracellular pH by color film histophotometry of frozen *in situ* rat brain, *in* "Oxygen Transport to Tissue. VIII. Advances in Experimental Medicine and Biology, vol. 200" (I. S. Longmuir, ed.), pp. 253–259, Plenum Publishing Corp., New York.

LaManna, J. C., Sick, T. J., Pikarsky, S. M., and Rosenthal, M., 1987, Detection of an oxidizable fraction of cytochrome oxidase in intact rat brain, *Am. J. Physiol.* **253:**C477–C483.

LaManna, J. C., McCracken, K. A., and Strohl, K. P., 1989, Changes in regional cerebral blood flow and sucrose space after 3–4 weeks of hypobaric hypoxia (0.5 atm), *in* "Oxygen Transport to Tissue. XI. Advances in Experimental Medicine and Biology, vol. 247" (K. Rakusan, G. P. Diro, T. K. Goldstick, and Z. Turek, eds.), pp. 471–477, Plenum Publishing Corp., New York.

Lassen, N. A., and Vorstrup, S., 1984, Ischemia penumbra results in incomplete infarction: Is the sleeping beauty dead?, *Stroke* **15**:755–756.

Lothman, E., LaManna, J. C., Cordingley, G., Rosenthal, M., and Somjen, G., 1975, Responses of electrical potential, potassium levels, and oxidative metabolic activity of the cerebral neocortex of cats, *Brain Res.* **88**:15–36.

Lowry, O. H., and Passonneau, J. V., 1972, "A Flexible System of Enzymatic Analysis," Academic Press, New York.

Lust, W. D., Feussner, G. K., Barbehenn, E. K., and Passonneau, J. V., 1981, The enzymatic measurement of adenine nucleotides and P-creatine in picomole amounts, *Anal. Biochem.* **110**: 258–266.

Mohamed, A. A., Gotoh, O., Graham, D. I., Osborne, K. A., McCulloch, J., Mendelow, A. D., Teasdale, G. M., and Harper, A. M., 1985, Effect of pretreatment with the calcium antagonist nimodipine on local cerebral blood flow and histopathology after middle cerebral artery occlusion, *Ann. Neurol.* **18**:705–711.

Moossy, J., 1979, Morphological validation of ischemic stroke models, *in* "Cerebrovascular Diseases" (T. R. Price and E. Nelson, eds.), pp. 3–10, Raven Press, New York.

Motti, E. D. F., Imhof, H.-G., and Yasargil, M. G., 1986, The terminal vascular bed in the superficial cortex of the rat, *J. Neurosurg.* **65**:834–846.

Mrsulja, B. B., Lust, W. D., Mrsulja, B. J., and Passonneau, J. V., 1976, Postischemic changes in certain metabolites following prolonged ischemia in the gerbil cerebral cortex, *J. Neurochem.* **26**:1099–1103.

Nakayama, H., Dietrich, W. D., Watson, B. D., Busto, R., and Ginsberg, M. D., 1988, Photothrombotic occlusion of rat middle cerebral artery: Histopathological and hemodynamic sequelae of acute recanalization, *J. Cereb. Blood Flow Metab.* **8**:357–366.

Nedergaard, M., Gjeddee, A., and Diemer, N. H., 1986, Focal ischemia of the rat brain: Autoradiographic determination of cerebral glucose utilization, glucose content, and blood flow, *J. Cereb. Blood Flow Metab.* **6**:414–424.

Nowicki, J.-P., Assumel-Lurdin, C., Duverger, D., and MacKenzie, E. T., 1988, Temporal evolution of regional energy metabolism following focal cerebral ischemia in the rat, *J. Cereb. Blood Flow Metab.* **8**:462–473.

Olsson, A.-L., Westergren, I., and Johansson, B. B., 1989, Brain edema after middle cerebral artery occlusion, *Acta Neurol. Scand* **80**(1):12–16.

Osborne, K. A., Shigeno, T., Balarsky, A. M., Ford, I., McCulloch, J., Teasdale, G. M., and Graham, D. I., 1987, Quantitative assessment of early brain damage in a rat model of focal cerebral ischaemia, *J. Neurol. Neurosurg. Psychiatry* **50**:402–410.

Payan, H. M., and Conard, J. R., 1977, Carotid ligation in gerbils. Influence of age, sex and gonads, *Stroke*, 194–201.

Ponten, U., Ratcheson, R. A., Salford, L. G., and Siesjö, B. K., 1973, Optimal freezing conditions for cerebral metabolites in rats, *J. Neurochem.* **21**:1127–1216.

Raichle, M. E., 1983, The pathophysiology of brain ischemia, *Ann. Neurol.* **13**:2–10.

Rapoport, S. I., Lust, W. D., and Fredericks, W. R., 1986, Effects of hypoxia on rat brain metabolism: unilateral *in vivo* carotid infusion, *Exp. Neurol.* **91**:319–330.

Ratcheson, R. A., and Ferrendelli, J. A., 1980, Regional cortical metabolism in focal ischemia, *J. Neurosurg.* **52**:755–763.

Rieke, G. K., Bowers, D. E., Jr., and Penn, P., 1981, Vascular supply pattern to rat caudatoputamen and globus pallidus: Scanning electron microscopic study of vascular endocasts of stroke-prone vessels, *Stroke* **12**:840–847.

Robins, M., and Baum, H. M., 1981, The NINCDS report on the national survey of stroke: Chapter 4, Incidence, *Stroke* **12**(Suppl. I):I-45–I-55.

Robinson, R. G., 1981, A model for the study of stroke using the rat, *Stroke* **104**:103–105.

Rosenthal, M., and LaManna, J. C., 1975, Effect of ouabain and phenobarbital on the kinetics of cortical metabolic transients associated with evoked potentials, *J. Neurochem.* **24**:111–116.

Rosner, G., and Heiss, W.-D., 1983, Survival of cortical neurons as a function of residual flow and duration of ischemia, *J. Cereb. Blood Flow Metab.* **3**(Suppl. 1):S393–S394.

Rossen, R., Kabat, H., and Anderson, J. P., 1943, Acute arrest of cerebral circulation in man, *Arch. Neurol. Psychiatry* **50**:510–528.

Rubino, G. J., and Young, W., 1988, Ischemic cortical lesions after permanent occlusion of individual middle cerebral artery branches in rats, *Stroke* **19**:870–877.

Sako, K., Kobatake, K., Yamamoto, Y. L., and Diksic, M., 1985, Correlation of local cerebral blood flow, glucose utilization, and tissue pH following a middle cerebral artery occlusion in the rat, *Stroke* **16**:828–834.

Schuier, F. J., and Hossmann, K.-A., 1980, Experimental brain infarcts in cats. 2. Ischemic brain edema, *Stroke* **11**:593–600.

Selman, W. R., VanDerVeer, C., Whittingham, T. S., LaManna, J. C., Lust, D., and Ratcheson, R. A., 1987, Visually defined zones of focal ischemia in the rat brain, *Neurosurgery* **21**:825–830.

Shigeno, T., Teasdale, G. M., McCulloch, J., and Graham, D. I., 1985, Recirculation model following MCA occlusion in rats: Cerebral blood flow, cerebrovascular permeability, and brain edema, *J. Neurosurg.* **63**:272–277.

Shockley, R. P., and LaManna, J. C., 1988, Determination of rat cerebral cortical blood volume changes by capillary mean transit time analysis during hypoxia, hypercapnia, and hyperventilation, *Brain Res.* **454**:170–178.

Siesjö, B. K., 1978, "Brain Energy Metabolism," John Wiley & Sons, Chichester, U.K.

Siesjö, B. K., 1981, Cell damage in the brain: A speculative synthesis, *J. Cereb. Blood Flow Metab.* **1**: 155–185.

Siesjö, B. K., 1984, Cerebral circulation and metabolism, *J. Neurosurg.* **60**:883–908.

Strong, A. J., Tomlinson, B. E., Venables, G. S., Gibson, G., and Hardy, A., 1983a, The cortical ischaemic penumbra associated with occlusion of the middle cerebral artery in the cat. 2. Studies of histopathology, water content, and in vitro neurotransmitter uptake, *J. Cereb. Blood Flow Metab.* **3**:97–108.

Strong, A. J., Venables, G. S., and Gibson, G., 1983b, The cortical ischemic penumbra associated with occlusion of the middle cerebral artery in the cat. 1. Topography of changes in blood flow, potassium ion activity and EEG, *J. Cereb. Blood Flow Metab.* **3**:86–96.

Sundt, T. M., Jr., Sharbrough, F. W., Anderson, R. E., and Michenfelder, J. D., 1974, Cerebral blood flow measurements and electroencephalograms during carotid endarterectomy, *J. Neurosurg.* **41**:310–320.

Symon, L., Pasztor, E., and Branston, N. M., 1974, The distribution and density of reduced cerebral blood flow following acute middle cerebral artery occlusion: An experimental study by the technique of hydrogen clearance in baboons, *Stroke* **5**:355–364.

Tamura, A., Graham, D. I., McCulloch, J., and Teasdale, G. M., 1981, Focal cerebral ischaemia in the rat. 1. Description of technique and early neuropathological consequences following middle cerebral artery occlusion, *J. Cereb. Blood Flow Metab.* **1**:53–60.

Tyson, G. W., Teasdale, G. M., Graham, D. I., and McCulloch, J., 1984, Focal cerebral ischemia in the rat: Topography of hemodynamic and histopathological changes, *Ann. Neurol.* **15**:559–567.

Veech, R. L., 1980, Freeze blowing of brain and the interpretation of the meaning of certain metabolite levels, *in* "Cerebral Metabolism and Neural Function" (J. V. Passonneau, R. A. Hawkins, W. D. Lust, and F. A. Welsh, eds.), pp. 34–41, Williams & Wilkins, Baltimore.

Walker, E. A., Robins, M., and Weinfeld, F. D., 1981, The NINCDS report on the national survey of stroke: Clinical findings, *Stroke* **12**(Suppl. I):I-13–I-31.

Weinstein, P. R., Anderson, D. G., and Telles, D. A., 1986, Neurological deficit and cerebral infarction after temporary middle cerebral artery occlusion in unanesthetized cats, *Stroke* **17**:318–324.

Weiss, H. R., 1988, Measurement of cerebral capillary perfusion with a fluorescent label, *Microvasc. Res.* **36:**172–180.

Welsh, F. A., 1984, Regional evaluation of ischemic metabolic alterations, *J. Cereb. Blood Flow Metab.* **4:**309–316.

Wolf, P. A., Kannel, W. B., and McGee, D. L., 1986, Epidemiology of strokes in North America, *in* "Stroke: Pathology, Diagnosis and Management" (H. J. M. Barnett, J. P. Moir, B. M. Stein, and F. M. Yatsu, eds.), pp. 19–29, Churchill Livingstone, Edinburgh.

Yamori, Y., Horie, R., Handa, H., Sato, M., and Fukase, M., 1976, Pathogenetic similarity of strokes in stroke-prone spontaneously hypertensive rats and humans, *Stroke* **7:**46–53.

Zea Longa, E., Weinstein, P. R., Carlson, S., and Cummins, R., 1989, Reversible middle cerebral artery occlusion without craniectomy in rats, *Stroke* **20:**84–91.

CHAPTER 3

ROLE OF PYRUVATE DEHYDROGENASE IN ISCHEMIC INJURY

FRANK A. WELSH

1. MOLECULAR MECHANISMS OF INJURY

Molecular mechanisms of ischemic brain damage remain poorly understood. To develop effective therapeutic agents, it is important to identify the primary neurochemical determinants of ischemic injury. Within the past decade, several attractive mechanisms of ischemic injury have been proposed (Siesjö, 1981; Raichle, 1983). First, loss of calcium homeostasis may be a major factor leading to cellular damage (Siesjö, 1988). During ischemia, depletion of energy reserves causes membrane failure, resulting in rapid entry of calcium into the cell (Harris *et al.*, 1981; Hansen, 1985). In addition, release of calcium from intracellular stores may contribute to an overwhelming increase in intracellular calcium concentration $[Ca]_i$. Although the increase in $[Ca]_i$ is reversible, even a transient rise may trigger secondary alterations that cause permanent cellular injury. A

FRANK A. WELSH • Division of Neurosurgery, University of Pennsylvania, Philadelphia, Pennsylvania.

Neurochemical Correlates of Cerebral Ischemia, Volume 7 of Advances in Neurochemistry, edited by Nicolas G. Bazan, Pierre Braquet, and Myron D. Ginsberg. Plenum Press, New York, 1992.

number of targets of increased $[Ca]_i$ have been postulated, but definitive proof implicating a specific target in cellular injury is lacking. Indeed, a causative relationship between increased $[Ca]_i$ and ischemic injury has not been established (Siesjö, 1988).

A second pathogenic factor is intracellular acidosis caused by the ischemic accumulation of lactic acid. Researchers in several laboratories, including our own, have demonstrated that hyperglycemia enhances the accumulation of lactate and exacerbates the degree of ischemic injury (Myers, 1979; Welsh *et al.*, 1980; Rehncrona *et al.*, 1981). Mitochondrial function is inhibited at low pH (Hillered *et al.*, 1984*a*); thus, acidosis may interfere directly with postischemic recovery of energy metabolism. However, regeneration of high-energy phosphates is substantial even when lactate accumulation exceeds 30 mmol/kg (Welsh *et al.*, 1978*a*, 1983). The additional increment in lactate that is associated with grossly impaired energy metabolism is small (Welsh *et al.*, 1983), and it has been suggested that acidification differs greatly in specific compartments of brain tissue (Kraig *et al.*, 1986). Acidosis may influence a number of other processes, such as calcium sequestration, cell swelling, and free-radical formation (Siesjö, 1985; Siesjö *et al.*, 1985). As discussed below, acid-catalyzed destruction of NADH may impair cellular energy metabolism.

In recent years, attention has focused on excitotoxic mechanisms of ischemic injury. First proposed by Olney (1969), the possibility that glutamate is toxic to neurons has been recently reviewed (Rothman and Olney, 1986). The ischemic depolarization of neurons causes a release of glutamate into the extracellular space (Benveniste *et al.*, 1984). Glutamate accumulates to high levels because reuptake systems are blocked by the ischemic energy failure. Exposure of neurons to glutamate in cell culture causes neuronal injury that is dependent on extracellular calcium (Choi, 1985). Furthermore, antagonists of specific receptors for glutamate diminish the degree of cellular damage caused by ischemia (Simon *et al.*, 1984; Ozyurt *et al.*, 1988). In particular, antagonists of *N*-methyl-D-aspartate (NMDA) receptors, which are linked to calcium-permeable channels, are reported to protect neurons against anoxic injury (Gill *et al.*, 1987). Although the intracellular mechanism by which excitatory substances injure cells is unknown, excessive entry of calcium through receptor-linked channels is an attractive possibility. Alternatively, persistent excitation of neurons may create a metabolic load that outstrips the capacity of the cells to produce high-energy phosphates and, thus, precipitates cellular energy failure.

2. REGIONAL HETEROGENEITY

Identification of pathologic mechanisms in vivo is severely impeded by the regional heterogeneity of brain tissue. To define the mechanisms of ischemic injury, it is critical to distinguish the biochemical changes in injured cells from those in recovering cells. Cerebral ischemia causes metabolic alterations that vary greatly in different regions of the brain (Welsh, 1984). Even in the most uniform of ischemic episodes, i.e., complete cessation of flow, metabolic changes are regionally inhomogeneous (Gatfield *et al.*, 1966). Furthermore, the patchy perfusion that characterizes incomplete ischemia accentuates the heterogeneity of the ischemic metabolic response (Welsh *et al.*, 1978*b*). Finally, in focal ischemia, metabolic perturbations in the ischemic focus are both quantitatively and qualitatively different from those in bordering regions (Ratcheson and Ferrendelli, 1980). Therefore, it is imperative that studies of cerebral ischemia employ methods with the highest spatial resolution.

Early studies of global ischemia and reperfusion failed to detect regions with impaired recovery of energy metabolism (Ljunggren *et al.*, 1974; Marshall *et al.*, 1975), possibly owing to inadequate regional resolution of the methods used. However, with the development of regional mapping methods for NADH (Welsh and Rieder, 1978), ATP (Kogure and Alonso, 1978), glucose (Paschen *et al.*, 1981), and pH (Kogure *et al.*, 1980; Csiba *et al.*, 1983), it was possible to detect small regions with impaired energy metabolism within a large mass of recovering tissue (Welsh *et al.*, 1978*a*, 1982). These regions were characterized by low levels of ATP and phosphocreatine (PCr), high levels of lactate, low pH, and paradoxically low levels of NADH and NAD^+ (Welsh *et al.*, 1982). Indeed, the diminution of the NAD pool suggested that defective oxidation-reduction of the NAD^+/NADH redox couple may have contributed to the permanent energy failure.

3. IMPAIRED GENERATION OF NADH

NAD^+ and NADH participate in oxidation-reduction reactions that are essential for oxidative phosphorylation. Thus, insufficient generation of NADH from NAD^+ would severely impair the production of high-energy phosphates. A number of lines of evidence indicate a defect in NADH metabolism during postischemic recirculation. First, postischemic regions with an impaired energy state exhibit decreased rather than increased levels of NADH (Welsh *et al.*, 1982). Second, in vivo fluorometry of NADH and spectroscopy of cytochrome $a-a_3$ demonstrates a hyperoxidation during postischemic reperfusion (Duckrow *et al.*, 1981). Third, the rate of formation of NADH during anoxia is markedly decreased in postischemic brain tissue (Welsh *et al.*, 1982). Indeed, complete cessation of flow to regions with energy failure did not elicit the expected rise in NADH level (Welsh *et al.*, 1978*a*). These results indicate impaired generation of NADH in regions undergoing energy failure.

Additional evidence suggests that a primary metabolic defect may limit the recovery of the brain following ischemia. Mitochondria isolated from post ischemic brain tissue exhibited a significant decrease in their maximal rate of respiration (Rehncrona *et al.*, 1979). Indeed, in several models of transient ischemic there was a good correlation between recovery of high-energy phosphate levels in vivo and the function of mitochondria in vitro (Hillered *et al.*, 1984*b*, 1985). Similarly, recent studies have demonstrated a postischemic decline in mitochondrial respiration in selectively vulnerable regions (striatum), with no change in a resistant area of cerebral cortex (Sims and Pulsinelli, 1987). Therefore, regions experiencing permanent energy failure appear to have defective mito-chondria.

Finally, postischemic regions with impaired energy metabolism exhibit an abnormally high concentration of glucose (Paschen *et al.*, 1983; Tanaka *et al.*, 1985). Although alterations of glucose transport cannot be excluded, it is likely that the increase in glucose content reflects a primary inhibition of glucose utilization. During prolonged focal ischemia in rat brain, increased tissue levels of glucose occurred prior to the deterioration of the energy state (Nowicki *et al.*, 1988). Therefore, it is possible that a primary inhibition of glucose metabolism limits the supply of reducing equivalents (NADH) needed for oxidative phos-phorylation.

4. ACID-CATALYZED DESTRUCTION OF NADH

During the oxidation of glucose, NADH is generated by glyceraldehyde-3-P dehydrogenase, pyruvate dehydrogenase (PDH), and the dehydrogenases of the citric acid cycle. Inhibition at any of these sites would limit the ability of the brain to produce high-energy phosphates. Furthermore, a critical decrement in the NAD pool would depress the generation of NADH at many of the dehydrogenases. As noted above, there is good evidence that the NAD pool is substantially diminished in regions with impaired energy metabolism (Welsh *et al.*, 1982). Thus, a decrease in the NAD pool may inhibit the generation of NADH and impair energy metabolism.

NADH is unstable at low pH, especially in the presence of P_i (Lowry *et al.*, 1961). Since ischemia causes a decrease in pH and an increase in NADH and P_i levels, acid-catalyzed destruction of NADH might account for the observed decrease in the NAD pool following ischemia. The effect of acid on NADH might also explain the exacerbation of ischemic injury when the accumulation of lactic acid is enhanced by hyperglycemia. Therefore, it was important to determine whether the NAD pool is degraded more rapidly during ischemic insults that generate high concentrations of lactic acid.

Low-lactate ischemia was produced by decapitation of mice. The severed heads were incubated at 37 to 38°C for 2 hr. At various times, the brains were frozen and samples of the cerebral cortex were analyzed for ATP, lactate, NAD^+, and NADH by enzymatic, fluorometric methods (Welsh *et al.*, 1987). As expected, complete ischemia depleted levels of ATP by 10 min, at which time the lactate level had increased to a plateau of 13 to 14 mmol/kg (Table 1). The NADH level rose progressively during the first hour of ischemia to a maximum of 250 μmol/kg before declining. During the first 10 min, the increase in NADH was matched by the decrease in NAD$^+$, but thereafter the NAD pool decreased steadily, reaching 50% of control levels by 2 hr. Thus, complete ischemia causes a marked degradation of the NAD pool.

The effect of complete ischemia on the NAD pool was compared with that of incomplete, focal ischemia, which generates higher concentrations of lactic acid. Focal ischemia was produced by occluding the middle cerebral artery in the mouse for 1 or 2 hr. To compare the results with those for complete ischemia, animals were selected for study only if ATP levels were depleted in the ischemic focus. Although lactate accumulated to levels twice those found during complete ischemia, the decline in the NAD pool during focal ischemia was slower than that observed during complete ischemia (Table 2). Thus, enhanced accumulation of lactate per se did not promote degradation of the NAD pool. Of course, since pH was not measured, it is possible that focal ischemia does not enhance the decrease in pH as much as it enhances the increase in lactate. Furthermore, the smaller increase in the NADH level during focal ischemia (to only 100 μmol/kg) may have limited the acid-catalyzed degradation. During focal ischemia, collateral flow delivers small amounts of oxygen, which may prevent maximal reduction of the NADH-NAD$^+$ redox couple. Since acid-catalyzed destruction of NADH is a function of both H$^+$ and NADH concentrations, the limited increase in the NADH level during focal ischemia may have offset any enhancement of lactic acidosis.

5. EFFECT OF HYPERGLYCEMIA ON THE NAD POOL

Hyperglycemia is known to impair the recovery of cerebral energy metabolism and to exacerbate the degree of ischemic injury (Myers and Yamaguchi, 1977;

TABLE 1. Effect of Complete (Low-Lactate) Ischemia on the NAD Pool[a]

Duration of ischema	No. of animals	Level (mean ± SEM)				
		ATP (mmol/kg)	Lactate (mmol/kg)	NADH (μmol/kg)	NAD$^+$ (μmol/kg)	NAD pool (μmol/kg)
Controls	6	2.46 ± 0.03	1.9 ± 0.5	51 ± 5	466 ± 23	517 ± 23
10 min	4	0.10 ± 0.02	13.0 ± 1.0	178 ± 7	327 ± 10	505 ± 12
30 min	4	0.03 ± 0.02	13.6 ± 1.2	208 ± 8	242 ± 12	450 ± 15
60 min	6	0.10 ± 0.03	13.5 ± 0.4	253 ± 8	129 ± 10	381 ± 4
120 min	6	0.03 ± 0.01	13.4 ± 1.3	174 ± 6	80 ± 4	254 ± 7

[a]Data reprinted from Welsh et al. (1987) with permission of Raven Press.

TABLE 2. Effect of Focal (High-Lactate) Ischemia on the NAD Pool[a]

Duration of ischema	No. of animals	ATP (mmol/kg)	Lactate (mmol/kg)	NADH (μmol/kg)	NAD+ (μmol/kg)	NAD pool (μmol/kg)
			Level (mean ± SEM)			
Sham	6	2.34 ± 0.07	2.1 ± 0.7	22 ± 2	447 ± 18	469 ± 18
60 min	6	0.24 ± 0.06	24.7 ± 3.2	96 ± 13	343 ± 15	442 ± 10
120 min	6	0.11 ± 0.02	32.9 ± 3.9	93 ± 16	291 ± 21	385 ± 27

[a]Data reprinted from Welsh et al. (1987) with permission of Raven Press.

Welsh et al., 1980; Rehncrona et al., 1981; Pulsinelli et al., 1982c). Furthermore, systemic administration of glucose impairs postischemic recovery of energy metabolism in a dose-dependent manner (Welsh et al., 1983). If the adverse effects of hyperglycemia were due to enhanced destruction of NADH by lactic acid, the NAD pool should suffer an earlier and more pronounced diminution in hyperglycemic animals.

Mice were pretreated with glucose (20 mmol/kg) or saline and subjected to unilateral hypoxia-oligemia produced by occlusion of one carotid artery and exposure to an atmosphere containing 10% O_2 (Welsh et al., 1983). After 30 min, the carotid occlusion was reversed and the animals were returned to room air for a recovery period of 15 or 60 min. Samples of the cerebral cortex ipsilateral to the carotid occlusion were analyzed for metabolite levels in animals frozen at 0, 15, or 60 min of recovery following the 30-min insult (Table 3).

At 30 min of hypoxia-oligemia (no recovery time), tissue levels of ATP in the ipsilateral cortex were nearly depleted in both saline- and glucose-pretreated

TABLE 3. Effect of Hyperglycemia on the NAD Pool Following a 30-Min Insult[a]

Recovery period	Treatment	ATP (mmol/kg)	Lactate (mmol/kg)	NADH (μmol/kg)	NAD+ (μmol/kg)	NAD pool (μmol/kg)
			Level (mean ± SEM)[b,c]			
0 min	Saline	0.19 ± 0.04	30.5 ± 2.0	77 ± 15	483 ± 10	560 ± 6
	Glucose	0.17 ± 0.07	39.6 ± 1.3*	72 ± 5	492 ± 7	564 ± 7
15 min	Saline	1.67 ± 0.18	12.4 ± 0.7	36 ± 7	449 ± 13	486 ± 17
	Glucose	1.05 ± 0.24	40.0 ± 2.0*	34 ± 12	473 ± 13	508 ± 14
60 min	Saline	1.77 ± 0.38	3.5 ± 0.8	45 ± 12	415 ± 12	461 ± 11
	Glucose	0.14 ± 0.14*	30.7 ± 4.2*	37 ± 16	350 ± 22	387 ± 35

[a]Data reprinted from Welsh et al. (1987) with permission of Raven Press.
[b]There were six animals per group.
[c]Asterisks indicate that the result was significantly different from saline ($P < 0.01$).

groups. Lactate accumulated to 30 and 40 mmol/kg in saline-pretreated and glucose-pretreated animals, respectively. However, glucose pretreatment had no effect on cortical levels of NADH, NAD$^+$, or the NAD pool. Indeed, the NAD pool was not significantly diminished from control values in either group.

After 15 min of recovery (Table 3), ATP levels were restored to 59% of control levels in saline-pretreated animals, compared with 36% of control levels following glucose-pretreatment. However, this difference was not statistically significant. Lactate levels showed substantial recovery in the saline group; in contrast, there was no recovery of lactate in glucose-pretreated animals. Despite these differences in lactate levels, the decrease in the NAD pool was nearly the same (10 to 13%) in both groups.

After 60 min of recovery, cortical levels of ATP were maintained at 65% of control levels in the saline group, whereas ATP levels exhibited a secondary decline in glucose-pretreated animals. Lactate levels remained grossly elevated in the glucose group, but returned nearly to normal in saline-pretreated animals. The NAD pool was diminished by 31% in the glucose group and by 18% in the saline group, but the difference between the groups was not statistically significant.

These results demonstrate that administration of glucose increases the accumulation of lactate, impairs the recovery of ATP and lactate, but has no early (15 min) effect on the size of the NAD pool. Only after 60 min of recovery was there a tendency for the NAD pool to be smaller in hyperglycemic animals. Furthermore, ATP levels were already severely depleted after 60 min of recovery; consequently, we could not establish that a diminution of the NAD pool preceded the secondary energy failure.

In summary, the results of the experiments described above do not support the hypothesis that acid-catalyzed destruction of NADH causes a premature diminution of NAD pool that might impair energy metabolism. Although a pathologic role for the destruction of NADH in acid is not ruled out, we must conclude that the pyridine nucleotide pool is not especially vulnerable during ischemic insults that permit a large accumulation of lactic acid.

6. ROLE OF PYRUVATE DEHYDROGENASE

PDH occupies a key position in the pathways of energy metabolism. A mitochondrial enzyme, PDH catalyzes the oxidative decarboxylation of the glycolytic end product, pyruvate. Coupled to the oxidation of pyruvate is the reduction of NAD$^+$ to NADH. Another product of the PDH reaction, acetyl coenzyme A (acetyl-CoA), is oxidized in the citric acid cycle and thus generates additional NADH equivalents. Since a continuous supply of NADH is required for oxidative phosphorylation, PDH activity is essential for energy metabolism. As a key enzyme, PDH is highly regulated and is therefore one of the rate-limiting enzymes of energy metabolism.

PDH is a complex of several polypeptides which are organized to carry out the separate steps of the overall reaction (Reed and Yeaman, 1987). PDH is inhibited by phosphorylation of the α-subunit and is activated by dephosphorylation. Associated with the PDH complex are the enzymes PDH kinase and PDH phosphatase, which catalyze phosphorylation and dephosphorylation of the α-subunit. The kinase and phosphatase, in turn, are activated or inhibited by a variety of solutes, including K^+, Mg^{2+}, Ca^{2+}, NADH, acetyl-CoA, ADP, and pyruvate. Thus, concentrations of these effectors in vivo finely control the rate of reaction to meet the energy needs of the cell.

In addition to its role in supplying reducing equivalents, PDH is important in metabolizing the lactate that accumulates during ischemia. Therefore, during postischemic recirculation, lactate is reoxidized to pyruvate, which then becomes a substrate for PDH. Since the concentration of lactic acid may be an important determinant in ischemic injury, activation of PDH might accelerate the post-ischemic clearance of lactate and thus reduce the extent of ischemic injury.

7. EFFECTS OF DICHLOROACETATE

Dichloroacetate (DCA) is known to activate PDH by inhibiting its kinase (Whitehouse and Randle, 1973). Recently, Dimlich and coworkers administered DCA to rats to determine whether brain levels of lactate could be reduced following an ischemic insult (Biros et al., 1986; Kaplan et al., 1987). DCA, administered either pre- or postischemically, was reported to diminish lactate levels measured at 30 min of recirculation following 30 min of global ischemia in rat brain.

Using a similar model, we determined whether pretreatment with DCA would diminish the accumulation of lactate during the ischemic insult (Colohan et al., 1986). Rats were pretreated with glucose to increase the ischemic accumulation of lactate. Following administration of DCA, cerebral ischemia was produced by occluding both carotid arteries while reducing arterial pressure to 50 mmHg by arterial hemorrhage. After 15 min of ischemia, the brain was frozen in situ with liquid nitrogen and the cerebral cortex was assayed for ATP, PCr, and lactate.

Pretreatment with DCA did not alter the changes in ATP, PCr, or lactate during the 15-min period of ischemia (Table 4). The lack of effect of DCA on brain lactate during ischemia is most probably due to limitation of substrate (NAD^+ or pyruvate) rather than the phosphorylation state of the enzyme. Indeed, PDH is known to be fully activated during cerebral ischemia (Jope and Blass, 1976); consequently, DCA would have little effect on PDH activity even with adequate availability of substrates.

TABLE 4. Effect of DCA on Ischemia Changes
in ATP, PCr, and Lactate[a]

Treatment	No. of animals	Level (mean ± SEM)		
		ATP (mmol/kg)	PCr (mmol/kg)	Lactate (mmol/kg)
Control	6	2.75 ± 0.03	3.60 ± 0.24	2.4 ± 0.4
Saline	6	0.87 ± 0.30	0.49 ± 0.24	29.5 ± 2.2
DCA	6	0.47 ± 0.21	0.31 ± 0.22	32.0 ± 1.8

[a]Data reprinted from Colohan et al. (1986) with permission of the American Heart Association.

8. EFFECT OF ISCHEMIA AND REPERFUSION ON PDH ACTIVITY

In a brief report, the expected activation of PDH was demonstrated during ischemia in the rat brain (Wieloch and Koide, 1987). However, recirculation led to an inhibition of PDH activity, which persisted for 6 hr postischemia. Inhibition of PDH could interfere with recovery of energy metabolites, including ATP and PCr, as well as lactate. In addition, inhibition of PDH could impair the generation of NADH. Since DCA activates PDH, it may be possible to overcome this inhibition by administering DCA. Therefore, we used a model of transient ischemia in the gerbil to determine whether administration of DCA improved the recovery of energy metabolism.

9. EFFECT OF DCA ON METABOLITE RECOVERY

Transient cerebral ischemia was produced in gerbils by using bilateral carotid artery occlusion. Animals were pretreated by intraperitoneal (i.p.) administration of DCA (2.3 mmol/kg), and control animals were given an equivalent dose of acetate. Both groups were also pretreated with glucose to increase the accumulation of lactate during ischemia. After 20 min of bilateral occlusion, the carotid arteries were reopened to permit postischemic reperfusion for up to 4 hr. Animals surviving for 4 hr were given a second dose of DCA at 2 hr postischemia. At various times, the brain was quick-frozen in liquid nitrogen and samples from the cerebral cortex and caudate nucleus were assayed for ATP, PCr, and lactate. Separate samples were assayed for PDH activity using a spectrophotometric method (Hinman and Blass, 1981).

Tissue levels of ATP were depleted during the 20-min insult in cortex and caudate in both DCA- and acetate-pretreated groups (Figure 1). During the first 60

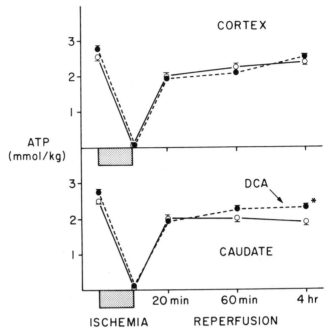

FIGURE 1. Effect of DCA on ATP levels in the cerebral cortex and caudate nucleus. Animals were pretreated with DCA (●) or acetate (○) and subjected to cerebral ischemia (20 min) followed by reperfusion for up to 4 hr. Two to four samples per animal were dissected from the cortex and caudate and assayed for ATP. Each point is the mean ± SEM for five to seven animals. The asterisk indicates a significant difference from acetate-treated controls ($P < 0.05$). Reprinted from Katayama and Welsh (1989) with permission of Raven Press.

min of reperfusion, ATP levels were restored to 70 to 80% of control levels in both regions. DCA pretreatment did not alter the recovery of ATP during the first 60 min of recirculation. However, at 4 hr, ATP levels in the caudate nucleus were significantly higher in DCA-treated animals, although the difference was small (+21%). ATP levels in the cerebral cortex were the same in both treatment groups (91 to 94% of preischemic values).

A similar time course was observed for levels of PCr (Figure 2). Nearly depleted during ischemia, PCr was restored to normal levels (or above) after 20 and 60 min of reperfusion in both regions, with no significant differences between treatment groups. However, at 4 hr, the PCr level was significantly higher in the cortex (+23%) and caudate (+84%) in DCA-treated animals. Indeed, in acetate-treated animals, PCr exhibited a secondary decline, which was especially evident in the caudate nucleus.

Changes in lactate levels during ischemia and reperfusion were consistent

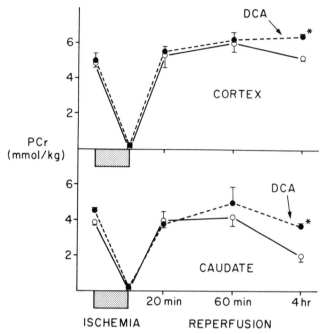

FIGURE 2. Effect of DCA on PCr levels in the cerebral cortex and caudate nucleus. Animals were pretreated with DCA (●) or acetate (○) and subjected to cerebral ischemia (20 min) followed by reperfusion for up to 4 hr. Two to four samples per animal were dissected from the cortex and caudate and assayed for PCr. Each point is the mean ± SEM for five to seven animals. Asterisks indicate significant differences from acetate-treated controls ($P < 0.05$). Reprinted from Katayama and Welsh (1989) with permission of Raven Press.

with those of the high-energy phosphates (Figure 3). Thus, lactate levels rose to 25 to 27 mmol/kg during ischemia in both regions and both treatment groups. During the first 60 min of reperfusion, recovery of lactate was somewhat slower in the caudate nucleus, but there was no difference between treatment groups in either region. However, at 4 hr, lactate levels in the caudate were significantly lower in DCA-treated animals than in acetate-treated animals. Indeed, there was a secondary increase in the level of lactate in the acetate group.

The activity of PDH also changed markedly during ischemia and reperfusion (Figure 4). Prior to ischemia, PDH was activated threefold in both regions by DCA pretreatment. During ischemia, PDH activity increased in the acetate group to values similar to those of the DCA-treated group. Presumably, this activity represents nearly full activation of the PDH complex. Remarkably, reperfusion caused a profound inhibition of PDH in both regions and in both treatment groups. During 4 hr of recirculation, PDH was reactivated in DCA-treated animals,

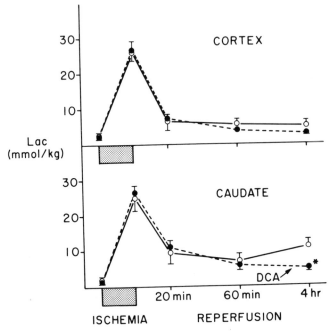

FIGURE 3. Effect of DCA on lactate (Lac) levels in the cerebral cortex and caudate nucleus. Animals were pretreated with DCA (●) or acetate (○) and subjected to cerebral ischemia (20 min) followed by reperfusion for up to 4 hr. Two to four samples per animal were dissected from the cortex and caudate and assayed for lactate. Each point is the mean ± SEM for five to seven animals. The asterisk indicates significant difference from acetate-treated controls ($P < 0.05$). Reprinted from Katayama and Welsh (1989) with permission of Raven Press.

contrasting with persistent inhibition in the acetate group. Thus, after 60 min and 4 hr of reperfusion, PDH activity was three- to fourfold higher in DCA-treated animals.

In summary, these results demonstrate that administration of DCA activated PDH and prevented the secondary deterioration of metabolite levels, which was most evident in the caudate nucleus. This finding suggests that PDH activity in acetate-treated animals was not sufficient to maintain the tissue energy state after 4 hr of reperfusion. Thus, persistent inhibition of PDH activity may be a limiting factor in the recovery of energy metabolism following cerebral ischemia.

The inhibition of PDH observed at 20 min of reperfusion was not affected by DCA pretreatment. Since PDH was significantly activated at 60 min of recovery with no additional administration of DCA, the failure to activate at 20 min cannot be attributed to decreased brain levels of DCA. Rather, the activation of PDH by DCA may be overshadowed by inhibitory effectors of PDH activity at 20 min of reperfusion. However, the mechanism of PDH inhibition is unknown.

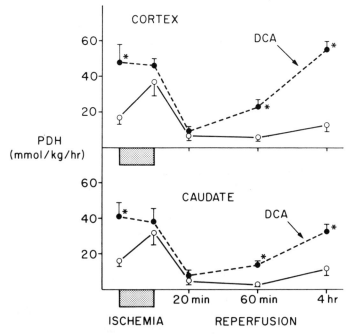

FIGURE 4. Effect of DCA on PDH activity in the cerebral cortex and caudate nucleus. Animals were pretreated with DCA (●) or acetate (○) and subjected to cerebral ischemia (20 min) followed by reperfusion for up to 4 hr. Two samples per animal were dissected from the cortex and caudate and assayed for PDH activity. Each point is the mean ± SEM for five to seven animals. Asterisks indicate significant differences from acetate-treated controls ($P < 0.05$). Reprinted from Katayama and Welsh (1989) with permission of Raven Press.

Despite the inhibition of PDH at 20 min of reperfusion, there was substantial recovery of metabolite levels. Since the metabolic demand is likely to be low immediately after ischemia, even a reduced activity of PDH may be sufficient restore levels of energy metabolites. However, when the metabolic demand returns to normal (at 4 hr), the capacity to generate high-energy phosphates may be limited by the inhibition of PDH, resulting in a secondary failure of energy metabolism.

10. MITOCHONDRIAL FAILURE AND CELL DEATH

The secondary deterioration of energy metabolites described above is similar to that observed in the dorsolateral striatum of the rat brain following 30 min of four-vessel occlusion (Pulsinelli and Duffy, 1983). However, in the rat model, energy metabolites continued to recover for 6 hr before showing secondary failure, measured at 24 hr. The secondary decline in metabolite levels paralleled the onset of morphologic change in the striatum as determined by light microscopy (Pulsinelli *et al.*, 1982*a*). In addition, the maximal rate of respiration of mitochondria in microhomogenates from striatum showed a similar decline after 6 hr of reperfusion (Sims and Pulsinelli, 1987). Therefore, there is good evidence that energy metabolism in the caudate nucleus recovers well during the first few hours of reperfusion, only to suffer a secondary deterioration that is associated with neuronal death.

The mechanism for the delayed energy failure in the caudate nucleus remains unknown. In the four-vessel rat model noted above, sequential changes in blood flow and glucose utilization in the caudate were measured during postischemic recirculation (Pulsinelli *et al.*, 1982*b*). Blood flow to the caudate was initially hyperemic, but subsided to 50% of preischemic values at 30 and 60 min postischemia. Thereafter, flow rose gradually to normal values at 6 hr and higher than normal at 24 and 48 hr postischemia. Therefore, it is not likely that hypoperfusion can explain the secondary energy failure after 6 hr. Glucose utilization in the dorsolateral striatum (the region showing greatest injury) returned to approximately 60% of control at 1, 3, and 6 hr, but fell to 40% of control at 24 and 48 hr. Thus, the rate of glucose utilization failed to indicate a progressive increase in metabolic demand that might contribute to delayed energy failure. However, the rate of glucose utilization will not accurately reflect the metabolic demands of the tissue if glucose metabolism is inhibited, for example, by PDH. Therefore, with the information presently available, the relative contributions of increased energy demand and decreased energy production to the delayed deterioration of energy state cannot be adequately assessed.

11. MECHANISM OF DELAYED ENERGY FAILURE: A HYPOTHESIS

To delineate the mechanisms of ischemic injury, the biochemical changes that occur within the first few hours of reperfusion must be more clearly defined. However, if speculation is permitted at present, what follows may serve as a working hypothesis for delayed energy failure.

The initial depletion of energy metabolites caused by ischemia produces widespread depolarization of neurons, release of neuroactive substances (such as glutamate), and a dramatic increase of Ca_i. As a result, Ca-dependent protein kinases are induced to phosphorylate a variety of proteins when resupplied with ATP during postischemic recirculation. Among the proteins that may become abnormally phosphorylated is PDH. Inhibition of PDH as a result of increased phosphorylation results in a decreased capacity to generate reducing equivalents (NADH) needed for oxidative phosphorylation. Energy metabolism is, in effect, substrate limited. Despite the decreased capacity for oxidative phosphorylation, the tissue energy state remains unimpaired as long as the cellular metabolic demand is low. However, as soon as metabolic demand exceeds the maximum capacity of PDH, tissue levels of energy metabolites will be diminished. Furthermore, abnormal phosphorylation of other proteins, such as ion channels, may cause long-lasting increases in ion permeability that lead to increased metabolic demand. Therefore, with the return of excitatory input, enhanced ion flux may place an abnormally large energy burden on specific neurons. Coupled with a persistent inhibition of PDH, these neurons will experience an energy crisis that leads to cell death. The selective vulnerability of specific neurons will then be dependent on the degree of inhibition of PDH as well as on the extent of excitatory input.

REFERENCES

Benveniste, H., Drejer, J., Schousboe, A., and Diemer, N. H, 1984, Elevation of extracellular concentrations of glutamate and aspartate in rat hippocampus during transient cerebral ischemia monitored by intracerebral dialysis, *J. Neurochem.* **43**:1369–1374.

Biros, M. H., Dimlich, R. V. W., and Barsan, W. G, 1986, Postinsult treatment of ischemia-induced cerebral lactic acidosis in the rat, *Ann. Emerg. Med.* **15**:397–404.

Choi, D. W, 1985, Glutamate neurotoxicity in cortical cell culture is calcium dependent, *Neurosci. Lett.* **58**:293–297.

Colohan, A. R. T., Welsh, F. A., Miller, E. D., and Kassell, N. F, 1986, The effect of dichloroacetate on brain lactate levels following incomplete ischemia in the hyperglycemic rat, *Stroke* **17**:525–528.

Csiba, L., Paschen, W., and Hossmann, K.-A, 1983, A topographic quantitative method for measuring brain tissue pH under physiological and pathophysiological conditions, *Brain Res.* **289**: 334–337.

Duckrow, R. B., LaManna, J. S., and Rosenthal, M, 1981, Disparate recovery of resting and stimulated oxidative metabolism following transient ischemia, *Stroke* **12**:677–686.

Gatfield, P. D., Lowry, O. H., Schulz, D. W., and Passonneau, J. V, 1966, Regional energy reserves in mouse brain and changes with ischaemia and anaesthesia, *J. Neurochem.* **13**:185–195.

Gill, R., Foster, A. C., and Woodruff, G. N, 1987, Systemic administration of MK-801 protects against ischemic-induced hippocampal degeneration in the gerbil, *J. Neurosci.* **7**:3343–3349.

Hansen, A. J, 1985, Effect of anoxia on ion distribution in the brain, *Physiol. Rev.* **65**:101–148.

Harris, R. J., Symon, L., Branston, N. M., and Bayhan, M, 1981, Changes in extracellular calcium activity in cerebral ischemia, *J. Cereb. Blood Flow Metab.* **1**:203–209.

Hillered, L., Ernster, L., and Siesjö, B. K, 1984a, Influence of in vitro lactic acidosis and hypercapnia on respiratory activity of isolated rat brain mitochondria, *J. Cereb. Blood Flow Metab.* **4**: 430–437.

Hillered, L., Siesjö, B. K., and Arfors, K.-E, 1984b, Mitochondrial response to transient forebrain ischemia and recirculation in the rat, *J. Cereb. Blood Flow Metab.* **4**:438–446.

Hillered, L., Smith, M.-L., and Siesjö, B. K, 1985, Lactic acidosis and recovery of mitochondrial function following forebrain ischemia in the rat, *J. Cereb. Blood Flow Metab.* **5**:259–266.

Hinman, L. M., and Blass, J.P, 1981, An NADH-linked spectrophotometric assay for pyruvate dehydrogenase complex in crude tissue homogenates, *J. Biol. Chem.* **256**:6584–6586.

Jope, R., and Blass, J. P, 1976, The regulation of pyruvate dehydrogenase in brain in vivo, *J. Neurochem.* **26**:709–714.

Kaplan, J., Dimlich, R. V. W., and Biros, M. H, 1987, Dichloroacetate treatment of ischemic cerebral lactic acidosis in the fed rat, *Ann. Emerg. Med.* **16:**298–304.

Katayama, Y., and Welsh, F. A, 1989, Effect of dichloroacetate on regional energy metabolites and pyruvate dehydrogenase activity during ischemia and reperfusion in gerbil brain, *J. Neurochem.* **52:**1817–1822.

Kogure, K., and Alonso, O. F, 1978, A pictorial representation of endogenous brain ATP by a bioluminescent method, *Brain Res.* **154:**273–284.

Kogure, K., Alonso, O. F., and Martinez, E, 1980, A topographic measurement of brain pH, *Brain Res.* **195:**95–109.

Kraig, R. P., Pulsinelli, W. A., and Plum, F, 1986, Carbonic acid buffer changes during complete brain ischemia, *Am. J. Physiol.* **250:**R348–R357.

Ljunggren, B., Ratcheson, R. A., and Siesjö, B. K, 1974, Cerebral metabolic state following complete compression ischemia, *Brain Res.* **73:**291–307.

Lowry, O. H., Passonneau, J. V., and Rock, M. K, 1961, The stability of the pyridine nucleotides, *J. Biol. Chem.* **236:**2756–2759.

Marshall, L. F., Welsh, F. A., Durity, F., Lounsbury, R., Graham, D. I., and Langfitt, T. W, 1975, Experimental cerebral oligemia and ischemia produced by intracranial hypertension. 3. Brain energy metabolism, *J. Neurosurg.* **43:**323–328.

Myers, R. E, 1979, A unitary theory of causation of anoxic and hypoxic brain pathology, *Adv. Neurol.* **26:**195–213.

Myers, R. E., and Yamaguchi, S, 1977, Nervous system effects of cardiac arrest in monkeys. Preservation of vision, *Arch. Neurol.* **34:**65–74.

Nowicki, J.-P., Assumel-Lurdin, C., Duverger, D., and MacKenzie, E. T, 1988, Temporal evolution of regional energy metabolites following focal cerebral ischemia in the rat, *J. Cereb. Blood Flow Metab.* **8:**462–473.

Olney, J. W, 1969, Brain lesions, obesity and other disturbances in mice treated with monosodium glutamate, *Science* **164:**719–721.

Ozyurt, E., Graham, D. I., Woodruff, G. N., and McCulloch, J, 1988, Protective effect of the glutamate antagonist, MK-801 in focal cerebral ischemia in the cat, *J. Cereb. Blood Flow Metab.* **8:**138–143.

Paschen, W., Niebuhr, I., and Hossmann, K.-A, 1981, A bioluminescence method for the demonstration of regional glucose distribution in brain slices, *J. Neurochem.* **36:**513–517.

Paschen, W., Hossmann, K.-A., and van den Kerckhoff, W, 1983, Regional assessment of energy-producing metabolism following prolonged complete ischemia of cat brain, *J. Cereb. Blood Flow Metab.* **3:**321–329.

Pulsinelli, W. A., and Duffy, T. E, 1983, Regional energy balance in rat brain after transient forebrain ischemia, *J. Neurochem.* **40:**1500–1503.

Pulsinelli, W. A., Brierley, J. B., and Plum, F, 1982a, Temporal profile of neuronal damage in a model of transient forebrain ischemia, *Ann. Neurol.* **11:**491–498.

Pulsinelli, W. A., Levy, D. E., and Duffy, T. E, 1982b, Regional cerebral blood flow and glucose metabolism following transient forebrain ischemia, *Ann. Neurol.* **11:**499–509.

Pulsinelli, W. A., Waldman, S., Rawlinson, D., and Plum, F, 1982c, Moderate hyperglycemia augments ischemic brain damage: A neuropathologic study in the rat, *Neurology* **32:**1239–1246.

Raichle, M. E, 1983, The pathophysiology of brain ischemia, *Ann. Neurol.* **13:** 2–10.

Ratcheson, R. A., and Ferrendelli, J. A, 1980, Regional cortical metabolism in focal ischemia, *J. Neurosurg.* **52:** 755–763.

Reed, L. J., and Yeaman, S. J, 1987, Pyruvate dehydrogenase, in "The Enzymes, vol. XVIII" (P. D. Boyer and E. G. Krebs, eds.), pp. 77–95, Academic Press, New York.

Rehncrona, S., Mela, L., and Siesjö, B. K, 1979, Recovery of brain mitochondrial function in the rat after complete and incomplete cerebral ischemia, *Stroke* **10:**437–446.

Rehncrona, S., Rosén, I., and Siesjö, B. K, 1981, Brain lactic acidosis and ischemic cell damage. 1. Biochemistry and neurophysiology, *J. Cereb. Blood Flow Metab.* **1**:297–311.

Rothman, S. M., and Olney, J. W, 1986, Glutamate and the pathophysiology of hypoxic-ischemic brain damage, *Ann. Neurol.* **19**:105–111.

Siesjö, B. K, 1981, Cell damage in the brain: A speculative synthesis, *J. Cereb. Blood Flow Metab.* **1**: 155–185.

Siesjö, B. K, 1985, Acid-base homeostasis in the brain: Physiology, chemistry, and neurochemical pathology, *Prog. Brain Res.* **63**:121–154.

Siesjö, B. K, 1988, Calcium, ischemia, and death of brain cells, *Ann. N. Y. Acad. Sci.* **522**:638–661.

Siesjö, B. K., Bendek, G., Koide, T., Westerberg, E., and Wieloch, T, 1985, Influence of acidosis on lipid peroxidation in brain tissues in vitro, *J. Cereb. Blood Flow Metab.* **5**:253–258.

Simon, R. P., Swan, J. H., Griffiths, T., and Meldrum, B. S, 1984, Blockage of N-methyl-D-aspartate receptors may protect against ischemic damage in the brain, *Science* **226**:850–852.

Sims, N. R., and Pulsinelli, W. A, 1987, Altered mitochondrial respiration in selectively vulnerable brain subregions following transient forebrain ischemia in the rat, *J. Neurochem.* **49**:1367–1374.

Tanaka, K., Welsh, F. A., Greenberg, J. H., O'Flynn, R., Harris, V. A., and Reivich, M, 1985, Regional alterations in glucose consumption and metabolite levels during postischemic recovery in cat brain, *J. Cereb. Blood Flow Metab.* **5**:502–511.

Welsh, F. A, 1984, Regional evaluation of ischemic metabolic alterations, *J. Cereb. Blood Flow Metab.* **4**:309–316.

Welsh, F. A., and Rieder, W, 1978, Evaluation of in situ freezing of cat brain by NADH fluorescence, *J. Neurochem.* **31**:299–309.

Welsh, F. A., Ginsberg, M. D., Rieder, W., and Budd, W. W, 1978a, Diffuse cerebral ischemia in the cat. II. Regional metabolites during severe ischemia and recirculation, *Ann. Neurol.* **3**:493–501.

Welsh, F. A., O'Connor, M. J., and Marcy, V. R, 1978b, Effect of oligemia on regional metabolite levels in cat brain, *J. Neurochem.* **31**:311–319.

Welsh, F. A., Ginsberg, M. D., Rieder, W., and Budd, W. W, 1980, Deleterious effect of glucose pretreatment on recovery from diffuse cerebral ischemia in the cat, *Stroke* **11**:355–363.

Welsh, F. A., O'Connor, M. J., Marcy, V. R., Spatacco, A. J., and Johns, R. L, 1982, Factors limiting regeneration of ATP following temporary ischemia in cat brain, *Stroke* **13**:234–242.

Welsh, F. A., Sims, R. E., and McKee, A. E, 1983, Effect of glucose on recovery of energy metabolism following hypoxia-oligemia in mouse brain: Dose-dependence and carbohydrate specificity, *J. Cereb. Blood Flow Metab.* **3**:486–492.

Welsh, F. A., Sakamoto, T., McKee, A. E., and Sims, R. E, 1987, Effect of lactacidosis on pyridine nucleotide stability during ischemia in mouse brain, *J. Neurochem* **49**:846–851.

Whitehouse, S., and Randle, P. J, 1973, Activation of pyruvate dehydrogenase in perfused rat heart by dichloroacetate, *Biochem. J.* **134**:651–653.

Wieloch, T., and Koide, T, 1987, Pyruvate dehydrogenase is inhibited in the recirculation period following transient cerebral ischemia, *J. Cereb. Blood Flow Metab.* **7**(Suppl. 1):S75.

CHAPTER 4

DISTURBANCES OF PROTEIN AND POLYAMINE METABOLISM AFTER REVERSIBLE CEREBRAL ISCHEMIA

K.-A. HOSSMANN and W. PASCHEN

1. INTRODUCTION

The high sensitivity of the brain to ischemia is generally attributed to the misrelationship between the high metabolic demands and the low energy reserves of this organ. In fact, complete cessation of blood flow in the nonanesthetized normothermic brain leads to complete depletion of energy reserves and a cessation of all endergonic metabolic processes within less than 5 min (Lowry *et al.*, 1964). However, experimental observations from our and other laboratories have clearly

K.-A. HOSSMANN and W. PASCHEN • Department of Experimental Neurology, Max Planck Institute for Neurological Research, D-5000 Cologne 41, Germany.

Neurochemical Correlates of Cerebral Ischemia, Volume 7 of *Advances in Neurochemistry*, edited by Nicolas G. Bazan, Pierre Braquet, and Myron D. Ginsberg. Plenum Press, New York, 1992.

established that this process is not irreversible. Provided that a no-reflow can be prevented, reoxygenation of the brain will result in a reactivation of energy metabolism after complete cerebrocirculatory arrest of as long as 1 hr (Hossmann and Kleihues, 1973; Pluta, 1987). However, it has also been shown that the recovery of energy metabolism correlates closely with the restoration of the electrophysiological function of the brain (Schmidt-Kastner *et al.*, 1986). Most ischemic experiments exceeding a duration of 5 to 10 min nevertheless result in more or less severe brain injury when the animals are allowed to survive for some time (Siesjö, 1988*b*). The foci of ischemic cell injury are accentuated in the so-called selectively vulnerable areas of the brain, i.e., the third layer of the cerebral cortex, hippocampal subfields CA1 and CA4, the dorsolateral aspect of the striate nucleus, and, under conditions of hyperglycemia, the pars reticulata of the substantia nigra (Pulsinelli *et al.*, 1982; Kirino and Sano, 1984; M. L. Smith *et al.*, 1988).

It is widely held that the lesions in the selectively vulnerable areas are induced by enhanced ischemic and/or postischemic calcium fluxes across voltage- and/or agonist-activated calcium channels (Siesjö, 1988*a*). However, ischemia causes numerous other metabolic and functional disturbances, and it is difficult to decide which of the various observed abnormalities are mediators or epiphenomena of the pathophysiological process.

In this chapter, we discuss disturbances of two metabolic pathways which are particularly sensitive to ischemia and which may be involved in the process of selective vulnerability: protein synthesis and polyamine metabolism. Both pathways are markedly deranged after ischemia of as short as 5 min, the changes outlast the postischemic disturbances of energy metabolism for hours or days, and the pathways do recover in the resistant but not in the selectively vulnerable regions of the brain (Bodsch *et al.*, 1985; Paschen *et al.*, 1987*b*). Disturbances of either polyamine or protein synthesis will not immediately result in cell death. However, in view of the long delay of the pathological process, their involvement in the maturation of ischemic injury should be considered.

2. PROTEIN METABOLISM

A detailed analysis of protein metabolism after ischemia suffers from the enormous complexity of this pathway and is far from being completed. In particular, no systematic investigations have been carried out in which the whole metabolic pathway of a given protein has been analyzed in a standardized ischemic experiment, i.e., the complete sequela from the transcription of the gene to the catabolism of the synthesized protein. Most of the available data concern global aspects of ischemic or postischemic protein synthesis, and the methodologies of many studies allow only indirect conclusions about the functional activity of the protein-synthesizing machinery. The following description, therefore, is not a comprehensive review of protein synthesis but is a discussion of selected aspects which reflect the historical and methodological developments in this field.

2.1. Ribosomal Aggregation

The molecular site of protein synthesis is the ribosome, which translates the genetic code of the mRNA into a newly synthesized polypeptide chain. Single ribosomes are called monosomes, agglomerations of a few ribomes attached to the same RNA molecules are called oligosomes, and agglomerations of many ribosomes are polysomes. It is well established that the degree of ribosomal aggregation correlates with the activity of the protein-synthesizing machinery (Clark-Walker, 1973). This relationship occurs because the rate of protein synthesis can be accelerated by attaching an increasing number of ribosomes to the same mRNA molecule.

The aggregational state of ribosomes can be assessed by two different methods: qualitatively by electron microscopy and quantitatively by fractional ultracentrifugation of ribosomes on sucrose gradients (Figures 1 and 2). Both methods have been applied to cerebral ischemia and revealed essentially the same findings. (1) During complete ischemia ribosomal aggregation does not change, although the depletion of energy reserves results in the complete cessation of (energy-dependent) protein synthesis (see below). (2) After ischemia restitution of flow causes a long-lasting disaggregation of ribosomes, which is dissociated from the much faster recovery of the energy metabolism (Kleihues and Hossmann, 1971; Burda et al., 1980; Petito and Pulsinelli, 1984).

This sequela is relatively independent of the duration of ischemia: ribosomes remain aggregated during ischemia of either 5 or 60 min, and they disaggregate after the beginning of recirculation irrespective of the length of ischemia (Kleihues et al., 1975; Munekata et al., 1987). There is also no difference between neurons and glial cells (Yanagihara, 1976).

The dissociation of ribosomal aggregation and cessation of protein synthesis during ischemia has been explained by the rapid breakdown of energy metabolism, which results in the simultaneous inhibition of all steps of polypeptide synthesis, i.e., polypeptide chain initiation, elongation, and termination. As a consequence, the ribosomes remain attached to the mRNA molecule although translation is completely blocked ("ischemic freeze" [Kleihues et al., 1975]). This interpretation is supported by the observation that under conditions of incomplete ischemia where some energy metabolism persists, ribosomes disaggregate during the ischemic period (Hartmann et al., 1973).

The reason for the postischemic disaggregation of ribosomes is not fully understood. A breakdown of the polyribosomal complex by increased RNAse activity has been excluded (Kleihues et al., 1975). The disaggregation into mono-

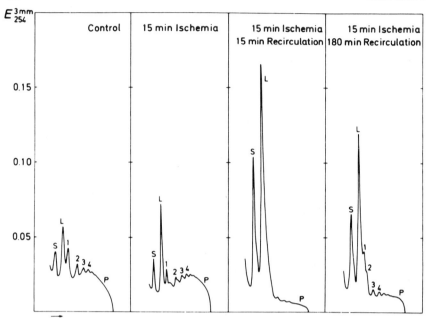

FIGURE 1. Cerebral polysome profiles from rats subjected to 15 min of complete ischemia and different times of recirculation. The postmitochondrial supernatant was analyzed on an exponential (15 to 55%) sucrose gradient. P, polyribosomes; 2 to 4, oligosomes; 1, monosomes; L and S, large and small ribosomal subunits, respectively. Note the preservation of polyribosomes at the end of the ischemic period. (From Cooper *et al.*, 1977).

somes therefore seems to result from a dissociation between the ongoing inhibition of polypeptide chain initiation and a recovery of elongation and termination. This interpretation is supported by an experiment in which the influence of specific inhibitors of polypeptide chain initiation was studied in vitro (Cooper *et al.*, 1977). Using ribosomes from normal or ischemic brains, these inhibitors reduce protein synthesis, as expected. However, in vitro protein synthesis of ribosomes which have been sampled after a brief period of postischemic recirculation is not influenced by these inhibitors. This has been interpreted as evidence that polypeptide chain initiation was already maximally inhibited as a consequence of the pathological process.

After several hours of postischemic recirculation, ribosomes gradually reaggregate provided that the brain is adequately reperfused after ischemia (Figures 1 and 3). Following 5 min of ischemia in gerbils (Munekata *et al.*, 1987) or 60 min of ischemia in monkeys (Kleihues *et al.*, 1975) or cats (Kleihues and Hossmann, 1971), reaggregation was completed after 24 h. As shown by morphometric evaluations of electron micrographs, the time course does not differ greatly

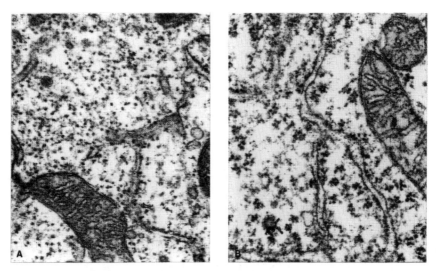

FIGURE 2. Electron microscopic evaluation of ribosomal aggregation in the neuronal cytoplasm of a gerbil. (A) Normal aggregation in control brain. (B) Complete disaggregation after 5 min of ischemia and 1 hr of recirculation. Magnification × 20,000. (From Munekata *et al.*, 1987)

between various brain regions except for the vulnerable CA1 subfield of the hippocampus, in which disaggregation was irreversible (Munekata *et al.*, 1987) (Figure 3). These findings are in line with the results of regional investigations of amino acid incorporation into brain proteins, which demonstrate a gradual recovery of protein synthesis in the areas in which ribosomes reaggregate but not in the selectively vulnerable regions (see below).

2.2. Amino Acid Incorporation into Brain Proteins

A more direct way to evaluate the function of the protein-synthesizing machinery is the biochemical or autoradiographic measurement of the incorporation of labeled amino acids into brain proteins. Although this approach requires a critical analysis of tracer kinetics (see below), it confirmed the previous observations of ribosomal aggregation. During ischemia, amino acid incorporation into brain proteins is completely suppressed, as shown by direct injection of labeled amino acids into brain tissue (Kleihues and Hossmann, 1971). However, ribosomes do not disaggregate, and they exhibit normal protein synthesis in vitro (Cooper *et al.*, 1977). Suppression of protein synthesis in vivo is therefore due to the

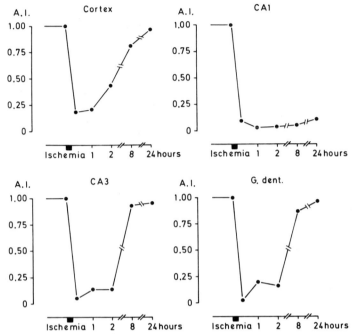

FIGURE 3. Aggregation index (A. I.) of neurons from parietal cortex, the CA1 and CA3 sectors of the hippocampus, and the dentate gyrus before and at different recirculation times after 5 min of ischemia in gerbils. Ribosomal aggregation index was determined morphometrically on electron micrographs. (From Munekata *et al.*, 1987).

breakdown of energy metabolism and not to a failure of the protein-synthesizing machinery.

When the brain is recirculated with blood, amino acid incorporation remains severely inhibited, although energy metabolism quickly recovers (Figure 4). Nowak *et al.* (1985) reported a reduction of protein synthesis to about 10% of control levels after 5 to 20 min of ischemia and 10 min of recirculation. Following 5 min of ischemia in gerbils, the incorporation of a mixture of five tritiated neutral amino acids was reduced in the frontal cortex to about 50% of control levels after 2 hr of recirculation (Munekata *et al.*, 1987). In cats submitted to 60 min of ischemia, cortical [14C] leucine incorporation was 6% of control levels after 30 min and about 50% after 2 hr of recirculation (Kleihues and Hossmann, 1971). In monkeys the incorporation of tritiated amino acids into brain proteins was reduced to 15% after 90 min of reflow (Bodsch *et al.*, 1986). At these recirculation times the energy state usually has completely recovered, indicating that the suppression of protein synthesis is not the consequence of energy failure.

Control   45 min   6 hours   24 hours

A

B

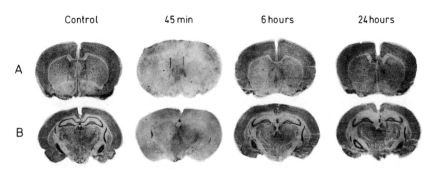

FIGURE 4. Autoradiographic evaluation of amino acid incorporation in brain proteins of gerbils before (control) and at different recirculation times after 5 min of ischemia. Brain sections were prepared at the level of the striate nucleus (A) and the dorsal hippocampus (B). Note the global decrease of radioactivity shortly after ischemia and the gradual recovery in all regions except the CA1 sector of hippocampus. (Reproduced by courtesy of Dr. R. Widmann.)

With longer recirculation times, protein synthesis gradually recovers, but not in all animals and not in all brain regions (Figure 4). The prerequisite for the individual recovery in different animals is the prevention of a no-reflow phenomenon. In the presence of reflow, protein synthesis returns to normal within 24 hr in most regions of the brain irrespective of the duration of ischemia: after 5 to 20 min of ischemia in gerbils (Nowak et al., 1985) and after 60 min of ischemia in cats (Kleihues and Hossmann, 1971) or monkeys (Bodsch et al., 1986). In animals without adequate reperfusion, energy metabolism is not restored and protein synthesis does not recover (Kleihues et al., 1975).

The regional pattern of amino acid incorporation in animals without flow impairment reflects the pattern of selective vulnerability and corresponds to that described above for the reaggregation of ribosomes (Figure 4). In gerbils submitted to 5 min of global ischemia, amino acid incorporation is irreversibly suppressed in hippocampal subfield CA1, although it returns to normal in the rest of the brain (Bodsch et al., 1986; Thilmann et al., 1986a). After 10 min of ischemia or longer, the other hippocampal sectors—except the dentate gyrus—may also be involved (Dienel et al., 1980). This pattern does not change much after 1 hr of ischemia. In a cat surviving for 1 year after cerebrocirculatory arrest of 60 min, permanent suppression of protein synthesis, and hence cell death, was present in the hippocampus and parts of the striate nucleus. The "resistent" parts of the brain, i.e., the cerebral cortex, thalamus, dentate gyrus, cerebellum, and brain stem, exhibited a normal regional pattern of protein synthesis (Hossmann et al., 1987).

Although regional recovery of amino acid incorporation correlates both with the pattern of ribosomal reaggregation and with the morphological preservation of the brain, some caveats must be expressed concerning the interpretation of these data in terms of quantitative protein synthesis. A reliable estimate of protein synthesis from tracer incorporation studies requires a precise determination of the tissue-integrated specific activity of the precursor pool, i.e., the aminoacyl-tRNA. For methodological reasons this is not easily done, even if the pathological process can be standardized to such a degree that tissue samples from multiple experiments can be combined to establish the time course of the precursor pool. A kinetic approach from which the time course of the precursor is calculated from radio-activity in the blood must consider up to 10 rate constants which may vary not only in different brain regions but also under different pathological conditions (C. B. Smith *et al.*, 1988). Quantification of the postischemic protein synthesis rate by in vivo tracer incorporation studies is therefore most problematic. It is, however, possible to determine the direction of the error which occurs when conventional measurements of amino acid incorporation are carried out. If at the end of the incorporation period the specific activity of either the aminoacyl-tRNA or the free amino acid pool is higher than under control conditions, the changes of amino acid incorporation into proteins overestimate the actual protein synthesis rate. Conversely, a decline in the specific activity of the precursor indicates an underestimation of protein synthesis. Application of this simple approach to the study of postischemic protein synthesis revealed a reciprocal relationship, i.e., an increase in the precursor specific activity when fractional incorporation of amino acids into proteins was inhibited and a decrease in the precursor activity when protein synthesis recovered (Bodsch *et al.*, 1986). The described biochemical or auto-radiographic determinations of postischemic amino acid incorporation can therefore be confidently interpreted as representing similar or even more pronounced alterations in protein synthesis rate.

2.3. Selective Gene Expression after Ischemia

Evaluations of either ribosomal aggregation or amino acid incorporation into proteins provide information about global protein metabolism but not about the expression of specific proteins. In fact, it has been shown that after ischemia, synthesis of different protein species is not inhibited to the same degree. The first indication of a difference between the synthesis rates of proteins with different half-lives came from measurements of ornithine decarboxylase (ODC) and *S*-adenosylmethionine decarboxylase (SAMDC) following 1 hr of global ischemia in the monkey brain (Kleihues *et al.*, 1975). The half-life of ODC is between 11 and 21 min and that of SAMDC between 35 and 120 min, whereas that of most other brain proteins is about 4 days. Because of the short half-lives, both the synthesis and degradation rates of ODC and SAMDC are higher than those of other proteins. During ischemia, synthesis and degradation are inhibited and the concentration does not change (Figure 5). After ischemia, degradation recovers earlier than

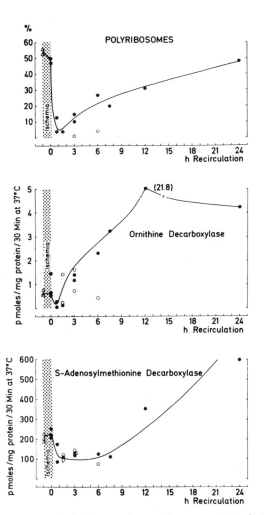

FIGURE 5. Relative amounts of polyribosomes (expressed as a percentage of total ribosomes plus ribosomal subunits) and activity of enzymes involved in polyamine synthesis before and at different recirculation times after 1 hr of ischemia in monkeys. Each value represents one experimental animal. Δ, controls; ○, monkeys without recovery of neuronal function. Note the gradual reaggregation of polyribosomes in animals with functional recovery and the differences in the postischemic induction of OCD and SAMDC. (From Kleihues *et al.*, 1975.)

synthesis and the concentration falls by about 50% within the first hour of recirculation. With longer recirculation times, synthesis is resumed after a delay that depends on the half-life of the proteins: ODC returned to normal within less than 3 hr and reached a peak of about 30 times control levels after 12 hr. SAMDC, which has a longer half-life began to recover between 6 and 12 hr and rose to three times control levels after 24 hr (Figure 5). This difference was even more pronounced after 30 min of ischemia in rats, after which SAMDC returned to control levels only after 5 days (Dienel *et al.*, 1985). The half-life of most other proteins is so long that the concentration does not change during the first days after ischemia, although protein synthesis is severely inhibited (see above).

Another example of selective gene expression is the postischemic synthesis of heat shock proteins. This has been investigated both in gerbils (Nowak, 1985) and in rats (Jacewicz *et al.*, 1985; Dienel *et al.*, 1986; Kiessling *et al.*, 1986). In both species heat shock proteins are expressed at high concentration during the period of general depression of protein synthesis. Recently, evidence has been provided that there is also a regional difference. In gerbils submitted to brief periods of ischemia, heat shock proteins were expressed in the resistant hippocampal subfield CA3 but not in the vulnerable CA1 sector (Nowak, 1988).

The consequences of selective expression of different proteins may be of considerable importance. An example of this is the above described dissociation between the induction of ODC and SAMDC (Kleihues *et al.*, 1975; Dienel *et al.*, 1985). This dissociation results in a substantial increase in the tissue content of putrescine, which, in turn, correlates with the degree of neuronal injury (see below). It is therefore conceivable that the dysregulation of postischemic protein synthesis is more important than the global inhibition because it triggers a secondary metabolic disturbance which may be directly involved in the pathogenesis of delayed neuronal death.

The mechanisms responsible for selective gene expression after ischemia have not been clarified, and it is not known whether ischemic or postischemic factors are responsible for this phenomenon. In a recent study in situ hybridization with cDNA probes was used to measure postischemic changes in various mRNA species. cDNA probes which hybridize with ribosomal or cytochrome *c* oxidase mRNA did not reveal any abnormalities, whereas β-actin and pre-A4 mRNA either increased or decreased (Xie *et al.*, 1989). Postischemic gene transcription, in consequence, varies in a complex way and may lead to equally complex interactions of various enzymatic systems. In view of the still poorly understood molecular mechanisms of ischemic cell injury, these processes deserve detailed analysis in the future.

2.4. Treatment of Postischemic Disturbances of Protein Synthesis

To our knowledge, only two experiments have been carried out with the intention of influencing postischemic protein synthesis by therapeutic interference. Thilmann *et al.* (1986*b*) used cycloheximide in gerbils to prevent the synthesis of proteins which are selectively expressed during the early post-ischemic recirculation period and which may trigger the pathological process leading to irreversible ischemic injury (see above). As a result, protein synthesis uniformly recovered and morphological lesions were absent. However, this effect could have been caused by the temperature drop which is induced by the drug, and it cannot be excluded that ischemic injury did not reach the threshold of neuronal vulnerability.

The other investigation was carried out in our laboratory (Xie *et al.*, in preparation). In this study gerbils were treated after 5 min of global ischemia with barbiturates, which previously have been shown to prevent morphological lesions in hippocampal CA1 sector (Hallmayer *et al.*, 1985). In this study hippocampal protein synthesis was normal after 2 days of recirculation. Two hours after ischemia, however, inhibition of protein synthesis was equal to or even more pronounced than in untreated animals. Barbiturate therapy, in consequence, promoted the recovery of protein synthesis but did not prevent the initial post-ischemic disturbance.

2.5. Disturbances of Protein Synthesis and Ischemic Cell Death

It is obvious that the irreversible suppression of protein synthesis must lead to the death of the cell. The close correlation between persistent inhibition of protein synthesis and morphological injury in the hippocampus strongly suggests that this disturbance is the final reason for postischemic delayed neuronal death. However, it cannot be excluded that this relationship is indirect. In fact, shortly after ischemia all neurons suffer a similar degree of polysomal disaggregation and inhibition of amino acid incorporation, but this disturbance is irreversible only in a few anatomically well-defined neuronal populations, which also differ from the rest of the brain in other respects. It is therefore possible that the irreversible suppression of protein synthesis in these neurons reflects a pathological process which is triggered by different molecular mechanisms and which is lethal irrespective of the functional state of the protein-synthesizing machinery (Hossmann, 1985). Several such mechanisms are conceivable. One of these is the much-discussed relationship between the ischemic or postischemic release of excito-toxins, which is thought to result in postischemic neuronal hyperexcitability, and cytosolic calcium flooding (Siesjö, 1988*b*). Another mechanism is the disturbance in polyamine metabolism, which seems to result from the selective dissociation of gene expression, as described in detail below. Finally, the activation of various calcium-dependent protein kinases may be able to trigger a variety of pathological events (Taft *et al.*, 1988; Louis *et al.*, 1988). It is therefore not possible to predict whether the therapeutic reversal of postischemic inhibition of protein synthesis in selectively vulnerable neurons would be able to protect these cells against delayed injury. The above-described effects of barbiturates can, in fact, be interpreted in two different ways: the initial aggravation of the disturbance of protein synthesis and the later recovery speak against and for a causal relationship, respectively.

In conclusion, the available experimental data unequivocally demonstrate that irreversible ischemic cell injury is associated with severe inhibition of protein synthesis. It has not been established whether this disturbance is the reason for or the consequence of the pathological process. However, it is obvious that the mechanisms of this disturbance must be clarified in order to understand the molecular causes of ischemic cell death.

3. POLYAMINE METABOLISM

In mammals the only route to putrescine is by decarboxylating the amino acid ornithine, a reaction which is catalyzed by ODC. A scheme of the synthesis of the polyamines putrescine, spermidine, and spermine is given in Figure 6; for simplicity, the diamine putrescine, which is the precursor of spermidine and spermine, will be included as one of the polyamines throughout the review. Two aminopropyl moieties are then added to putrescine to form spermidine and spermine, respectively. These aminopropyl moieties are made available from decarboxylated S-adenosylmethionine, a reaction catalyzed by SAMDC. The interconversion of spermine and spermidine to spermidine and putrescine, respectively, is achieved by the enzymes spermine/spermidine N-acetyltransferase and polyamine oxidase.

Polyamines play an important role in cellular growth processes, including cell proliferation, differentiation, regeneration, and cancer growth (for reviews, see Jänne et al., [1979]; Canellakis et al., [1979]; Williams-Ashman and Canellakis [1979]; Heby [1981]; Seiler [1981]; Pegg and McCann [1982]; and Pegg [1986]). In the brain, polyamine metabolism is markedly changed during perinatal cell growth (for a review, see Slotkin and Bartolome [1986]). The most pronounced changes are observed in ODC activity and putrescine levels immediately after birth. During birth, both ODC activity and putrescine levels are high, but decrease sharply within the first few days, reaching the levels in adult animals about 1 month after birth. Perinatal changes in spermidine and spermine levels are much smaller than those of putrescine. Treatment of animals with the specific ODC inhibitor α-difluoromethylornithine (DFMO) significantly delayed the development of the brain: brain DNA, RNA, and protein synthesis was markedly reduced in comparison with that in untreated animals, and the behavioral development was retarded.

In the brain of adult animals, basal ODC activity and putrescine levels are low, amounting to about 0.3 to 1 nmol/g per hr and 5 to 10 nmol/g, respectively. Stimulation of the brain with nerve growth factor or glucocorticoids (Lewis et al., 1978; Cousin et al., 1982) or regeneration after nerve transection (Gilad and Gilad, 1983) induces a significant increase in ODC activity. It has been suggested,

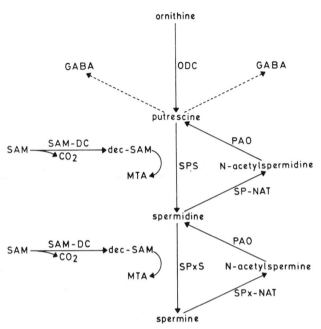

FIGURE 6. Scheme of synthesis and interconversion of the polyamines putrescine, spermidine, and spermine. In mammals the only route to putrescine is by decarboxylation of ornithine by ODC. Putrescine is converted to spermidine and spermine, respectively, by adding two aminopropyl groups which are taken from decarboxylated *S*-adenosylmethionine (dec-SAM). SPS, spermidine synthase; SPxS, spermine synthase; SAM, *S*-adenosylmethionine; MTA, methylthioadenosine; SPx-NAT, spermine *N*-acetyltransferase; SP-NAT, spermidine *N*-acetyltransferase; PAO, polyamine oxidase. (From Paschen *et al.*, 1987*b*.)

therefore, that activation of polyamine metabolism is necessary for the recovery process (Gilad and Gilad, 1983). In these studies, however, polyamine profiles have not been measured.

Because of the low basal ODC activity and putrescine levels, highly sensitive assays are necessary to be able to identify changes in the levels of both compounds in the adult brain. ODC activity is usually determined in tissue samples by measuring the release of $^{14}CO_2$ from L-[1-^{14}C]ornithine (Pegg *et al.*, 1970), permitting an ODC activity of about only 4 mg (wet weight) to be quantified in tissue samples (Paschen *et al.*, 1988*d*). For measuring regional polyamine profiles, tissue samples were extracted with perchloric acid, and neutralized with KOH-KCl, and polyamines in the neutralized extracts were derivatized with *o*-phthalaldehyde (Paschen *et al.*, 1987*a*; Djuricic *et al.*, 1988). Fluorescent polyamine derivatives were then separated chromatographically by using high-pressure liquid chromatography (HPLC) and quantified with a fluorescence detector and external standard solutions. This procedure permits the measurement of polyamine profiles of less than 1 mg (wet weight) in tissue samples (Djuricic *et al.*, 1988).

Under pathological conditions an increase in ODC activity seems to be a common response to cellular stress (Dienel and Cruz, 1984). Different pathological stimuli such as drilling a burr hole in the cranium, noxic chemicals, thermal injury, or metabolic stress induced a marked activation of ODC synthesis. This activation of polyamine metabolism was most pronounced following severe metabolic stress such as reversible ischemia (Kleihues *et al.*, 1975; Dienel and Cruz, 1984; Dienel *et al.*, 1985; Paschen *et al.*, 1988*a*; Dempsey *et al.*, 1988). Regional profiles of ODC activity have been studied in detail in rats during and after 30 min of four-vessel occlusion (Dienel *et al.*, 1985; Paschen *et al.*, 1988*a*) (Figure 7): ODC activity is unchanged during cerebral ischemia, decreased during the first 2 hr of recirculation, and increased considerably following prolonged recirculation, peaking first at about 8 to 10 hr of recirculation and again (but significantly less) after about 2 to 3 days of recirculation. In contrast to the situation with global cerebral ischemia, ODC activity was already markedly changed during the focal cerebral ischemia produced by unilateral middle cerebral artery occlusion in cats (Dempsey *et al.*, 1985): Within the ischemic core, in which the blood flow was below 20 ml/100 g per min, ODC activity was significantly below that measured in the contralateral hemisphere, whereas ODC

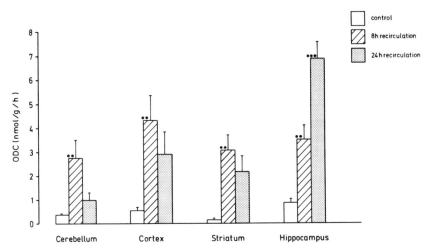

FIGURE 7. ODC activity in reversible cerebral ischemia of rats. Cerebral ischemia was produced by using the four-vessel occlusion model. After 30 min of ischemia, brains were recirculated for 8 or 24 hr. (From Paschen *et al.*, 1988*a*, with modifications.)

synthesis was significantly activated in the ischemic border zone, exhibiting blood flow rates of about 30 to 40 ml/100 g per min.

The increase in ODC activity observed after cerebral ischemia is not followed by an activation of the synthesis of SAMDC, the second key enzyme in polyamine metabolism. In contrast, SAMDC activity is considerably decreased following cerebral ischemia (Dienel *et al.*, 1985). These results clearly indicate that reversible cerebral ischemia induces pathological disturbances in polyamine metabolism: only the first step in polyamine synthesis (the ODC step) is activated, whereas the second step (the SAMDC step) is severely inhibited. It is therefore unlikely that the activation of polyamine synthesis after cerebral ischemia is similar to that observed after nerve transection (Gilad and Gilad, 1983), namely an indication of the repair mechanisms activated after stress. Reversible cerebral ischemia is known to induce proliferation of glial cells (Petito and Babiak, 1982), and the activation of polyamine metabolism may reflect the active and proliferative changes occurring in glial cells after ischemia. It has been shown, however, that the increase in ODC activity after cerebral ischemia is apparent in neurons rather than in glial cells (Dempsey *et al.*, 1988), illustrating that the observed changes indicate ischemia-induced pathological disturbances in neurons, not activation of physiological processes in glial cells.

Ischemia-induced alterations in the activity of both key enzymes in polyamine metabolism (ODC and SAMDC) cause significant changes in the pattern of regional polyamine profiles (Paschen *et al.*, 1987*a*, *b*, 1988*a*–*d*). The extent of the observed disturbances depended on the period of cerebral ischemia and the brain region examined. Disturbances were most severe following 30 min of forebrain ischemia and more pronounced in vulnerable brain structures than in invulnerable ones. The most prominent change observed was an increase in the putrescine level, which was already detectable during early recirculation. Spermidine and spermine levels, in contrast, did not change during early recirculation but were significantly reduced during prolonged recirculation (Paschen *et al.*, 1987*a*, *b*). In the following sections, disturbances in polyamine profiles will be discussed in relation to the animal model used, namely the four-vessel occlusion model (Pulsinelli and Brierley, 1979) and the gerbil model (Kirino, 1982).

3.1. Polyamines after Cerebral Ischemia in Rats

At the end of 30 min of forebrain ischemia in rats, no change in the levels of putrescine, spermidine, or spermine could be detected (Paschen *et al.*, 1987*a*), indicating that polyamine profiles are stable during ischemia. These results are in line with the observation that the activity of ODC and SAMDC is unchanged during vascular occlusion (Kleihues *et al.*, 1975; Dienel *et al.*, 1985). Following cerebral ischemia, tissue putrescine levels rose considerably in all brain structures studied; up to about 7-fold and 17-fold after 8 and 24 hr of recirculation, respectively (Figure 8). The increase in the putrescine level was most pronounced in the vulnerable striatum and significantly less in the less vulnerable cerebral cortex (Paschen *et al.*, 1987*a*). A decrease in spermidine and spermine levels was detectable only in the striatum after 24 hr of recirculation at a time when most neurons were already severely necrotic in this region. Results from a recent series of experiments (Paschen *et al.*, 1989) in which regional polyamine profiles were measured after 2 or 4 hr of recirculation following 30 min of forebrain ischemia indicate that the putrescine level has already significantly (about 2.5- to 3-fold) increased after 2 hr of recirculation, i.e., at a time when the neurons are still alive.

Postischemic treatment of animals with the specific ODC inhibitor DFMO reversed the ischemia-induced increase in ODC activity almost completely (Paschen *et al.*, 1988*a*). The effect of DFMO on ODC activity was most pronounced in the hippocampus, where the ODC activity of treated animals was identical to (8 hr of recirculation) or even below that (24 hr of recirculation) found in control animals. In contrast, DFMO produced only a slight decrease in putrescine levels after 8 hr of recirculation. In the cerebellum, cerebral cortex, and striatum putrescine levels in treated animals were only slightly (not significantly) lower

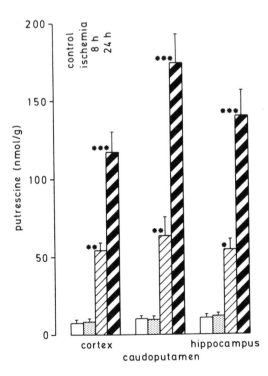

FIGURE 8. Regional putrescine levels in reversible cerebral ischemia of rats. Ischemia was produced by using the four-vessel occlusion model. Putrescine levels were measured in tissue samples taken from control animals at the end of 30 min of forebrain ischemia and after 8 or 24 hr of recirculation. (From Paschen *et al.*, 1988*e*.)

than those found in untreated ones, whereas in the hippocampus putrescine levels were identical in untreated and DFMO-treated animals (Paschen *et al.*, 1988*a*). These results clearly indicate that the postischemic increase in ODC activity is not the only cause of the overshoot in putrescine formation.

To study whether the postischemic increase in putrescine formation takes place in neurons (and may thus be involved in the pathological process of ischemic neuronal necrosis, as discussed below), synaptosomes, representing nerve endings, were isolated from rat brains subjected to 30 min of ischemia and 24 hr of recirculation (Röhn *et al.*, 1988, 1989). Putrescine levels were significantly increased after cerebral ischemia in synaptosomes; changes were most pronounced in synaptosomes isolated from the vulnerable striatum (an increase from 117 to 663 pmol/mg of protein) but significantly less pronounced in the less-vulnerable cerebral cortex (from 79 to 348 pmol/mg of protein).

3.2. Polyamines after Cerebral Ischemia in Gerbils

Ischemia-induced disturbances in polyamine metabolism have been studied in detail by using Mongolian gerbils (Paschen *et al.*, 1987*b*, 1988*b–d*) (the results are summarized in Figure 9). Similarly to the results of the rat experiments,

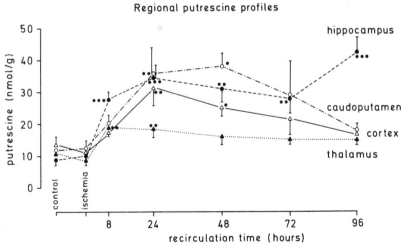

FIGURE 9. Regional putrescine levels in reversible cerebral ischemia of Mongolian gerbils. Ischemia was produced by occluding both common carotid arteries. Putrescine levels were measured in tissue samples taken from the cortex, caudoputamen, hippocampus (CA1 subfield), and thalamus of control animals at the end of 5 min of cerebral ischemia and after recirculation times of 8 to 96 hr. Note the only small transient increase in putrescine in the thalamus and the marked stable increase in the hippocampal CA1 subfield. (From Paschen *et al.*, 1988*e*.)

polyamine profiles did not change during cerebral ischemia, but changed only afterwards (Paschen et al., 1987b). In the CA1 subfield of the hippocampus putrescine levels were already about 2.5- to 3-fold above control values after 5 min of cerebral ischemia and 8 hr recirculation, i.e., at a time when the cells of the hippocampal CA1 sector were still morphologically, functionally, and metabolically preserved (Kirino 1982; Mies et al., 1983; Suzuki et al., 1983; Arai et al., 1986). After 24 hr of recirculation, the putrescine content was considerably increased in all forebrain structures studied. Following prolonged recirculation, putrescine levels declined to near control values in invulnerable brain structures such as the cerebral cortex or thalamus, but remained markedly elevated in the vulnerable hippocampal CA1 subfield (Paschen et al., 1987b). In the striatum both, postischemic putrescine levels and the density of ischemic neuronal necrosis varied considerably from animal to animal. However, in all animals exhibiting severe cell necrosis in the striatum after 4 days of recirculation, putrescine levels were severalfold above control levels but nearly identical to control levels in animals without severe cell damage (Table 1). A similar relationship between putrescine levels and cell damage was observed in the hippocampal CA1 subfield. About 20% of animals subjected to bilateral common carotid artery occlusion did not develop cell damage in the hippocampus. Putrescine levels in the CA1 subfield in these animals were similar to those found in control animals.

The postischemic increase in putrescine levels correlated with the period of vascular occlusion: when animals were subjected to 10 min of cerebral ischemia, putrescine levels measured after 24 hr recirculation were about twice as high as those found in animals after 5 min of ischemia (Paschen et al., 1987b). In contrast to putrescine, spermidine and spermine levels did not change during recirculation, with the exception of levels in the severely damaged regions, which were significantly reduced (Paschen et al., 1987b).

In the hippocampal CA1 subfield the density of neuronal necrosis can be

TABLE 1. Putrescine Levels in the Lateral
Striatum of Mongolian Gerbils after 5 Min
of Cerebral Ischemia and 96 hr Recirculation
in Relation to the Extent of Neuronal Necrosis

Putrescine levels (nmol/g)[a]		
	Ischemic gerbils	
Controls	Without injury	With injury
12.0 ± 1.0	13.1 ± 1.1	53.5 ± 10.3*[b]

[a]Values are the means ± SEM of 5 determinations.
[b]The asterisk denotes statistically significant differences between experimental groups and controls ($P \leq 0.001$).

quantified simply by counting microscopically the number of necrotic neurons per millimeter of stratum pyramidale. By comparing the density of neuronal necrosis with putrescine levels in the hippocampal CA1 subfield after 5 min of cerebral ischemia and 4 days of recirculation, a close threshold relationship was observed (Figure 10) (see also Paschen *et al.* [1988c]). In all animals in which putrescine levels were below 20 nmol/g, fewer than 5% of neurons were necrotic, whereas more than 90% of neurons were severely damaged in animals with putrescine levels above 30 nmol/g.

Postischemic treatment of gerbils with either the calcium antagonist nimodipine or the barbiturate pentobarbital markedly reduced the postischemic increase in putrescine and the density of neuronal necrosis (Paschen *et al.*, 1988*b*, *c*). Barbiturate significantly inhibited the increase in putrescine and the development of neuronal necrosis in both the vulnerable lateral striatum and hippocampal CA1 subfield, whereas nimodipine had a significant effect in the striatum but not in the hippocampus.

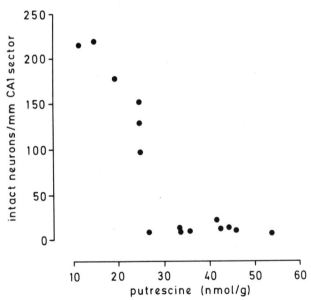

FIGURE 10. Relationship between putrescine levels and density of ischemic neuronal necrosis in the hippocampal CA1 subfield of Mongolian gerbils. Animals were subjected to 4 min of cerebral ischemia and 96 hr of recirculation. The density of ischemic neuronal necrosis was quantified in the CA1 subfield by counting the total number of neurons and the number of intact and necrotic neurons per millimeter of stratum pyramidale. Values obtained were correlated with putrescine levels measured in the CA1 subfield of the same animals. Note the close thresholdlike relationship between the two parameters. (From Paschen *et al.*, 1988*c*.)

3.3. Disturbance of Polyamine Metabolism and Ischemic Cell Death

The disturbances in polyamine metabolism observed during and after cerebral ischemia can be summarized as follows. (1) Polyamine metabolism does not change during global cerebral ischemia but only following recirculation. In focal cerebral ischemia, in contrast, ODC activity is significantly increased in the border zone in which blood flow is moderately reduced. (2) Following the onset of recirculation ODC and SAMDC activities are severely suppressed. ODC activity recovers, and the synthesis of ODC is considerably activated, peaking after about 8 to 10 hr of recirculation, whereas SAMDC activity remains markedly reduced for up to several days after ischemia. (3) During early recirculation the putrescine content is considerably increased in all brain structures studied. Following prolonged recirculation the putrescine levels normalize in invulnerable brain structures but remain high in vulnerable ones. Within in brain region the density of ischemic cell damage is related to putrescine levels. This is most prominent in the hippocampal CA1 subfield in which a close thresholdlike relationship is observed between the two parameters. (4) A marked increase in the putrescine level is apparent in synaptosomes isolated from the vulnerable striatum. (5) Spermidine or spermine levels are significantly reduced in necrotic regions. (6) Therapeutic intervention inhibiting the development of neuronal necrosis also inhibits the postischemic increase in putrescine levels. (7) The postischemic increase in putrescine levels precedes the development of neuronal necrosis. This is most prominent in the hippocampal CA1 subfield.

It is still not fully understood whether the postischemic disturbances in polyamine metabolism play a role in the manifestation of ischemic cell damage (Paschen *et al.*, 1987*a*, *b*) or whether these changes are independent of ischemic neuronal necrosis. Assuming that a direct relationship exists between the postischemic increase in putrescine levels and the development of neuronal necrosis, it is mandatory to illustrate that the observed increase in putrescine may be deleterious for the cell. In fact, over the last few years putrescine has been shown to exhibit important functions besides its role as a precursor of the polyamines spermidine and spermine: polyamines, and especially putrescine, have been found (1) to influence cellular calcium homeostasis (Koenig *et al.*, 1983*a*, *b*), (2) to modulate the release of neurotransmitters from synaptosomes (Iqbal and Koenig, 1985; Bondy and Walker, 1986; Komulainen and Bondy, 1987), (3) to evoke electrical hyperactivity (Nistico *et al.*, 1980), and (4) to be involved in the breakdown of the blood-brain barrier (Koenig *et al.*, 1983*c*, 1989; Trout *et al.*, 1986). Since disturbances in the homeostasis of calcium ions and excitatory neurotransmitters and electrical hyperactivity of neurons have been found to contribute to the manifestation of ischemic neuronal necrosis, the possible involvement of putrescine in this process will be discussed in detail below.

As regards point 1, under physiological conditions a small transient increase in the putrescine level contributes to the influx of calcium ions into the cell and efflux from mitochondria observed after activation. β-Adrenergic stimulation of the tissue, leading to an increase in the activity of cytosolic Ca^{2+} ions, also produces a transient increase in ODC activity and in the levels of putrescine, spermidine, and spermine (Koenig et al., 1983a, b). It has been suggested, therefore, that polyamines play an important role in stimulus-response coupling by generating a calcium signal after stimulus binding to a receptor on the cell surface. The influx of calcium ions into the cell and efflux from mitochondria after hormonal activation can be prevented by inhibiting ODC with DFMO, and this inhibition of calcium fluxes is reversed in the presence of putrescine. These results support the hypothesis that putrescine is directly involved in this process. The disturbances in the calcium homeostasis after cerebral ischemia may similarly result from the high putrescine levels, which are stable for several hours or even days.

As regards point 2, depolarization of synaptosomes triggers an influx of calcium ions into the cell and subsequent release of neurotransmitters. These reactions are accompanied by a small transient increase in ODC activity and polyamine levels (Iqbal and Koenig, 1985; Bondy and Walker, 1986; Komulainen and Bondy, 1986). The influx of calcium ions and the release of neurotransmitters from synaptosomes were markedly reduced after inhibiting ODC with DFMO, and this inhibition was reversed in the presence of putrescine. Interestingly, the DFMO effect could be reversed only after adding putrescine, whereas spermidine or spermine had no effect (Bondy and Walker 1986; Komulainen and Bondy, 1986), indicating that this is a putrescine-specific reaction. These results support the hypothesis that the release of excitatory neurotransmitters which may be involved in ischemic cell damage (Benveniste et al., 1984; Rothman, 1984; Choi, 1985; Wieloch, 1985) is triggered by putrescine.

As regards point 3, reversible cerebral ischemia induces an electrical hyper-activity of vulnerable neurons during the first day of recirculation. This hyper-activity has been observed in the hippocampal CA1 subfield of gerbils subjected to 5 min of cerebral ischemia (Suzuki et al., 1983) and in the striatum and hippocampus of rats after 30 min of ischemia (Pulsinelli, 1985). It has been suggested that the electrical hyperactivity of vulnerable neurons reflects an overactivation of the cell, which then dies as a result. Putrescine, when injected into the ventricle of chicken brains, causes a depletion of mid-brain γ-amino-butyric acid (GABA) levels and triggers electrical hyperactivity in the cerebral cortex (Nistico et al., 1980). It is therefore conceivable that putrescine contributes to the electrical hyperactivity in vulnerable brain structures after cerebral ischemia.

4. CONCLUSION

In conclusion, disturbances of polyamine metabolism are clearly associated with the manifestation of ischemic cell injury and therefore must be correlated with other metabolic dysfunctions which may also be involved in this process. As shown in this review, it is possible to establish correlations with disturbances of different metabolic and physiological functions such as protein synthesis, neurotransmitter metabolism, calcium-mediated processes, and the blood-brain barrier. It is still unknown whether these or any other disturbances trigger the pathological cascade leading to postischemic cell death and at which steps this cascade can be interrupted. Further analysis of the disturbances of protein or polyamine metabolism should be directed toward this goal.

REFERENCES

Arai, H., Passonneau, J. V., and Lust, W. D., 1986, Energy metabolism in delayed neuronal death of CA1 neurons of the hippocampus following transient ischemia in the gerbil, *Metab. Brain Dis.* **1:** 263–278.

Benveniste, H., Drejer, J., Schousboe, A., and Diemer, N., 1984, Elevation of the extracellular concentrations of glutamate and aspartate in rat hippocampus during transient cerebral ischemia monitored by intracerebral microdialysis, *J. Neurochem.* **43:**1369–1374.

Bodsch, W., Takahashi, K., Barbier, A., Grosse Ophoff, B., and Hossmann, K.-A., 1985, Cerebral protein synthesis and ischemia, *Prog. Brain Res.* **63:**197–210.

Bodsch, W., Barbier, A. Oehmichen, M., Grosse Ophoff, B., and Hossmann, K.-A., 1986, Recovery of monkey brain after prolonged ischemia, *J. Cereb. Blood Flow Metab.* **6:**22–33.

Bondy, S. C., and Walker, C. H., 1986, Polyamines contribute to calcium-stimulated release of aspartate from brain particulate fraction, *Brain Res.* **371:**96–100.

Burda, J., Chavko, M., and Marsala, J., 1980, Changes in ribosomes from ischemic spinal, *Coll. Czech.* **45:**2566–2571.

Canellakis, E. S., Viceps-Madore, D., Kyriakidis, D. A., and Heller, J. S., 1979, The regulation and function of ornithine decarboxylase and of the polyamines, *Curr. Top. Cell. Regul.* **15:**155–202.

Choi, D. W., 1985, Glutamate neurotoxicity in cortical cell cultures is calcium dependent, *Neurosci. Lett.* **58:**293–297.

Clark-Walker, G. D., 1973, Translation of messenger RNA, *in* "The Ribonucleic Acids" (P. R. Stewart and D. S. Letham, eds.), pp. 135–149, Springer-Verlag, New York.

Cooper, H. K., Zalewska, T., Kawakami, S., Hossmann, K.-A., and Kleihues, P., 1977, The effect of ischaemia and recirculation on protein synthesis in the rat brain, *J. Neurochem.* **28:**929–934.

Cousin, M. A., Lando, D., and Moguilewsky, M., 1982, Ornithine decarboxylase induction by glucocorticoids in brain and liver of adrenalectomized rats, *J. Neurochem.* **38:**1296–1304.

Dempsey, R. J., Roy, M. W., Meyer, K., Tai, H. H., and Olson, J. W., 1985, Polyamine and prostaglandin markers in focal cerebral ischemia, *Neurosurgery* **17:**635–640.

Dempsey, R. J., Maley, B. E., Cowen, D., and Olson, J. W., 1988, Ornithine decarboxylase activity and immunohistochemical location in postischemic brain, *J. Cereb. Blood Flow Metab.* **8:**843–847.

Dienel, G. A., and Cruz, N. F., 1984, Induction of brain ornithine decarboxylase during recovery from metabolic, mechanical, thermal or chemical injury, *J. Neurochem.* **42:**1053–1061.

Dienel, G. A., Pulsinelli, W. A., and Duffy, T. E., 1980, Regional protein synthesis in rat brain following acute hemispheric ischemia, *J. Neurochem.* **35:**1216–1226.

Dienel, G. A., Cruz, N. F., and Rosenfeld, S. J., 1985, Temporal profiles of proteins responsive to transient ischemia, *J. Neurochem.* **44:**600–610.

Dienel, G. A., Kiessling, M., Jacewicz, M., and Pulsinelli, W. A., 1986, Synthesis of heat shock proteins in rat brain cortex after transient ischemia, *J. Cereb. Blood Flow Metab.* **6:**505–510.

Djuricic, B. M., Paschen, W., and Schmidt-Kastner, R., 1988, Polyamines in the brain: HPLC analysis and its application in cerebral ischemia, *Jugosl. Physiol. Pharmacol. Acta* **24:**9–17.

Gilad, G. M., and Gilad, V. H., 1983, Early rapid and transient increase in ornithine decarboxylase activity within sympathetic neurons after axonal injury, *Exp. Neurol.* **81:**158–166.

Hallmayer, J., Hossmann, K.-A., and Mies, G., 1985, Low dose of barbiturates for prevention of hippocampal lesions after brief ischemic episodes, *Acta Neuropathol.* **68:**27–31.

Hartmann, J. F., Becker, R. A., and Cohen, M. M., 1973, Cerebral ultrastructure in experimental hypoxia and ischemia, *Monogr. Neurol. Sci.* **1:**50–64.

Heby, O., 1981, Role of polyamines in the control of cell proliferation and differentiation, *Differentiation* **19:**1–20.

Hossmann, K.-A., 1985, Post-ischemic resuscitation of the brain: Selective vulnerability versus global resistance, *Prog. Brain Res.* **63:**3–17.

Hossmann, K.-A., and Kleihues, P., 1973, Reversibility of ischemic brain damage, *Arch. Neurol.* **29:** 375–384.

Hossmann, K.-A., Schmidt-Kastner, R., and Grosse Ophoff, B., 1987, Recovery of integrative central nervous function after one hour global cerebro-circulatory arrest in normothermic cat, *J. Neurol. Sci.* **77:**305–320.

Iqbal, Z., and Koenig, N. H., 1985, Polyamines appear to be second messengers in mediating Ca^{2+} fluxes and neurotransmitter release in potassium-stimulated synaptosomes, *Biochem. Biophys. Res. Commun.* **133:**563–573.

Jacewicz, M., Kiessling, M., and Pulsinelli, W. A., 1985, Selective gene expression in focal cerebral ischemia, *Ann. Neurol.* **18:**126.

Jänne, J., Pösö, H., and Raina, A., 1979, Polyamine in rapid growth and cancer, *Biochim. Biophys. Acta* **473:**241–293.

Kiessling, M., Dienel, G. A., Jacewicz, M., and Pulsinelli, W. A., 1986, Protein synthesis in postischemic rat brain: A two-dimensional electrophoretic analysis, *J. Cereb. Blood Flow Metab.* **6:**642–649.

Kirino, T., 1982, Delayed neuronal death in the gerbil hippocampus following ischemia, *Brain Res.* **239:**57–69.

Kirino, T., and Sano, K., 1984, Selective vulnerability in the gerbil hippocampus following transient ischemia, *Acta Neuropathol.* **62:**201–208.

Kleihues, P., and Hossmann, K.-A., 1971, Protein synthesis in the cat brain after prolonged cerebral ischemia, *Brain Res.* **35:**409–418.

Kleihues, P., Hossmann, K.-A., Pegg, A. E., Kobayashi, K., and Zimmermann, V., 1975, Resuscitation of the monkey brain after one hour complete ischemia. III. Indications of metabolic recovery, *Brain Res.* **95:**61–73.

Koenig, H., Goldstone, A., and Lu, C. Y., 1983*a*, Polyamines regulate calcium fluxes in a rapid membrane response, *Nature* (London) **305:**530–534.

Koenig, H., Goldstone, A., and Lu, C. Y., 1983*b*, β-Adrenergic stimulation of Ca^{2+}-fluxes, endocytosis, hexose transport, and amino acid transport in mouse kidney is mediated by polyamine synthesis, *Proc. Natl. Acad. Sci. USA* **80:**7210–7214.

Koenig, H., Goldstone, A., and Lu, C. Y., 1983*c*, Blood brain barrier breakdown in brain edema following cold injury is mediated by microvascular polyamines, *Biochem. Biophys. Res. Commun.* **116:**1039–1048.

Koenig, K., Goldstone, A. D., and Lu, C. Y., 1989, Blood-brain barrier breakdown in cold-injured brain is linked to biphasic stimulation of ornithine decarboxylase and polyamine synthesis: Both are coordinately inhibited by verapamil, dexamethasone, and aspirin, *J. Neurochem.* **52:** 101–109.

Komulainen, H., and Bondy, S. C., 1987, Transient elevation of intrasynaptosomal free calcium by putrescine, *Brain Res.* **401:**50–54.

Lewis, M. E., Lakshamanan, K., Nagaiah, K., MacDonnell, P. C., and Guroff, G., 1978, Nerve growth factor increases activity of ornithine decarboxylase in rat brain, *Proc. Natl. Acad. Sci. USA* **75:** 1021–1023.

Louis, J.-C., Magal, E., and Yavin, E., 1988, Protein kinase C alterations in the fetal rat brain after global ischemia, *J. Biol. Chem.* **263**:19282–19285.

Lowry, O. H., Passonneau, J. V., Hasselberger, F. X., and Schulz, D. W., 1964, Effect of ischemia on known substrates and cofactors of the glycolytic pathway in brain, *J. Biol. Chem.* **239**:18–30.

Mies, G., Paschen, W., Hossmann, K.-A., and Klatzo, I., 1983, Simultaneous measurement of regional blood flow and metabolism during maturation of hippocampal lesions following short-lasting cerebral ischemia in gerbils, *J. Cereb. Blood Flow Metab.* **3**(Suppl. 1):S329–S330.

Munekata, K., Hossmann, K.-A., Xie, Y., Seo, K., Oschlies, U ., 1987, Selective vulnerability of hippocampus: Ribosomal aggregation, protein synthesis, and tissue pH, *in* "Cerebrovascular Diseases" (M. E. Raichle and W. J. Powers, eds.), pp. 107–118, Raven Press, New York.

Nistico, G., Jentile, R., Rotiroti, D., and Di Giorgio, R. M., 1980, GABA depletion and behavioral changes produced by intraventricular putrescine in chicks, *Biochem. Pharmacol.* **29**:954–957.

Nowak, T. S., Jr., 1985, Synthesis of a stress protein following transient ischemia in the gerbil, *J. Neurochem.* **45**:1635–1641.

Nowak, T. S., Jr., 1988, NMDA-receptor antagonist MK-801 blocks postischemic HSP70 induction: Evidence that the heat shock (stress) response is a component of excitotoxic pathology in gerbil hippocampus, *J. Neuropathol. Exp. Neurol.* **47**:363.

Nowak, T. S., Jr., Fried, R. L., Lust, W. D., and Passonneau, J. V., 1985, Changes in brain energy metabolism and protein synthesis following transient bilateral ischemia in the gerbil, *J. Neurochem.* **44**:487–494.

Paschen, W., Schmidt-Kastner, R., Djuricic, B., Meese, C., Linn, F., and Hossmann, K. A., 1987*a*, Polyamine changes in reversible cerebral ischemia, *J. Neurochem.* **49**:35–37.

Paschen, W., Hallmayer, J., and Mies, G., 1987*b*, Regional profile of polyamines in reversible cerebral ischemia of Mongolian gerbils, *Neurochem. Pathol.* **7**:143–156.

Paschen, W., Röhn, G., Meese, C. O., Djuricic, B., and Schmidt-Kastner, R., 1988*a*, Polyamine metabolism in reversible cerebral ischemia: Effect of α-difluoromethylornithine, *Brain Res.* **453**:9–16.

Paschen, W., Hallmayer, J., and Röhn, G., 1988*b*, Relationship between putrescine content and density of ischemic cell damage in the brain of mongolian gerbils: Effect of nimodipine and barbiturate, *Acta Neuropathol.* **76**:388–394.

Paschen, W., Hallmayer, J., and Röhn, G., 1988*c*, Regional changes of polyamine profiles after reversible cerebral ischemia in Mongolian gerbils: Effects of nimodipine and barbiturate, *Neurochem. Pathol.* **8**:27–41.

Paschen, W., Röhn, G., Hallmayer, J., and Mies, G., 1988*d*, Polyamine metabolism in reversible cerebral ischemia of Mongolian gerbils, *Metab. Brain Dis.* **3**:297–302.

Paschen, W., Schmidt-Kastner, R., Hallmayer, J., and Djuricic, B., 1988*e*, Polyamines in cerebral ischemia, *Neurochem. Pathol.* **9**:1–20.

Paschen, W., Röhn, G., Kocher, M., and Hallmayer, J., 1989, Disturbances in polyamine metabolism in reversible cerebral ischemia, *New Trends in Clin. Neuropharmacol.* **3**:99.

Pegg, A. E., 1986, Recent advantages in the biochemistry of polyamines in eukaryotes, *Biochem. J.* **234**:249–262.

Pegg, A. E., and McCann, P. P., 1982, Polyamine metabolism and function, *Am. J. Physiol.* **243**:C212–C221.

Pegg, A. E., Lockwood, D. H., and Williams-Ashman, H. G., 1970, Concentration of putrescine and polyamines and their enzymatic synthesis during androgen-induced prostatic growth, *Biochem. J.* **117**:17–31.

Petito, C. K., and Babiak, T., 1982, Early proliferative changes in astrocytes in postischemic noninfarcted rat brain, *Ann. Neurol.* **11**:510–518.

Petito, C. K., and Pulsinelli, W. A., 1984, Sequential development of reversible and irreversible neuronal damage following cerebral ischemia, *J. Neuropathol. Exp. Neurol.* **43**:141–153.

Pluta, R., 1987, Resuscitation of the rabbit brain after acute complete ischemia lasting up to one hour:

Pathophysiological and pathomorphological observations, *Resuscitation* **15**:267–287.

Pulsinelli, W. A., 1985, Selective neuronal vulnerability: Morphological and molecular characteristics, *Prog. Brain Res.* **63**:29–37.

Pulsinelli, W. A., and Brierley, J., 1979, A new model of bilateral hemispheric ischemia in unanesthetized rat, *Stroke* **10**:267–272.

Pulsinelli, W. A., Brierley, J. B., and Plum, F., 1982, Temporal profile of neuronal damage in a model of transient forebrain ischemia, *Ann. Neurol.* **11**:491–498.

Röhn, G., Kocher, M., Oschlies, U., and Paschen, W., 1988, Distribution of putrescine in subcellular fractions of rat brain after reversible cerebral ischemia, *Biol. Chem. Hoppe-Seyler* **396**:1210.

Röhn, G., Paschen, W., Kocher, M., Oschlies, U., and Hossmann, K.-A., 1989, Subcellular distribution of putrescine in reversible cerebral ischemia of rat brain, *in* "Cerebral Vascular Disease, vol. 7" (J. S. Meyer, H. Lechner, M. Reivich, and E. O. Ott, eds.), pp. 269–272, Excerpta Medica, Amsterdam.

Rothman, S., 1984, Synaptic release of excitatory amino acid neurotransmitter mediates anoxic neuronal death, *J. Neurosci.* **4**:1884–1891.

Schmidt-Kastner, R., Hossmann, K.-A., and Grosse Ophoff, B., 1986, Relationship between metabolic recovery and the EEG after prolonged ischemia of cat brain, *Stroke* **17**:1164–1169.

Seiler, N., 1981, Polyamine metabolism and function in the brain, *Neurochem. Int.* **3**:95–110.

Siesjö, B. K., 1988*a*, Mechanisms of ischemic brain damage, *Crit. Care Med.* **16**:954–963.

Siesjö, B. K., 1988*b*, Historical overview: Calcium, ischemia and death of brain cells, *Ann. N.Y. Acad. Sci.* **522**:638–661.

Slotkin, T. A., and Bartolome, J., 1986, Role of ornithine decarboxylase and the polyamines in nervous system development: A review, *Brain Res. Bull.* **17**:307–320.

Smith, C. B., Deibler, G. E., Eng, N., Schmidt, K., and Sokoloff, L., 1988, Measurement of local cerebral protein synthesis in vivo: Influence of recycling of amino acids derived from protein degradation, *Proc. Natl. Acad. Sci. USA* **85**:9341–9345.

Smith, M.-L., Kalimo, H., Warner, D. S., and Siesjö, B. K., 1988, Morphological lesions in the brain preceding the development of postischemic seizures, *Acta Neuropathol.* **76**:253–264.

Suzuki, R., Yamaguchi, T., Li, C. L., and Klatzo, I., 1983, The effects of 5-minutes ischemia in Mongolian gerbils. II. Changes in spontaneous neuronal activity in cerebral cortex and CA1 sector of hippocampus, *Acta Neuropathol.* **60**:217–222.

Taft, W. C., Tennes-Rees, K. A., Blair, R. E., Clifton, G. L., and DeLorenzo, R. J., 1988, Cerebral ischemia decreases endogenous calcium-dependent protein phosphorylation in gerbil brain, *Brain Res.* **447**:159–163.

Thilmann, R., Xie, Y., Kleihues, P., and Kiessling, M., 1986*a*, Persistent inhibition of protein synthesis precedes delayed neuronal death in postischemic gerbil hippocampus, *Acta Neuropathol.* **71**:88–93.

Thilmann, R., Xie, Y., Kleihues, P., and Kiessling, M., 1988*b*, Delayed ischemic cell death in gerbil hippocampus: Suppression and recovery of protein synthesis and the protective effect of cycloheximide, *Clin. Neurol.* **5**:107.

Trout, J. J., Koenig, H., Goldstone, A. D., and Lu, C. Y., 1986, Blood-brain barrier breakdown by cold injury. Polyamine signals mediate acute stimulation of endocytosis, vesicular transport, and microvillus formation in rat cerebral capillaries, *Lab. Invest.* **55**:622–631.

Wieloch, T., 1985, Neurochemical correlates to selective neuronal vulnerability, *Progr. Brain Res.* **63**:69–85.

Williams-Ashman, H. G., and Canellakis, Z. N., 1979, Polyamines in mammalian biology and medicine, *Perspect. Biol. Med.* **22**:421–438.

Xie, Y., Herget, T., Hallmayer, J., Starzinski-Powitz, A., and Hossmann, K.-A., 1989, Determination of RNA content in post-ischemic gerbil brain by in situ hybridization, *Metab. Brain Dis.* **4**:239–251.

Yanagihara, T., 1976, Cerebral anoxia: Effect on neuron-glia fractions and polysomal protein synthesis, *J. Neurochem.* **27**:539–543.

CHAPTER 5

OXYGEN DEPENDENCE OF NEURONAL METABOLISM

DAVID F. WILSON

1. INTRODUCTION

In the brain, as in many other tissues, the delivery of oxygen is highly regulated and the tissue oxygen pressure is normally maintained within a narrow range. Periods of hypoxia and/or ischemia followed by reoxygenation/reperfusion present a complex series of stresses to cellular and vascular physiology. Depending on the duration and severity of the initial period of hypoxia/ischemia and the succeeding reoxygenation protocol, there are various degrees of irreversible damage to cells. The primary cause of the damage is oxygen deprivation, which results in a deficiency in the metabolic energy available for cellular maintenance and repair. Energy-deprived cells in the central nervous system (CNS) first undergo progressive dissipation of the cellular ionic balance, including a very rapid (seconds) increase in intracellular Na^+ levels and decrease in intracellular K^+ levels, membrane depolarization with attendant increased intracellular Ca^{2+} levels, and release of neurotransmitters such as the excitatory amino acids. After longer

DAVID F. WILSON • *Department of Biochemistry and Biophysics, Medical School, University of Pennsylvania, Philadelphia, Pennsylvania.*

Neurochemical Correlates of Cerebral Ischemia, Volume 7 of *Advances in Neurochemistry*, edited by Nicolas G. Bazan, Pierre Braquet, and Myron D. Ginsberg. Plenum Press, New York, 1992.

periods (minutes) there is progressive lipolysis and proteolysis. In the first minutes of this process it may be fully reversible, and reoxygenation leads to essentially complete recovery. As the duration of the hypoxic/ischemic episode increases, however, the extent of recovery progressively decreases. The physiological basis for the irreversible component of the recovery remains poorly understood, although it has been reported that hyperglycemia exacerbates the damage (Meyers and Yamaguchi, 1977; Rehncrona *et al.*, 1981; Welsh *et al.*, 1983) and that many factors, including excitatory amino acid neurotransmitters released during the hypoxic episode (see, for example Olney [1978]; Watkins and Evans [1981]) and oxygen radicals produced during reperfusion, may be important contributors to the lack of recovery (Siesjö, 1981; Bazan and Rodriguez de Turco, 1980; Yoshida *et al.*, 1980). The present review will focus on the initial metabolic consequences of oxygen depravation in the CNS and will highlight only key elements of the more complex recovery process.

2. OXYGEN DELIVERY TO CELLS AND OXYGEN DEPENDENCE OF MITOCHONDRIAL OXIDATIVE PHOSPHORYLATION

The utilization of oxygen by tissue requires three sequential steps. (1) The first is delivery of O_2 to the tissue through flow of blood from the lungs to the capillary bed of the tissue. The oxygen pressure in the blood entering the capillary bed is approximately 65 torr, while that in the veins is approximately 15 to 20 mmHg. (2) The second is net movement (diffusion) of the oxygen from the erythrocytes in the capillaries (mean pressure of approximately 40 mmHg) to the mitochondria in each cell, a movement which is powered by the oxygen pressure differences between the erythrocyte and the mitochondria. (3) The third is the oxygen pressure needed by the mitochondria to synthesize ATP at the rate and energy level ($[ATP]/[ADP][P_i]$) needed for cellular function. Recent data have substantially modified our understanding of tissue oxygen metabolism in two areas: the oxygen dependence of mitochondrial oxidative phosphorylation under normal cellular conditions, and the diffusion-induced oxygen pressure differences between the extracellular space surrounding individual cells and the mitochondria of that cell. These data will then be discussed in terms of their contributions to the pathology of periods of cerebral hypoxia/ischemia and reperfusion.

2.1. Oxygen Dependence of Mitochondrial Oxidative Phosphorylation in Suspensions of Isolated Mitochondria

There are substantial quantitative differences in the literature concerning the effects of oxygen pressure on oxidative phosphorylation. These differences exist in both the reported dependence of mitochondrial respiration on oxygen at low oxygen pressures (less than about 20 mmHg) and, more importantly, the oxygen dependence of the mitochondrial capacity to synthesize ATP. The data will fall into two fundamentally different categories.

(1) The respiration of the mitochondria is independent of oxygen pressure until very low values (less than 1 mmHg). The oxygen-dependent region of the respiratory rate is characterized by a pressure for half-maximal rate (P_{50}) of less than 0.1 mmHg for well-coupled mitochondria. This value increases when the mitochondria are uncoupled or the energy state is decreased, and the increase is proportional to the increase in respiratory rate. Similarly, as the oxygen pressure is lowered, the reduction of the chemical process of the cytochromes occurs at higher oxygen pressures for uncoupled mitochondria than for coupled mitochondria (Oshino et al., 1974; Sugano et al., 1974). This will be referred to as the "small-oxygen-dependence" model.

(2) The respiration of mitochondria is independent of oxygen pressure in the medium until the latter is less than approximately 6 mmHg. Below this pressure the respiration of suspensions of well-coupled mitochondria decreases with a P_{50} of approximately 0.6 mmHg. When the mitochondria are uncoupled or the energy state ($[ATP]/[ADP][P_i]$) is lowered, the P_{50} decreases to values less than 0.30 mmHg, although the respiratory rate increases severalfold. As the oxygen pressure is lowered, reduction of the cytochromes occurs at lower oxygen pressures for uncoupled mitochondria than for coupled mitochondria (Peterson et al., 1974; Wilson et al., 1979b, 1988; Wilson and Erecinska, 1985). This will be referred to as the "large-oxygen-dependence" model.

It is clearly important to our understanding of the oxygen dependence of cellular and tissue metabolism to determine which of the sets of experimental data is representative of the behavior of mitochondria in vivo. A more extensive review of the data and the methods used to obtain them has been presented elsewhere (Wilson et al., 1988; Robiolio et al., 1989), and only a brief summary will be presented here. The experimental support for the small-oxygen-dependence model is based primarily on experiments in which oxygen was continuously added to the mitochondrial suspension (Oshino et al., 1974; Sugano et al., 1974). This method, essentially that developed by Degn and Wohlrab (1971), has also been used, under similar conditions, to provide some of the data supporting the large-oxygen-dependence model (Petersen et al.,1974). The technique of continuous oxygen addition is particularly sensitive to errors introduced by failure to fully consider the time required to stir in the oxygen as it is added. A combination of the oxygen consumption rate in the suspension and the time required for the oxygen to be stirred in from the point of addition can generate substantial macroscopic oxygen pressure differences in the medium. These macroscopic oxygen pressure differences are dependent on the rate of oxygen consumption in the medium and can give rise to a range of possible oxygen dependences and/or errors in interpretation. The very divergent results reported for this method are indicative of the potential for error (compare Petersen *et al.*, [1974] with Oshino *et al.*, [1974] and Sugano *et al.*, [1974]). On the other hand, data supporting the large-oxygen-dependence model have been obtained by using various methods for measuring oxygen, some of which did not require continuous addition of oxygen to the medium in order to measure the oxygen dependence of the respiratory rate (see, for example, Wilson *et al.*, 1988). In our view, the large-oxygen-dependence model is the more consistent with available biochemical and physiological data. It will be used in further discussions of cellular metabolism in this paper.

The oxygen dependence of oxidative phosphorylation in suspensions of isolated mitochondria may be summarized as follows. The increases in cytochrome reduction which occur at oxygen pressures up to at least 30 mmHg for suspensions of isolated mitochondria at high energy levels (high extramitochondrial [ATP]/[ADP][P_i]) are indicative of adjustments in the redox components of the electron transport system in response to the changes in oxygen pressure. The redox changes thus report an oxygen dependence which extends throughout the range of oxygen pressures normally found in cells, i.e., pressures less than 30 mmHg. The oxygen dependence, with respect to both cytochrome reduction and respiratory rate, extends to higher oxygen pressures by 50-fold or more for suspensions of mitochondria at high energy levels than it does for suspensions of mitochondria at low energy levels.

2.2. Oxygen Dependence of Oxidative Phosphorylation in Cells Originating in the Central Nervous System

The oxygen dependence of mitochondrial oxidative phosphorylation has been measured for several types of cells originating from the CNS. The initial reports were for suspensions of C-1300 neuroblastoma cells (Wilson *et al.*, 1979*a*; Figure 2 of that paper is reproduced in this review as Figure 1). As the oxygen pressure in the cell suspension was lowered, reduction of cytochrome *c* was readily observed as the oxygen pressure fell below approximately 40 mmHg. This reduction progressively increased with further decrease in oxygen pressure. Direct measurements of cellular energy metabolism, as indicated by the [ATP]/[ADP] ratio, at various oxygen pressures confirmed that the oxygen dependence of cellular energy metabolism began at oxygen pressures above 40 mmHg. Many cells with high metabolic energy levels, such as glioma (M. Erecinska and D. F. Wilson, unpublished results) and human neuroblastoma (Robiolio *et al.*, 1989), have this characteristic oxygen dependence. These data suggest that the capacity of mitochondria in situ to synthesize ATP decreases as the oxygen pressure is lowered. This decrease is expressed as either a decrease in the cellular [ATP]/[ADP][P_i], reduction of cytochrome *c*, or a combination of the two. It should be noted that the effects of decreasing oxygen pressure on these cells, as expressed in their [ATP]/[ADP] ratio and in cytochrome *c* reduction, began at oxygen pressures well above those at which the respiratory rate began to decline.

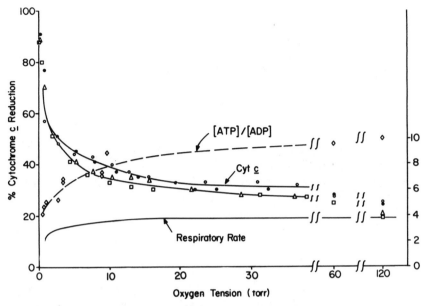

FIGURE 1. Oxygen dependence of cellular energy metabolism in neuroblastoma cells. The cells were suspended at 20 to 25 mg (wet weight)/ml in Hanks' medium and placed in a stirred spectrophotometer cuvette. Cytochrome c reduction was measured as the absorbance change at 550 nm minus that at 540 nm, and oxygen was measured with an oxygen electrode. At various oxygen pressures, aliquots of the suspension were ejected into cold perchloric acid solution. ATP and ADP were measured enzymatically in the neutralized acid extract. Individual points are placed on the cytochrome c reduction curves only to identify data from four separate experiments and thereby indicate the experimental reproducibility. (From Wilson *et al.*, 1979a.)

2.3. Oxygen Diffusion from the Extracellular Medium to the Mitochondria as a Factor in the Oxygen Dependence of Cellular Respiration

The oxygen utilized by the mitochondria in situ must diffuse from the extracellular medium to the mitochondria before it can be utilized for respiration. Since the net flow of oxygen occurs from regions of higher oxygen pressure to those of lower oxygen pressure, the oxygen pressure must be lower at the mitochondria than in the extracellular medium. The oxygen dependence of mitochondrial respiration can be used to quantitate the oxygen pressure difference between the mitochondria and the extracellular medium. The measured P_{50} for oxygen measured in suspensions of isolated, uncoupled mitochondria for oxygen is less than 0.03 mmHg. Thus, when intact cells are treated with uncoupler and the oxygen dependence of respiration is measured as a function of the extracellular oxygen pressure, the measured P_{50} reflects the oxygen dependence of the mito-chondria (P_{50} less than 0.03 mmHg) plus the difference in oxygen pressure between the extracellular medium and the mitochondria. A measured P_{50} of greater than 0.03 mmHg for uncoupler-treated cells is not, however, sufficient evidence that the P_{50} is determined by oxygen diffusion. The presence of such differences in oxygen pressure can be verified by measuring the P_{50} at various rates of cellular respiration. If the diffusion-induced difference in oxygen pressure within each cell is greater than 0.03 mmHg (and thus determines the P_{50}), the P_{50} should not only be greater than 0.03 mmHg but should also be proportional to the rate of oxygen consumption per unit volume of the cell. Intracellular oxygen pressure differences will, however, be independent of the number of cells per unit volume of the medium as long as the respiratory rate of each cell is unchanged. This behavior is in contrast to that of oxygen pressure dependencies resulting from the existence of macroscopic oxygen pressure differences in the suspending medium. In the latter case, the effects of varying the respiratory rate by changing the respiratory rate per cell and by changing the number of cells per unit volume of the medium are similar.

This method for evaluating the oxygen diffusion barrier for cells has been applied to human neuroblastoma cells (Robiolio *et al.*, 1989; Figure 4b of that paper is reproduced in this review, in modified form, as Figure 2). In these cells, the P_{50} was approximately 0.8 mmHg and the respiratory rate was approximately 4.5 nmol of O_2/min per mg of protein. Addition of uncoupler increased the respiratory rate by fourfold to 18 nmol of O_2/min per mg of protein. The P_{50} for cellular respiration decreased slightly to approximately 0.6 mmHg. The respira-tion of the uncoupler-treated cells was then systematically decreased by adding aliquots of Amytal, an inhibitor of the mitochondrial respiratory chain. The P_{50} for respiration decreased as the respiratory rate per cell decreased. the P_{50} was proportional to the respiratory rate, approaching zero (< 0.03 mmHg) as the respiratory rate approached zero. At a respiratory rate of the uncoupler-treated cells equal to that of normal cells, the P_{50} values were 0.15 and 0.8 mmHg, respectively. This establishes the oxygen diffusion barrier for this cell type (an approximately 10-μm-diameter cell) and the oxygen pressure difference induced by normal respiration. The diffusion of oxygen can be described as inducing an oxygen pressure difference between the extracellular medium and the mito-chondria in the human neuroblastoma cells of 0.07 mmHg/nmol of O_2 consumed per min per mg of cellular dry weight. This means the oxygen pressure difference from the extracellular medium to the mitochondria for their normal (high-oxygen) respiratory rate is approximately 0.3 mmHg (twice the P_{50} for uncoupled cells with the same high oxygen respiratory rate [0.15 mmHg]). When respiring at 50% of the high-oxygen rate, this would be only 0.15 mmHg, and the measured P_{50} for the respiration of normal cells of 0.8 mmHg is not substantially dependent on oxygen diffusion. Since much of the oxygen dependence of mitochondrial oxidative

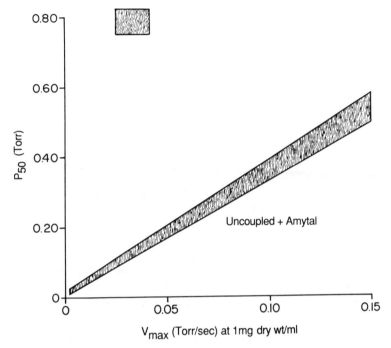

FIGURE 2. Oxygen pressure dependence of respiration in suspensions of human neuroblastoma cells. The oxygen pressure required for the half-maximal respiratory rate (P_{50}) was measured for normal cells ($\square$) and cells treated with uncoupler at levels 1.5 times that required for maximal stimulation of respiration. The uncoupler-treated cells were then titrated with Amytal, an inhibitor of the mitochondrial respiratory chain, and the P_{50} measured for each level of cellular respiration. These data were taken for three different cell concentrations. In this figure, the data for uncoupler-treated cells have been averaged and are represented as a single line. (The original data and figure are from Robiolio *et al.*, 1989.)

phosphorylation occurs at oxygen pressures greater than about 6 mmHg, limits set by diffusion are significant only in acute cellular abnormalities such as those resulting from oxygen deprivation or work rates exceeding maximal oxygen delivery rates.

These conclusions are in direct contrast to those of Jones (1984, 1986) and Jones and Kennedy (1982). These workers reported that isolated hepatocytes, cells of similar size and respiratory rate to the human neuroblastoma cells, had diffusion-induced oxygen pressure differences between the cytoplasm and the mitochondria of several mmHg. This interpretation was based on experiments in which aliquots of medium containing sufficient oxygen to give final oxygen pressures of up to about 15 mmHg were injected into stirred, anaerobic suspensions of hepatocytes and the redepletion of the oxygen was measured by using an oxygen electrode. The cells would be expected to be in an energy-depleted state when the oxygen was added. Thus, the respiratory rate is high immediately after oxygen addition because the ATP degraded during hypoxia must be resynthesized and the cellular ion balances reestablished. As the cellular ATP level and energy balance approach normal values, the respiratory rate would decline toward the aerobic steady state. For the conditions used in the experiments, this phase of energy-dependent respiration would merge with the phase of oxygen dependence. The authors interpreted all of the changes in respiratory rate as being due to oxygen pressure change, greatly overestimating the oxygen dependence of the cellular respiration. This, combined with interpretation by the small-oxygen-dependence model, led these authors to attribute the entire dependence to oxygen diffusion between the cytoplasm and the mitochondria. This interpretation required unreasonably large oxygen pressure differences between the extracellular medium and the mitochondria (by 5- to 10-fold) and even larger differences between the cytoplasm and the mitochondria (by > 50-fold). The role of oxygen diffusion in cellular respiration is also discussed by Katz *et al.* (1984), Clark and Clark (1985), Clark *et al.*, (1987), Wilson (1982), Wittenberg and Wittenberg (1985), Gayeski and Honig (1986), and Robiolio *et al.* (1989).

2.4. Comparison of the Oxygen Dependence of Mitochondrial Oxidative Phosphorylation in Vivo and in Vitro

The evidence reviewed above indicates that the oxygen pressure at the mitochondria of human neuroblastoma cells differs from that in the suspending medium by less than 1 mmHg. Thus, when the oxygen pressure in the suspending medium is above about 5 mmHg, the oxygen pressure dependence of mitochondria in situ can be directly compared with that of suspensions of isolated mitochondria. This comparison indicates that the mitochondria in situ behave similarly to those in vitro except that the dependence on oxygen pressure is slightly greater in situ. This is consistent with the fact that the isolation procedures, no matter how gently they are carried out, damage at least a fraction of the mitochondria isolated. Both in vivo and in vitro, any procedures which decrease the extramitochondrial energy level or the capacity of the mitochondria to synthesize ATP result in a decrease in the oxygen dependence of oxidative phosphorylation.

2.5. General Considerations Concerning the Onset of Hypoxia and Its Effect on Cellular Metabolism

Oxidative phosphorylation in normal cells is dependent on oxygen pressure throughout the range of oxygen pressures found in cells under physiological conditions. At first glance, this would seem to mean that the respiratory rate of cells would decrease as the oxygen pressure decreased. In cells, however, the rate of ATP utilization is independent of oxygen pressure per se, and if the oxygen pressure is decreased the use of ATP continues at an unchanged rate. The rate of synthesis of ATP must, as an average over time, equal the rate of ATP utilization or progressive metabolic failure will result. In the higher-oxygen-pressure region ($>$ 10 mmHg), when oxygen pressure is deceased, the mitochondrial oxidative phosphorylation only transiently fails to maintain the rate of ATP synthesis. The initial decrease in the rate of ATP synthesis results in a fall in ATP concentration and a rise in ADP and P_i concentrations, decreasing the cellular $[ATP]/[ADP][P_i]$ ratio. The latter stimulates the rate of ATP synthesis by the mitochondria (increased respiratory rate) and glycolysis until it again equals the rate of ATP utilization and the latter no longer decreases. Thus, a new steady state is rapidly generated in which the oxygen pressure and $[ATP]/[ADP][P_i]$ are lower but the respiratory rate is the same as for the higher oxygen pressure.

As the oxygen pressure in a suspension of cells is progressively decreased from high values ($>$ 10 mmHg) to low values, the cells may be thought of as progressing through a series of different metabolic states. When the oxygen pressures are greater than 10 mmHg, a decrease in the oxygen pressure results in a new metabolic state with the same rate of ATP utilization and synthesis. The other metabolic parameters, however, are modified and the cellular energy state usually decreases and/or the mitochondrial pyridine nucleotide reduction increases as the oxygen pressure decreases. These metabolic changes affect the overall metabolic status of the cell, but as long as the $[ATP]/[ADP][P_i]$ ratio is above a certain level, the cell remains viable. When the oxygen pressure is lowered to below the normal tissue levels, the $[ATP]/[ADP][P_i]$ ratio becomes too small to support the normal cellular ATP-consuming reactions. At this point the rate of ATP utilization, and therefore the rate of respiration, falls. A significant decrease in respiratory rate is the signal that the cell is no longer capable of continuing normal function, and damage, or at least modification of cellular function, results. The extent and nature of the damage are dependent on the extent of hypoxia, cell type, and other considerations.

Brain cells are normally exposed to oxygen pressures lower than those required to saturate the mitochondrial respiratory chain. This condition may be an important aspect of the mechanism(s) by which the local oxygen supply in brain tissue is regulated. It couples a direct and metabolically important response to changes in local oxygen pressure. This metabolic response can readily be translated into information (messengers) which modulates vascular resistance. This role of tissue energy metabolism has been most clearly shown in the heart. In the isolated perfused heart, a direct correlation between the tissue $[ATP]/[ADP][P_i]$ ratio and coronary flow was observed. This correlation was the same whether the increase in coronary flow was induced by increasing the cardiac metabolic rate or by limiting the mitochondrial respiratory capacity by inhibitors of the respiratory chain (Nuutinen *et al.*, 1982, 1983; Figure 9 of the latter reference is reproduced in this review as Figure 3). These data indicate that the tissue energy state is an important factor in determining local blood flow (oxygen delivery) in cardiac tissue. It is not oxygen pressure per se, but the products of oxygen metabolism by mitochondrial oxidative phosphorylation which provide the information used to regulate coronary resistance. The regulation of blood flow in the brain is very different from that in the heart, but some of the basic elements may be similar.

3. RECOVERY OF TISSUE FROM HYPOXIC/ISCHEMIC EPISODES AND THE CAUSE OF IRREVERSIBLE CELL DAMAGE

3.1. Microvascular Insufficiency during Recovery

Reperfusion with well-oxygenated blood, and the attendant reoxygenation of the tissue, is potentially capable of rapidly restoring the cellular metabolic energy supply ($[ATP]/[ADP][P_i]$) as long as the mitochondria remain functional. Restoration of total blood flow does not, however, guarantee reoxygenation of all regions of the brain tissue. In models of temporary cerebral ischemia, the recirculation is characterized by initial hyperemia, followed by a period of hypoperfusion (Marcy and Welsh, 1984; Kågström *et al.*, 1983*a*, *b*). It is not clear whether the hypoperfusion causes tissue ischemia or is the result of depressed tissue metabolism (Steen *et al.*, 1978; Pulsinelli *et al.*, 1982). Ginsberg *et al.* (1978) measured the effects of 15 and 30 min of carotid artery occlusion plus mild hypotension on the brain of pentobarbital-anesthetized cats. In this model, the reperfusion after 15 min of ischemia was fairly uniform but was depressed to 31 to 35% of control levels. After 30 min of ischemia there were marked heterogeneities in the local cerebral flow, with focal postischemic perfusion abnormalities. Marcy and Welsh (1984) reported that measurements of metabolites, particularly ATP, and H_2 clearance in local regions (0.5 to 1 mg of tissue) were consistent with the conclusion that the period of hypoperfusion following 30 min of ischemic insult is associated with below-normal metabolic rates. Longer ischemic periods (60 min) were, however, associated with significant impairment of recirculation. Kågström *et al.* (1983*a*, *b*) observed, by radiographic methods, local regions of no reflow (1 to 2 mm in diameter or larger) after 15-min periods of ischemia. These areas of no reflow appeared after 10 min and became more extensive at 15 and 30 min, but decreased after longer periods of reperfusion as flow returned to these areas.

The great diversity of the models and methods used makes generalizations difficult. In most of the published work, local flow is defined in terms of the anatomy of the brain and generally refers to regions of 1 mm in diameter or larger. This definition of local applies to rather larger areas than may be appropriate.

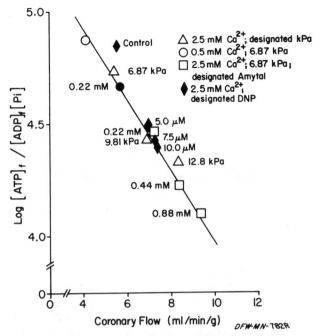

FIGURE 3. Relationship between coronary flow and $[ATP]_f/[ADP]_f[P_i]$ in isolated rat heart perfused under various conditions. The subscript f is used to indicate that the values are for the free cytosolic [ATP]/[ADP] ratio calculated from equilibrium of the creatine phosphokinase reaction. Data obtained from titrations with various levels of the uncoupler 2,4-dinitrophenol were added to the data for perfusion with low Ca^{2+} and various concentrations of Amytal, an inhibitor of the mitochondrial respiratory chain. (From Nuutinen *et al.*, 1983.)

Microoxygen electrode studies by Silver (1976, 1977, 1978) and by Moskalenko (1975) indicate that a sudden increase in cell activity leads to a change in the local PO_2 which is biphasic (decrease then increase) or monophasic (increase only). The fall is compensated within 1.5 to 3 sec by an increase in local blood flow. Most importantly, the changes in local flow did not extend beyond 250 μm from the site of increased activity (Silver, 1978). This observation was confirmed by using thioflavine S as an indicator of vascular perfusion. When this dye was injected into the vascular system during local stimulation, only parts of the endothelium of the capillary bed were stained (Silver, 1978). Since staining was associated with regions of high PO_2 and lack of staining with regions of low PO_2, this suggests that some but not all of the capillaries were perfused. This result is consistent with observations made under pathological conditions such as hypovolemic shock. Under these conditions, where regional or total blood flow can be maintained at low but critical levels, microelectrode measurements indicate the presence of regions of very low PO_2 surrounding regions of unusually high PO_2.

It would be useful to define local flow by the minimal region of vascular control, in this case units of at most a few hundred micrometers. The model for the arteriolar/capillary bed proposed by Silver (1978) and reproduced as Figure 4 may provide a valuable model for understanding the microvascular abnormalities occurring during reperfusion. It appears that the vascular system is particularly susceptible to damage at the level of the capillaries, and analysis on a larger scale may obscure the extent and severity of damage at this level. During the hypoxic episode, the vascular endothelium becomes injured and flow in the microcirculation may be blocked by any of several mechanisms. Macrophages may enter the capillaries and stick, platelets may adhere and aggregate, while extravasation into the extravascular space due to increased vascular permeability and cellular swelling may collapse the vessels by increasing external pressure. It has also been reported that there may be vasospasm, vasoparalysis, and even rupture of microvessels during periods of ischemia (Brandt et al., 1983; Garcia et al., 1983). Disruption of the microvasculature would give rise to areas of ischemia which persist after reperfusion. Initially the areas range from a few to hundreds of micrometers in diameter, but they expand with the severity of the vascular damage. These may be responsible for an early expression of irreversible damage, which appears on histological examination as shrunken cell bodies with triangular, darkly staining cytoplasm and loss of discrete Nissl substance with only widely scattered neurons affected (Tanaka et al., 1986) and development of focal areas of cell death. The reperfusion period immediately after the ischemic episode is probably associated with hypermetabolism as the cells attempt to recover their metabolic energy state and ion balances. In this initial period, the cells which have functional mitochondria try to reestablish their ion balance and at the same time many are hyperactive and therefore hypermetabolic owing to the presence of high concentrations of excitatory neurotransmitters (see below). It could be speculated that the following period of hypometabolism is associated with the death of significant populations of cells combined with loss of normal electrical activity of the cells which survive.

3.2. Role of the Excitatory Neurotransmitters in Recovery from Hypoxia/Ischemia

Modification of neuronal function begins within seconds of the onset of hypoxia, and anoxic depolarization occurs within 2.5 to 3 min (see, for example, Silver [1976, 1977, 1978]). The depolarization results in the release of neurotransmitters from the presynaptic terminals with resulting maximal stimulation of the postsynaptic membranes. These excitatory amino acid neurotransmitters (glutamate, aspartate, and cysteine sulfinate) are normally accumulated in the neurons to concentrations more than 10^4-fold greater than the extraneuronal

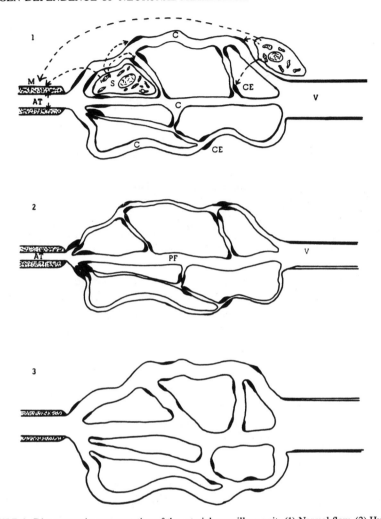

FIGURE 4. Diagrammatic representation of the arteriolar-capillary unit. (1) Normal flow. (2) Hypovolaemia with preferred route (PF) only perfused. (3) Hyperaemia, all vessels perfused. M, smooth muscle; AT, arteriole; S, sensor cell; C, capillary; CE, possible sites of flow controlling cells; PF, preferred route; V, venule. (From Silver, 1978.)

concentrations (> 1 mM versus < 0.1 μM). The transport system responsible is reversible, and the amino acids are cotransported with two Na^+ ions and one H^+ ion to give a net charge of $+2$. The high intraneuronal/extraneuronal concentration ratio is maintained by the combined energy in the Na^+ concentration difference and the membrane potential (see, for example, Erecinska *et al.* [1983] and Wilson and Pastuszko [1986]). Depolarization of the neurons causes the release of large numbers of these amino acids, and these accumulate in the extracellular space to concentrations up to hundreds of times those required for maximal stimulation of the postsynaptic membranes. When reoxygenation occurs, these amino acids must be removed from the extracellular medium, but first the membranes must be repolarized. For most of the time required for reaccumulation, these amino acids not only saturate the postsynaptic receptors but also may enhance calcium permeability by way of receptors on the neuronal cell bodies and presynaptic terminals (see Olney [1978] and Watkins and Evans [1981]). If, after a period of hypoxia, cells are exposed to limited quantities of oxygen, it is initially used by the mitochondria to accumulate calcium from the cytoplasm. With a full supply of oxygen, the cellular ATP levels rise and the calcium is pumped out of the cell, eventually removing the calcium accumulated by the mitochondria as well. As long as the oxygen supply remains smaller than that necessary to reestablish normally high [ATP]/[ADP][P_i] ratios, the calcium moved from the cytoplasm to the mitochondria is replaced by that leaking in from the extracellular medium. The longer these conditions persist, the higher the mitochondrial calcium levels rise and the worse the mitochondria are damaged. Failure of the energy to reach the levels needed to return the cytoplasmic calcium to physiologically low levels eventually leads to mitochondrial and cellular destruction.

3.3. Oxygen Radicals and Their Potential Role in Exacerbating Hypoxic/Ischemic Damage

The recovery is further jeopardized by oxygen itself because it results in, among other things, peroxidation of the unsaturated fatty acids released by lipase activity during the hypoxic episode. During hypoxic and ischemic insult there is substantial breakdown of the cellular lipids, resulting in elevated levels of free fatty acids (Bazan, 1970; Aveldano de Caldironi and Bazan, 1975; Marion and Wolfe, 1979; Abe *et al.*, 1987). The phospholipids of brain membranes are highly enriched in the unsaturated fatty acids arachidonate (20:4), adrenate (22:4), and docosohexanoate (22:6). Deacylation of the phospholipids by activated phospholipases A$_2$ and C (Edgar *et al.*, 1982; Wei *et al.*, 1982) gives rise to free fatty acids (arachidonate being the main component) in concentrations several orders of magnitude higher than the trace levels (< 0.01 µmol/g [wet weight]) found in normal brain (Horrocks, 1985). When the tissue oxygen pressure increases again as a result of reperfusion, there is a transient period during which the free fatty acids are exposed to oxygen pressures which may even exceed those normally found in tissue (Silver, 1978; Siesjö, 1981). The unsaturated free fatty acids are readily oxidized to hydroperoxides both directly by oxygen and by lipoxygenases, and this has been implicated in injury to the brain tissue (see, for example, Yoshida *et al.* [1980] and Watson *et al.* [1984]). Recently, evidence has been obtained that the lipid peroxides of unsaturated fatty acids are potent inhibitors of the reacylation process necessary for repair of lipid degradation which occurs during hypoxia (Zaleska and Wilson, 1989).

4. GENERAL OBSERVATIONS ON HYPOXIC/ISCHEMIC EPISODES AND RECOVERY

Although the processes involved in cellular degradation during periods of hypoxia/ischemia can be described qualitatively, the quantitative relationships are extremely variable, being dependent on the nature of the hypoxic/ischemic insult, cell type, and many other circumstances. The cause of the damage is the lack of oxygen during the hypoxic/ischemic period, and it is the effect on synaptic junctions of neurons which may be least likely to be reversible. When the hypoxic/ischemic episode is not too severe, the irreversible component of the damage may be due in large part to failure of the microvasculatures, resulting in local regions of persistent hypoxia. The extent of the vascular damage is exacerbated by high levels of excitatory amino acid neurotransmitters and damage to the membranes and to their capacity for repair induced by oxygen radicals.

ACKNOWLEDGMENTS

This work was supported by U.S. Public Health Service grants GM-21524 and NS-10939. The author is indebted to Dr. Anna Pastuszko and Dr. William L. Rumsey for their helpful comments and criticisms of the manuscript during its preparation.

REFERENCES

Abe, K., Kogure, K., Yamamoto, H., Imazawa, M., and Miyamoto, K., 1987, Mechanism of arachidonic acid liberation during ischemia in gerbil brain, *J. Neurochem.* **48**:503–509.

Aveldano de Caldironi, M., and Bazan, N. G., 1975, Rapid production of diacylglycerols enriched in arachidonate and stearate during early brain ischemia, *J. Neurochem.* **25**:919–920.

Bazan, N. G., 1970, Effects of ischemia and electroconvulsive shock on free fatty acid pool in the brain, *Biochim. Biophys. Acta.* **218**:1–10.

Bazan, N. G., and Rodriguez de Turco, E. B., 1980, Membrane lipids in the pathogenesis of brain edema: Phospholipids and arachidonic acid, the earliest membrane components changed at the onset of ischemia, *Adv. Neurol.* **28**:197–205.

Brandt, L., Ljunggren, B., Anderson, K. A., Edvinsson, L., MacKenzie, E., Tamura, A., and Teasdale, G., 1983, Effects of topical application of a calcium antagonist (nifedipine) on feline cortical pial microvascular diameter under normal conditions and in focal ischemia, *J. Cereb. Blood Flow Metab.* **3**:44–50.

Clark, A., Jr., and Clark, P. A. A., 1985, Local oxygen gradients near isolated mitochondria, *Biophys. J.* **48**:931–938.

Clark, A., Jr., Clark, P. A. A., Connett, R. J., Gayeski, T. E. J., and Honig, C. R., 1987, How large is the drop in P_{O_2} between cytosol and mitochondrion? *Am. J. Physiol.* **252:**C583–C587.

Degn, H., and Wohlrab, H., 1971, Measurement of steady-state values of respiratory rate and oxidation levels of respiratory pigments at low oxygen tensions: A new technique, *Biochim. Biophys. Acta* **245:**347–355.

Edgar, A. D., Strosznajder, J., and Sun, G. Y., 1982, Activation of ethanolamine phospholipase A_2 in brain during ischemia, *J. Neurochem.* **39:**1111–1116.

Erecinska, M., Wantorski, D., and Wilson, D. F., 1983, Aspartate transport in synaptosomes from rat brain, *J. Biol. Chem.* **258:**9067–9077.

Garcia, J. H., Lowry, S. L., and Briggs, L., 1983, Brain capillaries expand and rupture in areas of ischemia and reperfusion, *in* Cerebrovascular Diseases. Thirteenth Research (Princeton) Conference (M. Reivich and H. I. Hurtig, eds.), pp. 169–179, Raven Press, New York.

Gayeski, T. E., and Honig, C. R., 1986, O_2 gradients from the sarcolemma to cell interior in red muscle at maximal V_{O_2}, *Am. J. Physiol.* **251:**H789–H799.

Ginsberg, M. D., Budd, W. W., and Welsh, F., 1978, Diffuse cerebral ischemia in the cat. 1. Local blood flow during severe ischemia and recirculation, *Ann. Neurol.* **3:**482–492.

Horrocks, L. A., 1985, Metabolism and function of fatty acids in brain, *in* "Phospholipids in Nervous Tissue" (J. Eichberg, ed.), pp. 173–199, John Wiley & Sons, New York.

Jones, D. P., 1984, Effect of mitochondrial clustering on O_2 supply in hepatocytes, *Am. J. Physiol.* **247:**C83–C89.

Jones, D. P., 1986, Intracellular diffusion gradients of O_2 and ATP, *Am. J. Physiol.* **250:**C663–C675.

Jones, D. P., and Kennedy, F. G., 1982, Intracellular oxygen supply during hypoxia, *Am. J. Physiol.* **243:**C247–C253.

Kågström, E., Smith, M.-L., and Siesjö, B. K., 1983a, Local cerebral blood flow in the recovery period following complete cerebral ischemia in the rat, *J. Cereb. Blood Flow Metab.* **3:**170–182.

Kågström, E., Smith, M.-L., and Siesjö, B. K., 1983b, Recirculation in the rat brain following incomplete ischemia, *J. Cereb. Blood Flow Metab.* **3:**183–192.

Katz, I. R., Wittenberg, J. B., and Wittenberg, B. A., 1984, Monoamine oxidase, an intracellular probe of oxygen pressure in isolated cardiac myocytes, *J. Biol. Chem.* **259:**7504–7509.

Marcy, V. R., and Welsh, F. A., 1984, Correlation between cerebral blood flow and ATP content following tourniquet-induced ischemia in cat brain, *J. Cereb. Blood Flow Metab.* **4:**362–367.

Marion, J., and Wolfe, L. S., 1979, Origin of arachidonic acid release post mortem in the rat forebrain, *Biochim. Biophys. Acta* **547:**25–32.

Meyers, R. E., and Yamaguchi, S., 1977, Nervous system effects of cardiac arrest in monkeys, *Arch. Neurol.* **34:**65–74.

Moskalenko, Y. Y., 1975, Regional cerebral blood flow and its control at rest and during increased functional activity, *in* "Brain Work" (D. H. Ingvar and H. A. Lassen, eds.), pp. 133–141, Munskgaard, Copenhagen, Denmark.

Nuutinen, E. M., Nishiki, K., Erecinska, M., and Wilson, D. F., 1982, Role of mitochondrial oxidative phosphorylation in regulation of coronary blood flow, *Am. J. Physiol.* **243:**H157–H169.

Nuutinen, E. M., Nelson, D., Wilson, D. F., and Erecinska, M., 1983, Regulation of coronary blood flow: Effects of 2,4-dinitrophenol and theophylline, *Am. J. Physiol.* **244:**H396–H405.

Olney, J. W., 1978, Neurotoxicity of excitatory amino acids, *in* "Kainic Acid as a Tool in Neurobiology" (R. G. McGeer, J. W. Olney, and P. L. McGeer, eds.), pp. 95–121, Raven Press, New York.

Oshino, N., Sugano, T., Oshino, R., and Chance, B., 1974, Mitochondrial function under hypoxic conditions: The steady states of cytochromes a + a_3 and their relation to mitochondrial energy states, *Biochim. Biophys. Acta* **368:**298–310.

Petersen, L. C., Nicholls, P., and Degn, H., 1974, The effect of energization on the apparent Michaelis-Menten constant for oxygen in mitochondrial respiration, *Biochem. J.* **142:**249–252.

Pulsinelli, W. A., Waldman, S., Rawlinson, D., and Plum, F., 1982, Moderate hyperglycemia augments ischemic brain damage: A neuropathological study in the rat, *Neurology* **32**:1239–1246.

Rehncrona, S., Rosen, I., and Siesjö, B. K., 1981, Brain lactic acidosis and ischemic cell damage. 1. Biochemistry and neurophysiology, *J. Cereb. Blood Flow Metab.* **1**:297–311.

Robiolio, M., Rumsey, W. L., and Wilson, D. F., 1989, Oxygen diffusion and mitochondrial respiration in neuroblastoma cells, *Amer. J. Physiol.* **256**:C1207–C1213.

Siesjö, B. K., 1981, Cell damage in the brain: A speculative synthesis, *J. Cereb. Blood Flow Metab.* **1**: 155–185.

Silver, I. A., 1976, Tissue response to hypoxia, stroke and shock, *Adv. Exp. Med. Biol.* **75**:325–334.

Silver, I. A., 1977, Ion fluxes in hypoxic tissues, *Microvasc. Res.* **13**:409–420.

Silver, I. A., 1978, Cellular microenvironment in relation to local blood flow, *Ciba Found. Symp.* **56**: 49–67.

Steen, P. A., Milde, J. H., and Michenfelder, J. D., 1978, Cerebral metabolic and vascular effects of barbituate therapy following complete global ischemia, *J. Neurochem.* **31**:1317–1324.

Sugano, T., Oshino, N., and Chance, B., 1974, Mitochondrial functions under hypoxic conditions: The steady states of cytochrome c reduction and of energy metabolism, *Biochim. Biophys. Acta* **347**: 340–358.

Tanaka, K., Dora, E., Greenberg, J. H., and Reivich, M., 1986, Cerebral glucose metabolism during the recovery period after ischemia: Its relationship to NADH-fluorescence, blood flow, EcoG and histology, *Stroke* **17**:994–1004.

Watkins, J. C., and Evans, R. H., 1981, Excitatory amino acid transmitters, *Annu. Rev. Pharmacol. Toxicol.* **21**:165–204.

Watson, B. D., Busto, R., Goldberg, W. J., Santiso, S., Yoshida, S., and Ginsberg, M. D., 1984, Lipid peroxidation *in vivo* induced by reversible global ischemia in rat brain, *J. Neurochem* **23**:268–274.

Wei, E. P., Lamb, R. G., and Kontos, H. A., 1982, Increased phospholipase C activity after experimental brain injury, *J. Neurosurg.* **56**:695–698.

Welsh, F. A., Sims, R. E., and McKee, A. E., 1983, Effect of glucose on recovery of energy metabolism following hypoxia-oligemia in mouse brain: Dose-dependent and carbohydrate specificity, *J. Cereb. Blood Flow Metab.* **3** 486–492.

Wilson, D. F., 1982, Regulation of *in vivo* mitochondrial oxidative phosphorylation, *in* "Membranes and Transport, vol. 1" (A. Martonosi, ed.), pp. 349–355, Plenum Press, New York.

Wilson, D. F., and Erecinska, M., 1985, Effect of oxygen concentration on cellular metabolism, *Chest* **88**:229–232.

Wilson, D. F., and Pastuszko, A., 1986, Transport of cysteate by synaptosomes isolated from rat brain: Evidence that it utilizes the same transporter as aspartate, glutamate, and cysteine sulfinate, *J. Neurochem.* **47**:1091–1097.

Wilson, D. F., Erecinska, M., Drown, C., and Silver, I. A., 1979a, The oxygen dependence of cellular energy metabolism, *Arch. Biochem. Biophys.* **195**:485–493.

Wilson, D. F., Owen, C. D., and Erecinska, M., 1979b, Quantitative dependence of mitochondrial oxidative phosphorylation on oxygen concentration: A mathematical model, *Arch. Biochem. Biophys.* **195**:494–504.

Wilson, D. F., Rumsey, W. L., Green, T. J., and Vanderkooi, J. M., 1988, The oxygen dependence of mitochondrial oxidative phosphorylation measured by a new optical method for measuring oxygen concentration, *J. Biol. Chem.* **263**:2712–2718.

Wittenberg, B. A., and Wittenberg, J. B., 1985, Oxygen pressure gradients in isolated cardiac myocytes, *J. Biol. Chem.* **260**:6548–6554.

Yoshida, S., Inoh, S., Asano, T., Sano, K., Shimizaki, H., and Ueta, N., 1980, Effect of transient ischemia on free fatty acid levels and phospholipids in the gerbil brain. Lipid peroxidation as possible cause of post ischemic injury, *J. Neurosurg.* **53**:323–331.

Zaleska, M., and Wilson, D. F., 1989, Lipid hydroperoxides inhibit reacylation of phospholipids in neuronal membranes, *J. Neurochem.* **52**:255–260.

CHAPTER 6

DYSMETABOLISM IN LIPID BRAIN ISCHEMIA

KYUYA KOGURE and SHINICHI NAKANO

1. INTRODUCTION

Brain tissue has a high lipid content, as much as 40 to 65% of its dry weight (Lapentina *et al.*, 1968; O'Brien and Sampson, 1965), with phospholipids as the major structural component of membranes, whose integrity is a prerequisite for normal brain function. Most of the membrane phospholipids are in bilayer form, arranged with their ionic and polar heads in contact with water and with their nonpolar residues in the embedded parts (Singer and Nicolson, 1972). Biological membranes play a crucial role in almost all cellular functions such as energy production, active transport of various ions, and signal transmission or transduction. Considering the pathogenetic mechanism of ischemic cell damage as membrane injury, it is quite reasonable to assume that the alterations in lipid metabolism during and after brain ischemia are closely related to ischemic brain damage.

Recently the biochemical mechanism of ischemic brain damage has been divided into two main processes, (1) hypoxic injury during ischemia and (2) free-

KYUYA KOGURE and SHINICHI NAKANO • Department of Neurology, Institute of Brain Diseases, 1-1 Seiryo-Machi, Aoba-Ku, Sendai, Japan.

Neurochemical Correlates of Cerebral Ischemia, Volume 7 of *Advances in Neurochemistry*, edited by Nicolas G. Bazan, Pierre Braquet, and Myron D. Ginsberg. Plenum Press, New York, 1992.

radical injury after postischemic recirculation (Kogure *et al.*, 1979; Yoshida *et al.*, 1980).

In this article we will give an outline of ischemia-induced alterations in lipid metabolism in line with the two main processes mentioned above and will introduce our new findings on lipid metabolism long after postischemic recirculation.

2. DECOMPOSITION OF MEMBRANE PHOSPHOLIPIDS DURING ISCHEMIA

Accumulation of free fatty acids (FFAs) has been considered for many years to be related to the impairment of mitochondrial oxidative phosphorylation and subsequent brain edema (Hayaishi *et al.*, 1961; Sako *et al.*, 1969). In 1970, Bazan first demonstrated the accumulation of FFAs in the rat brain during postdecapitation ischemia (Bazan, 1970), and brain ischemia is known to induce hydrolytic breakdown of membrane phospholipids through activation of endogenous phospholipases (Abe *et al.*, 1987; Galli and Spagnuolo, 1976; Ikeda *et al.*, 1986; Yaruda *et al.*, 1985; Yoshida *et al.*, 1980). The major constituents of the membrane phospholipid bilayer are phosphatidylethanolamine (PE), and phosphatidylcholine (PC) (Rehncrona *et al.*, 1982). It is quite reasonable to assume that hydrolytic breakdown of these membrane structural phospholipids induced by prolonged ischemia causes membrane dysfunction and finally cell death.

Other experimental studies, however, suggest that cerebral ischemia initially induces a hydrolytic breakdown of membrane functional phospholipids such as inositol phospholipids through activation of phospholipase C, followed by the action of diacylglycerol (DG) and monoacylglycerol (MG) lipases (Bell *et al.*, 1979; Hee-Cheong *et al.*, 1985; Mauco *et al.*, 1978). This hypothesis is substantiated by the following evidence: (1) levels of polyphosphoinositides (PPIs) including triphosphoinositide (TPI) and diphosphoinositide (DPI) began to decrease only 20 to 30 sec after the onset of ischemia (Abe *et al.*, 1987; Ikeda *et al.*, 1986; Yoshida *et al.*, 1986), whereas membrane structural phospholipids such as PE or PC are hardly decomposed even after 15 min of ischemia (Abe *et al.*, 1987) (Figure 1); (2) PPIs are particularly rich in stearic and arachidonic acids (Baker and Thompson, 1972), which are the two major FFAs accumulated during the early period of ischemia (Abe *et al.*, 1987; Bazan, 1970; Ikeda *et al.*, 1986; Yoshida *et al.*, 1985) (Figure 2); and (3) the levels of 1,2-DG enriched in stearic and arachidonic acids increase during ischemia (Abe *et al.*, 1987; Ikeda *et al.*, 1986).

Considering that the metabolism of inositol phospholipids essentially plays a key role in signal transduction as well as cyclic AMP metabolism (Brown *et al.*, 1984), the breakdown of inositol phospholipids during the early period of ischemia

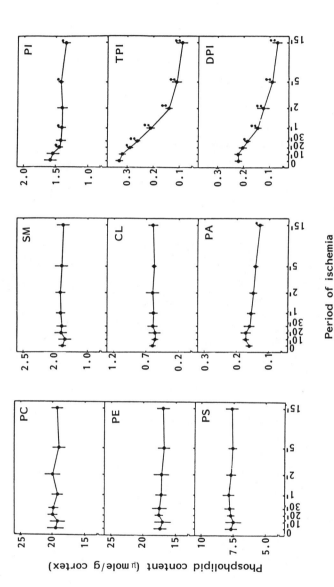

Period of ischemia

FIGURE 1. Changes in the amount of phospholipids during ischemia in gerbil frontoparietal cerebral cortices. The amounts of PC, PE, PS, SM, and CL do not change significantly throughout 15 min of ischemia. However, the amounts of inositol phospholipids begin to decrease significantly as early as 20 or 30 sec after the onset of ischemia (*$P < 0.05$, **$P < 0.01$, compared with a sham control). Abbreviations: PC, phosphatidylcholine; PE, phosphatidylethanolamine; PS, phosphatidylserine; SM, sphingo-myelin; CL, cardiolipin (diphosphatidylglycerol); PA, phosphatidic acid; PI, phosphatidylinositol; TPI, triphosphoinositide; DPI, diphosphoinositide.

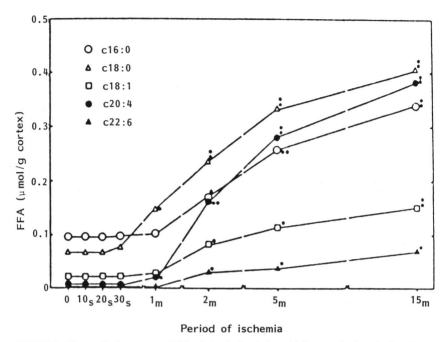

FIGURE 2. Changes in the contents of FFAs during ischemia in gerbil frontoparietal cerebral cortices. Stearic ($C_{18:0}$) and arachidonic ($C_{20:4}$) acids are the two major FFAs liberated during the early period of ischemia, and their liberation starts as early as 0.5 to 1 min after the onset of ischemia. The liberation of other FFAs also starts about 2 min after the onset of ischemia (*$P < 0.05$, **$P < 0.01$, compared with a sham control).

can be considered to be the result of the activation of the physiological signal-transducing systems.

2.1. Decomposition of Membrane Functional Phospholipids during the Early Period of Ischemia

It is well known that the primary effect induced by ischemia is the inhibition of mitochondrial function and inhibition of energy production, causing the rapid depletion of ATP (Astrup, 1982; Hansen 1985; Shaller *et al.*, 1980). The immediate effect of the lack of high-energy phosphate compounds is the inhibition of the ion-pumping ATPases, with the subsequent breakdown of transmembranous ionic gradients (Mela, 1979; Shaller *et al.*, 1980). Most notable is the inhibition of the Na,K-ATPase, which allows intracellular potassium ions to leak into the extracellular space and permits sodium and chloride ions to accumulate intracellularly.

This subsequently produces membrane depolarization, which induces transmembranous Ca^{2+} influx through activation of voltage-dependent Ca^{2+} channels (Meyer, 1989). Intracellular Ca^{2+} accumulation in the presynaptic neurons causes a nonspecific, nonphysiological release of neurotransmitters from the presynaptic terminals (Calderini *et al.*, 1978), which in turn facilitates receptor-mediated hydrolysis of inositol phospholipids through activation of phospholipase C. The immediate target is TPI located in the inner leaflet of the plasma membrane, even though this phospholipid is a very minor component of membranes (Nishizuka, 1984). As a consequence of this hydrolysis, TPI is cleaved into 1,2,-DG and inositol 1,4,5-triphosphate (IP_3), which serve as two independent second messengers (Berridge and Irvine, 1984; Nishizuka, 1984). IP_3 increases the intracellular Ca^{2+} concentration by releasing Ca^{2+} from the intracellular Ca^{2+} store, and a part of IP_3 is converted by IP_3 kinase to IP_4, which potentiates transmembranous Ca^{2+} influx from the extracellular space (Berridge and Irvine, 1984). The endoplasmic reticulum appears to be the major source of Ca^{2+} released by IP_3, perhaps through stimulation of the Ca^{2+}-ATPase or by opening of intracellular Ca^{2+} channels (Choquette *et al.*, 1984). On the other hand, 1,2-DG activates protein kinase C, which is a Ca^{2+}- and phosphatidylserine (PS)-dependent enzyme, to stimulate protein phosphorylation (Nishizuka, 1984). Under physiological conditions, both IP_3 and 1,2-DG are used in the resynthesis of inositol phospholipids (Figure 3). In the ischemic brain, however, neither protein phosphorylation nor reuse of 1,2-DG takes place, owing to the lack of ATP, and 1,2-DG is decomposed by DG and MG lipases, resulting in the liberation of FFAs (for the most part, stearic and arachidonic acids). These FFAs accumulated during ischemia can subsequently be the source of free radicals and can contribute to cell injury during postischemic recirculation.

2.2. Decomposition of Membrane Structural Phospholipids during the Later Period of Ischemia

In the postsynaptic neurons, in addition to voltage-dependent Ca^{2+} channel opening, receptor-operated Ca^{2+} channels are opened by some neurotransmitters such as glutamate and aspartate; this facilitates a marked increase in the cytosolic Ca^{2+} concentration combined with the Ca^{2+} mobilization by IP_3 and IP_4 described above (Meyer, 1989). This increase in the cytosolic Ca^{2+} concentration induces nonspecific activation of phospholipase A_2 and other phospholipases, which subsequently facilitates decomposition of membrane structural phospholipids such as PC and PE. Since PC and PE are rich in palmitic and docosahexaenoic acids, respectively (Marion and Wolfe, 1979; Rehncrona *et al.*, 1982), an increase in the concentration of these two FFAs indicates the decomposition of these membrane structural phospholipids. Although short periods of ischemia (less than 15 min) do not cause a significant decrease in the amount of membrane structural

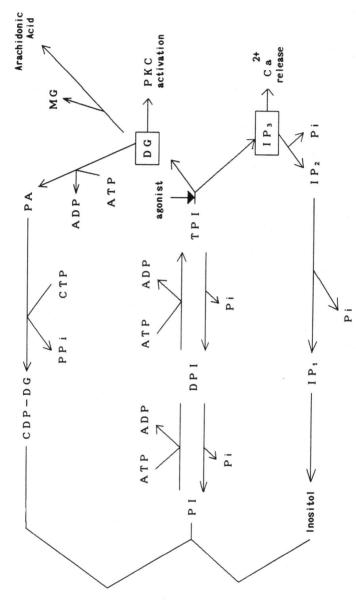

FIGURE 3. Inositol phospholipid metabolism and signal transduction. PI, phosphatidylinositol; DPI, diphosphoinositide; TPI, triphosphoinositide; DG, diacylglycerol; MG, monoacylglycerol; PA, phosphatidic acid; CDP-DG, CDP-diacylglycerol; IP$_3$, inositol triphosphate; IP$_2$, inositol diphosphate; IP$_1$, inositol phosphate.

phospholipids (Abe *et al.*, 1987) (Figure 1), the liberation of palmitic and docosahexaenoic acids, which indicates the decomposition of PC and PE, respectively, starts 2 to 3 min after the onset of ischemia (Abe *et al.*, 1987) (Figure 2). On the other hand, there have been reports that prolonged ischemia (as long as 30 min) decomposes 16% of membrane PE (Yoshida *et al.*, 1980) and that 37% of free arachidonic acid accumulated during 30 min of ischemia is released from membrane PC (Marion and Wolfe, 1979). The disruption of Ca^{2+} homeostasis induced by prolonged ischemia causes nonspecific activation of various lipases and proteases, which subsequently causes cell autolysis.

3. LIPID PEROXIDATION DURING POSTISCHEMIC RECIRCULATION

There are four possible pathways which cause a decrease in FFA levels: (1) vascular washout and diffusion into cerebrospinal fluid, (2) reacylation to form phospholipids, (3) β-oxidation as a substrate for energy production, and (4) peroxidation of free arachidonic acid (Yoshida *et al.*, 1980). Since the conversion of FFAs into acyl coenzyme A (acyl-CoA), an initial step required both for the resynthesis of phospholipids and B-oxidation processes, is an ATP-dependent reaction and since the enzymatic peroxidation of free arachidonic acid into prostaglandins or leukotrienes is an oxygen-dependent pathway, it is unlikely that all four pathways described above take place actively during ischemia. Therefore, the FFAs liberated during ischemia have to accumulate until the onset of postischemic recirculation.

It is well known that the increased FFA levels during ischemia return rapidly to the control level; this is assumed to be mainly due to vascular washout and diffusion into cerebrospinal fluid (Yoshida *et al.*, 1980). However, the level of free arachidonic acid decreases about three times faster than do the levels of other FFAs. This accelerated decline may be the result of arachidonic acid metabolism via the cyclooxygenase or lipoxygenase pathway. In fact, levels of eicosanoids, products of enzymatically peroxidized arachidonic acid, have been shown to increase markedly during the postischemic recirculation (Gaudet and Levine, 1979, 1980; Gaudet *et al.*, 1980; Kempski *et al.*, 1987). Eicosanoids are considered to contribute to the ischemic brain damage through regulation of cerebral blood flow, vascular permeability, and modulation of excitatory or inhibitory transmitter effects.

Under conditions in which high-energy phosphates are available, free arachidonic acid becomes readily incorporated into triacylglycerol-acyl residues at position 1 or 3, particularly in a synaptosomal fraction (MacDonald *et al.*, 1975; Sun and Foudin, 1984). This reacylation may also contribute to the selectively rapid disappearance of free arachidonic acid during the early period of postischemic recirculation (Yoshida *et al.*, 1980, 1983, 1986). On the other hand, nonenzymatic peroxidative processes are also operating in the decomposition of phospholipids. Flamm *et al.* (1978, 1979) and Demopoulos *et al.* (1977) have provided evidence of peroxidative damage to membrane lipids during cerebral ischemia. They postulated that peroxidative degradation of biomembranes was initiated by uncontrolled mitochondrial electron transport radicals derived from sudden oxygen deprivation at the terminus of the respiratory chain. Since then, however, many investigators have demonstrated that loss of oxygen as a result of ischemia alone cannot initiate peroxidative processes, which require restoration of oxygen supply (Folbergrova *et al.*, 1979; Kogure *et al.*, 1979). Peroxy radicals of free arachidonic acid are potent oxidants and are capable of abstracting hydrogen atoms at the α-methylene carbon position in polyunsaturated fatty acids to be transformed into less active hydroperoxyarachidonic acid. The resultant lipid alkyl radicals, together with resupplied oxygen molecules, could easily initiate and propagate the peroxidative chain reactions in the membrane matrix (Mead, 1976). It seems reasonable, therefore, to speculate that the peroxidative processes of nonesterified arachidonic acid may be closely linked to further catabolism and alterations of membrane lipids during the early period of postischemic recirculation. The further increase of all FFA levels except for free arachidonic acid during the early period of postischemic recirculation may be the result of these nonenzymatic peroxidative processes (Nakano *et al.*, 1990) (Figure 4). It is likely that the enzymatic and nonenzymatic peroxidation of polyunsaturated FFAs accounts, at least in part, for the ischemic brain damage.

4. ISCHEMIA-INDUCED ALTERATIONS IN LIPID METABOLISM LONG AFTER POSTISCHEMIC RECIRCULATION

4.1. Delayed Increase in FFA Levels

It is well known that FFA levels are increased and PPI levels are decreased during 15 to 45 min of ischemia and return to control levels within a few hours of postischemic recirculation, along with the recovery of high-energy phosphate (Yoshida *et al.*, 1986). In the gerbil model of a transient 5-min bilateral carotid artery occlusion, decreased PPI levels in the cerebral cortices return to control levels within only 30 min of postischemic recirculation (Abe *et al.*, 1989) (Figure 5). In the same experimental model, morphological brain damage is not observed in the cerebral cortices (Crain *et al.*, 1988). From these experimental data, it was concluded that impaired lipid metabolism during ischemia recovers rapidly along with the recovery of the high-energy phosphates.

Our recent experiments with the same model, however, disclosed that the FFA levels that had transiently returned to control levels began to increase again

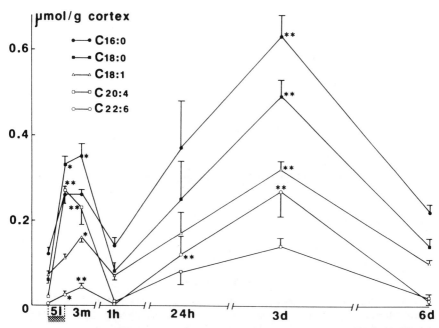

FIGURE 4. Time course of changes in the FFA levels accumulated during 5 min of ischemia (5i) and after various recirculation times. The FFA levels increase during ischemia and the early period of postischemic recirculation and return to control levels in 1 h. However, they increase again a few days after the onset of recirculation. Thereafter, the increased FFA levels return to the control levels after 6 days of recirculation (*P < 0.05, **P < 0.01, compared with a sham control).

after 24 h of recirculation and that the delayed increase in all FFA levels was clearly observed after 3 days of recirculation (Nakano *et al.*, 1990) (Figure 4). Taking the vascular washout and reacylation mechanism into consideration, the amount of liberated FFAs seemed to be quite considerable. Furthermore, the increased levels of FFAs contained large amounts of palmitic, oleic, and docosahexaenoic acids, suggesting that the main source of these liberated FFAs would be the membrane structural phospholipids other than inositol phospholipids. Considering the fatty acid composition of inositol phospholipids, they are only minor sources of free palmitic acid and their contribution to the production of free oleic acid is negligible. PC and PE may be decomposed by the combined action of phospholipase A_2 and lysophospholipase (Edgar *et al.*, 1982; Sun and Foudin, 1984). To our surprise, despite the liberation of such large amounts of FFAs, PPI was maintained at control levels (Abe *et al.*, 1989) (Figure 5). If this delayed increase in the FFA levels reflects the process of cell death or the result of epileptic seizure, PPI cannot be maintained at the control level. Since the cellular and subcellular

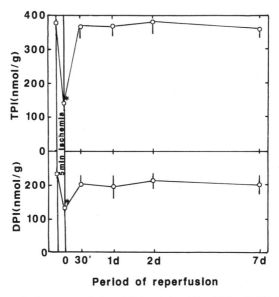

FIGURE 5. Changes in the amount of tri- and diphosphoinositides (TPI and DPI) during and after 5 min of ischemia in the parietal cortex. Both TPI and DPI levels return to the control levels within 30 min after the onset of recirculation (*$P < 0.01$, compared with a sham control).

origin of liberated FFAs in this period is not clear, the significance of the delayed increase in FFA levels remains unknown.

4.2. Postischemic Membrane Perturbation

As shown in Figure 4, the FFA levels that had shown a delayed increase returned to control levels 6 days after the onset of recirculation, suggesting that the perturbed lipid metabolism finally returns to normal conditions during this period. Of interest, however, is that the response of FFA liberation to the second 5-min period of ischemia in this postischemic recirculation period is quite different from that in the initial 5-min period of ischemia. In the second 5-min period of ischemia, the total amount of liberated FFAs was two or three times larger than the amount in the initial 5-min period, and their composition suggests that not only inositol phospholipids but also other membrane structural phospholipids are decomposed from the earlier period of ischemia (Figure 6; Table 1). Considering that the liberation of FFAs by ischemia is the result of receptor activation and subsequent increase in cytosolic Ca^{2+} concentration, this large response to the second period of ischemia probably reflects some alteration in membrane reactivity such as Ca^{2+} conductance or receptor sensitivity. It is likely that post-

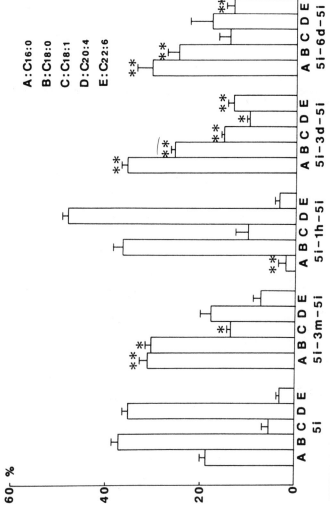

FIGURE 6. Changes in composition of the FFAs liberated during the initial or the second 5-min period of ischemia following various recirculation intervals (for durations, see Fig. 4). The response of FFA liberation to the second period of ischemia are quite different from that to the initial period ($*P < 0.05$, $**P < 0.01$, compared with a group undergoing a single 5-min period of ischemia).

TABLE 1. Changes in the Amount of FFAs Liberated During the Initial or the Second 5-Min Period of Ischemia Following at Various Recirculation Intervals

FFA	Concentration (nmol/g wet wt) of FFA after[a]				
	5i (n = 5)	5i-3m-5i (n = 8)	5i-1h-5i (n = 6)	5i-3d-5i (n = 6)	5i-6d-5i (n = 6)
Total	0.71 ± 0.05	1.79 ± 0.21	0.40 ± 0.03	10.78 ± 1.22**	1.89 ± 0.28
$C_{16:0}$	0.14 ± 0.02	0.56 ± 0.08	0.01 ± 0.01	3.80 ± 0.37**	0.60 ± 0.12
$C_{18:0}$	0.27 ± 0.02	0.54 ± 0.06	0.14 ± 0.02	2.78 ± 0.35**	0.48 ± 0.09
$C_{18:1}$	0.04 ± 0.01	0.25 ± 0.04	0.04 ± 0.01	1.65 ± 0.19**	0.26 ± 0.04
$C_{20:4}$	0.25 ± 0.01	0.30 ± 0.03	0.21 ± 0.02	1.06 ± 0.14*	0.31 ± 0.06
$C_{22:6}$	0.02 ± 0.00	0.14 ± 0.04	0.01 ± 0.00	1.50 ± 0.25**	0.26 ± 0.06

[a]Each FFA concentration was calculated by subtracting the prior mean accumulated FFA concentration from the individual FFA concentration at the end of the respective 5-min period of ischemia. The changes in FFA concentrations at the end of the single 5-min period of ischmia served as a control (*$P < 0.05$, **$P < 0.01$).
[b]Abbreviations: 5i, 5-min period of ischemia; 3m, 3 min; 1h, 1 hr; 3d and 6d, 3 and 6 days, respectively.

ischemic membrane perturbation may not recover even in such a later period of postischemic recirculation.

5. CONCLUSION

It is well known that the cellular response to many neurotransmitters is regulated by changes in the number of receptor sites and the conformation of membrane-bound enzymes. Membrane fluidity, which is closely related to the regulation of the number of receptor sites or the conformation of membrane-bound enzymes, is regulated by alteration in the membrane fatty acid composition. Since genetic, nutritional, and temperature manipulation has been found to alter membrane fluidity (Hiraka and Axelrod, 1978; Seiler and Hasselbach, 1971), it is quite reasonable to speculate that transient ischemia also alters membrane fluidity by changing the composition of membrane fatty acids. Is it a bold working hypothesis that the delayed increase in FFA levels in our experiment may reflect a process of alteration of membrane fluidity? Further investigations are needed to clarify the significance of these preliminary but provocative results.

REFERENCES

Abe, K., Kogure, K., Yamamoto, H., et al., 1987, Mechanism of arachidonic acid liberation during ischemia in gerbil cerebral cortex, *J. Neurochem.* **48:**503–509.

Abe, K., Yoshidomi, M., and Kogure, K., 1989, Arachidonic acid metabolism in ischemic neuronal damage, *Ann. N.Y. Acad. Sci.* **559:**259–268.

Astrup, J., 1982, Energy-requiring cell functions in the ischemic brain, *J. Neurosurg.* **56:**482–497.

Baker, R. R., and Thompson, W., 1972, Positional distribution and turnover of fatty acids in phosphatidic acid, phosphoinositides, phosphatidylcholine and phosphatidylethanolamine in rat brain in vivo, *Biochim. Biophys. Acta* **270**:489–503.

Bazan, N. G., 1970, Effects of ischemia nd electroconvulsive shock on free fatty acid pool in the brain, *Biochim. Biophys. Acta* **218**:1–10.

Bell, R. L., Kennerly, D. A., Stanford, N., et al., 1979, Digylceride lipase: A pathway for arachidonate release from human platelets, *Proc. Natl. Acad. Sci. USA* **76**:3238–3241.

Berridge, M. J., and Irvine, R. F., 1984, Inositol triphosphate, a novel second messenger in cellular signal transduction, *Nature* **312**:315–321.

Brown, E., Kendall, D. A., and Nahorski, S. R., 1984, Inositol phospholipid hydrolysis in rat cerebral cortical slices. I. Receptor characterization, *J. Neurochem.* **42**:1379–1387.

Calderini, G., Carlsson, A., and Nordstrom, C. H., 1978, Influence of transient ischemia on monoamine metabolism in the rat brain during nitrous oxide and phenobarbitone anaesthesia, *Brain Res.* **157**:303–310.

Choquette, D., Hakim, G., Filotep, A. G., et al., 1984, Regulation of plasma membrane Ca^{2+} ATPase by lipids of the phosphatidylinositol cycle, *Biochem. Biophys. Res. Commun.* **125**:908–915.

Crain, B. J., Westerkam, W. D., Harrison, A. H., et al., 1988, Selective neuronal death after transient forebrain ischemia in the Mongolian gerbil: A silver impregnation study, *Neuroscience* **27**:387–402.

Demopoulos, H. B., Flamm, E. S., Seligman, M. L., et al., 1977, Molecular pathology of lipids in CNS membranes, in "Oxygen and Physiological Function" (F. F. Jobsis, ed.), pp. 491–508, Professional Information Library, Dallas.

Edgar, A. D. Strosznajder, J., and Horrocks, L. A., 1982, Activation of ethanolamine phospholipase A_2 in brain during ischemia, *J. Neurochem.* **39**:1111–1116.

Flamm, E. S., Demopoulos, H. B., Seligman, M. L., et al., 1978, Free radicals in cerebral ischemia, *Stroke* **9**:445–447.

Flamm, E. S., Demopoulos, H. B., Seligman, M. L., et al., 1979, Barbiturates and free radicals, in "Neural Trauma" (A. J. Popp, R. S. Bourke, L. R. Nelson, et al., eds.), pp. 289–296, Raven Press, New York.

Folbergrova, J., Rehncrona, S., and Siesjö, B. K., 1979, Oxidized and reduced glutathione in the rat brain under normoxic and hypoxic conditions, *J. Neurochem.* **32**:1621–1627.

Galli, C., and Spagnuolo, C., 1976, The release of brain free fatty acids during ischemia in essential fatty acid-deficient rats, *J. Neurochem.* **26**:401–404.

Gaudet, R. J., and Levine, L., 1979, Transient cerebral ischemia and brain prostaglandins, *Biochem. Biophys. Res. Commun.* **86**:893–901.

Gaudet, R. J., and Levine, L., 1980, Effect of unilateral common carotid artery occlusion on levels of prostaglandin D_2, F_{2a} and 6-keto PGF_{1a} in gerbil brain, *Stroke* **11**:648–652.

Gaudet, R. J., Alam, I., and Levine, L., 1980, Accumulation of cyclooxygenase products of arachidonic acid metabolism in gerbil brain during reperfusion after bilateral common carotid artery occlusion, *J. Neurochem.* **35**:653–658.

Hansen, A. J., 1985, Effect of anoxia on ion distribution in the brain, *Physiol. Rev.* **65**:101–148.

Hayaisha, O., Ozawa, K., Araki, C., et al., 1961, Biochemistry of brain injury and brain edema (in Japanese), *Jpn. J. Med. Prog.* **48**:519–539.

Hee-Cheong, M., Fletcher, T., Kryski, S. K., et al., 1985, Diacylglycerol lipase and kinase activities in rat brain microvessels, *Biochim. Biophys. Acta* **833**:59–68.

Hirata, F., and Axelrod, J., 1978, Enzymatic methylation of phosphatidylethanolamine increases erythrocyte membrane fluidity, *Nature* **275**:219–220.

Ikeda, M., Yoshida, S., Busto, R., et al., 1986, Polyphosphoinositides as a probable source of brain free fatty acids accumulated at the onset of ischemia, *J. Neurochem.* **47**:123–132.

Kempski, O., Shohami, E., von Lubitz, D., et al., 1987, Postischemic production of eicosanoids in gerbil brain, *Stroke* **18**:111–119.

Kogure, K., Morooka, H., Busto, R., et al., 1979, Involvement of lipid peroxidation in postischemic brain damage, *Neurology* **29**:546.

Lapentina, E. G., Soto, E. F., and DeRobertis, E., 1968, Lipids and proteolipids in isolated subcellular membranes of rat brain cortex, *J. Neurochem.* **15**:437–445.

MacDonald, G., Baker, R. R., and Thompson, W., 1975, Selective synthesis of molecular classes of phosphatidic acid, diacylglycerol and phosphatidylinositol in rat brain, *J. Neurochem.* **24**: 655–661.

Marion, J., and Wolfe, L. S., 1979, Origin of the arachidonic acid released post-mortem in rat forebrain, *Biochim. Biophys. Acta* **574**:25–32.

Mauco, G., Chap, H., Simon, M. F., et al., 1978, Phosphatidic acid and lysophosphatidic acid production in phospholipase C and thrombin-treated platelets. Possible involvement of a platelet lipase, *Biochimie* **60**:653–661.

Mead, J. F., 1976, Free radical mechanisms of lipid damage and consequences for cellular membranes, *in* "Free Radicals in Biology," vol. 1 (W. A. Pryor, ed.), pp. 51–68, Academic Press, New York.

Mela, L., 1979, Mitochondrial function in cerebral ischemia and hypoxia: Comparison of inhibitory and adaptive responses, *Neurol. Res.* **1**:51–63.

Meyer, F. B., 1989, Calcium, neuronal hyperexcitability and ischemic injury, *Brain Res. Rev.* **14**: 227–243.

Nakano, S., Kogure, K., Abe, K., et al., 1990, Ischemia-induced alterations in lipid metabolism of the gerbil cerebral cortex. I. Changes in free fatty acid liberation, *J. Neurochem.* **54**:1911–1916.

Nishizuka, Y., 1984, The role of protein kinase C in cell surface signal transduction and tumor promotion, *Nature* **308**:693–698.

O'Brien, J. S., and Sampson, E. L., 1965, Lipid composition of the normal brain: Gray matter, white matter and myelin, *J. Lipid Res.* **6**:537–544.

Rehncrona, S., Westerberg, E., Akesson, B., et al., 1982, Brain cortical fatty acids and phospholipids during and following complete and severe incomplete ischemia, *J. Neurochem.* **38**:84–93.

Sato, K., Yamaguchi, M., Mullan, S., et al., 1969, Brain edema: A study of biochemical and structural alterations, *Arch. Neurol.* **21**:413–424.

Seiler, D., and Hasselbach, W., 1971, Essential fatty acid deficiency and the activity of the sarcoplasmic calcium pump, *Eur. J. Biochem.* **21**:385–387.

Shaller, C. A., Jacques, S., and Shelden, H., 1980, The pathophysiology of stroke: A review with molecular considerations, *Surg. Neurol.* **14**:433–443.

Singer, S. J., and Nicolson, G. L., 1972, The fluid mosaic model of the structure of cell membranes, *Science* **175**:720–731.

Su, K. L., and Sun, G. Y., 1977, The effects of carbamylcholine on incorporation in vivo of (1-^{14}C)arachidonic acid into glycerolipids of mouse brain, *J. Neurochem.* **29**:1059–1063.

Sun, G. Y., and Foudin, L. L., 1984, On the status of lysolecithin in rat cerebral cortex during ischemia, *J. Neurochem.* **43**:1081–1086.

Yasuda, H., Kishiro, K., Izumi, N., et al., 1985, Biphasic liberation of arachidonic and stearic acids during cerebral ischemia, *J. Neurochem.* **45**:168–172.

Yoshida, S., Inoh, S., Asano, T., et al., 1980, Effect of transient ischemia on free fatty acids and phospholipids in the gerbil brain: Lipid peroxidation as a possible cause of postischemic injury, *J. Neurosurg.* **53**:323–331.

Yoshida, S., Inoh, S., Asano, T., et al., 1983, Brain free fatty acids, edema and mortality in gerbils subjected to transient, bilateral ischemia and effect of barbiturate anesthesia, *J. Neurochem.* **40**: 1278–1286.

Yoshida, S., Ikeda, M., Busto, R., et al., 1986, Cerebral phosphoinositides, triacylglycerol and energy metabolism in reversible ischemia: Origin and fate of free fatty acids, *J. Neurochem.* **47**: 744–757.

CHAPTER 7

INVOLVEMENT OF CALCIUM, LIPOLYTIC ENZYMES, AND FREE FATTY ACIDS IN ISCHEMIC BRAIN TRAUMA

AKHLAQ A. FAROOQUI,
YUTAKA HIRASHIMA, TAHIRA FAROOQUI,
and LLOYD A. HORROCKS

1. INTRODUCTION

The onset of cerebral ischemia causes a series of metabolic changes in central nervous system (CNS) that lead to the depletion of energy reserves and the loss of neuronal function in a time-dependent manner (Siesjö, 1981, 1984; Siesjö and Wieloch, 1985). At early stages of ischemia, recirculation of blood flow restores

---

AKHLAQ A. FAROOQUI, YUTAKA HIRASHIMA, and LLOYD A. HORROCKS • Department of Medical Biochemistry, The Ohio State University, Columbus, Ohio.   TAHIRA FAROOQUI • Division of Pharmacology, College of Pharmacy, The Ohio State University, Columbus, Ohio.

Neurochemical Correlates of Cerebral Ischemia, Volume 7 of *Advances in Neurochemistry*, edited by Nicolas G. Bazan, Pierre Braquet, and Myron D. Ginsberg. Plenum Press, New York, 1992.

the energy reserves and neuronal functions, but there is a critical period of ischemia after which these functions are restored only partially upon reperfusion. Blood reflow under such conditions is assumed to be more harmful to the organ or tissue than is continued ischemia alone (Siesjö and Wieloch, 1985). In the past decade many potentially damaging factors such as ATP depletion, plasma membrane phospholipid degradation, loss of calcium homeostasis, cellular acidosis, superoxide-induced membrane damage, and mitochondrial dysfunction have been reported to play important role in ischemic injury (Siesjö, 1990; Bazan, 1976; Bazan *et al.*, 1986). Several studies have indicated that ischemic insult markedly affects membrane integrity and membrane-associated functions such as activities of membrane-bound enzymes, ion transport, oxidative phosphorylation, and synaptic transmission (Siesjö, 1984; Bazan *et al.*, 1986; Flynn *et al.*, 1989). The purpose of this article is to discuss and critically evaluate the biochemical events (such as changes in calcium homeostasis, turnover of membrane phospholipids, and activation of phospholipases) initiated by ischemia and their potential role in determining the survival of nerve cells.

2. ROLE OF CALCIUM IN ISCHEMIC BRAIN INJURY

In the central nervous system, propagation of the nerve impulses and the release of neurotransmitters require maintenance of an optimal ionic gradient across the plasma membrane. The ionic gradients (high extracellular Ca^{2+} and Na^+ and low K^+) are maintained by ion pumps and Na^+/Ca^{2+} exchangers, which penetrate the phospholipid bilayer of the plasma membrane (Siesjö, 1981, 1984, 1986). This membrane has low permeability for calcium ions. Under normal conditions the concentration of calcium in cytosol (10^{-7} M) is 10,000 times lower than in the extracellular spaces (10^{-3} M). Influx of calcium ions is brought about either by the binding of agonists to receptors or by the opening of voltage-operated channels. The low levels of calcium ions in cytosol are maintained by the Na^+/Ca^{2+} exchanger or by ATP-derived efflux which involves Ca^{2+}-dependent ATPases located in the plasma membrane. Furthermore, Ca^{2+}-dependent ATPase is also localized in the endoplasmic reticulum, and the calcium-binding protein calmodulin may also play an important role in maintaining low levels of calcium ions in cytosol (Klee *et al.*, 1980).

During ischemic insult, membrane depolarization causes a rise in the cytosolic concentration of calcium ions. Calcium ions disrupt cellular metabolism by uncoupling mitochondrial electron transport and enhancing anaerobic metabolism and lactic acidosis (Siesjö, 1981, 1984). These ions markedly affect activities of lipolytic and proteolytic enzymes (Table 1). The stimulation of these enzymes may result in cell death (Schanne *et al.*, 1979; Cheung *et al.*, 1986; Becker *et al.*, 1988). It must be emphasized here that the evidence that calcium is involved in cell

TABLE 1. Effect of Calcium Ions on Lipolytic and Proteolytic Enzymes

Enzyme	Effect of calcium	Reference
Phospholipase A_1	Stimulated	Farooqui and Horrocks (1988)
Phospholipase A_2	Stimulated	Farooqui and Horrocks (1988)
Phospholipase C	Stimulated	Farooqui and Horrocks (1988)
Diacylglycerol lipase	Stimulated	Bell et al. (1979), Farooqui et al. (1985)
Monoacylglycerol lipase	No effect	Farooqui and Horrocks (unpublished)
Plasmalogenase	Stimulated	Arthur et al., 1985
Proteinases	Stimulated	Schlaepfer and Zimmerman, 1985

necrosis is circumstantial and that some neurons are more vulnerable to calcium toxicity than others (Becker et al., 1988; Jenkins et al., 1986; Choi, 1988). At present very little is known about the factors that determine the selective vulnerability of neurons. However, it has been proposed that vulnerable neurons have a high density of dendritic calcium channels and that they are innervated by excitatory amino acids, making them targets for excitotoxic damage (Benveniste et al., 1984; Rothman, 1984; Wieloch, 1985; Choi 1988; Rothman and Olney, 1986; McDonald and Johnston, 1990). Thirty minutes of ischemia causes large increases in levels of extracellular amino acids (Hagberg et al., 1985). Glutamate and aspartate levels are increased 163- and 20-fold, respectively, over the basal level. It has been suggested that excitatory amino acids (glutamate and aspartate) are toxic because they open postsynaptic calcium channels and allow entry of extracellular calcium into the cell and the calcium ions induce lipolytic and proteolytic reactions in the vulnerable neurons (Choi, 1988; McDonald and Johnston, 1990). A speculative description of glutamate neurotoxicity has been recently proposed (Choi, 1990). Glutamate neurotoxicity may have three stages: first, induction, i.e. overstimulation of glutamate receptors leading to a set of immediate cellular derangements; second, amplification, i.e. events that intensify these derangements and promote the excitotoxic involvement of additional neurons; and third, expression, the destructive cascade directly responsible for neuronal cell degeneration (Choi, 1990).

3. PHOSPHOLIPID METABOLISM AND ACTIVITIES OF LIPOLYTIC ENZYMES DURING ISCHEMIC INSULT

A rise in the concentration of intracellular calcium ions may be involved in activation of lipolytic enzymes (phospholipases A_1, A_2, and C), the breakdown of membrane phospholipids, and the accumulation of free fatty acids, lysophospholipids, and diacylglycerols (Bazan, 1970, 1976; Edgar et al., 1982; Rordorf et al.,

1991). Phospholipases A_1 and A_2 liberate the fatty acid at the first and second carbons of the glycerol moiety. Phospholipase C hydrolyzes the phosphatidyl base group from phospholipids, liberating diacylglycerol. The diacylglycerol is hydrolyzed to free fatty acid and glycerol by diacylglycerol and monoacylglycerol lipases. Under normal conditions these metabolites are recycled through a series of energy-dependent reactions. As a result, the normal phospholipid content of cellular membranes is not altered and the intracellular concentrations of free fatty acids, lysophospholipids, and diacylglycerols are maintained at low levels; however, during ischemic insult, stimulation of lipolytic enzymes (Figures 1 and 2) causes the depletion of critical membrane phospholipids (Farber *et al.*, 1981; Edgar *et al.*, 1982; Hirashima *et al.*, 1984, 1989). The free fatty acids that accumulate during ischemia are arachidonate, stearate, palmitate, oleate, and docosahexaenoate.

Liberation of several free fatty acids indicates that more than one lipolytic enzyme may be involved in phospholipid degradation (Table 2). However, owing to the predominant accumulations of arachidonate and the enrichment of this fatty acid at the second carbon of glycerophospholipid, it was suggested (Bazan, 1971, 1976) that the activation of a phospholipase A_2 is involved during ischemic insult. It is becoming increasingly evident (Hsueh and Needleman, 1979) that mammalian tissues contain two types of phospholipase A_2. The highly specific phospholipase A_2 is hormone or agonist sensitive (such as to bradykinin), involves

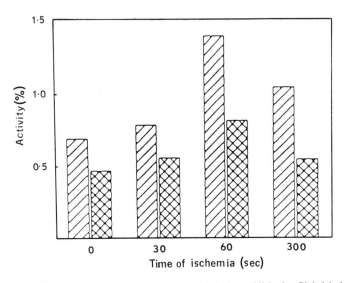

FIGURE 1. Specific activities of phospholipases A_1 and A_2 in gerbil brain. Global ischemia was induced by bilateral ligation of the carotid arteries PLA_1 (striped bars) and PLA_2 (cross-hatched bars). Data are from Edgar *et al.* (1982).

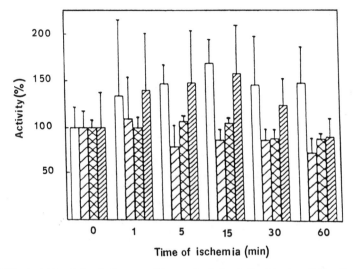

FIGURE 2. Activities of phospholipases and lipases after ischemic insult by decapitation. From left to right, results are shown for phospholipase A, lysophospholipase, phospholipase C, and diacylglycerol and monoacylglycerol lipases (*n* = 6).

receptor-mediated mechanism, and selectively liberates arachidonic acid from membrane phospholipids. This enzyme may be involved in ischemic injury at a early period, and damage produced by such mechanism is reversible. The other phospholipase A_2 nonspecifically responds to noxious stimuli (ischemia and trauma) and releases all fatty acids (including arachidonic, oleic, palmitic, and stearic acids) from the C-2 carbon of phospholipids. Under ischemic insult the latter type of phospholipase A_2 is probably activated (Hsueh and Needleman, 1979), and damage caused by the stimulation of this enzyme is irreversible.

TABLE 2. Effect of Ischemia on Lipolytic Enzymes

Enzyme	Effect of calcium	Reference
Phospholipase A_1	Stimulated	Edgar et al. (1982), Hirashima et al. (1984)
Phospholipase A_2	Stimulated	Edgar et al. (1982), Hirashima et al. (1984)
Phospholipase C	Stimulated	Hirashima et al. (1989)
Lysophospholipase	Stimulated	Hirashima et al. (1984), Sun and Fondin (1984)
Monoacylglycerol lipase	Not known	
Diacylglycerol lipase	Stimulated	Abe et al. (1987), Otani et al. (1988)
Triacylglycerol lipase	Inhibited	Alberghina et al. (1982)
Plasmalogenase	Stimulated	Horrocks et al. (1978)

Recently we have found a cytosolic calcium independent phospholipase A_2 in bovine brain (Hirashima *et al.*, 1991). It has been shown that this enzyme is also stimulated during myocardial ischemic events (Ford *et al.*, 1991).

Activation of phospholipase A_2 may affect cellular function in many ways. It causes destruction of synaptosomal membranes in vitro (Moskowitz *et al.*, 1984). Such degradation of synaptosomal membranes inactivates several membrane-bound enzymes (Fourcans and Jain, 1974; Farias *et al.*, 1975). The products of the phospholipase reaction, namely free fatty acids and lysophospholipids, can inhibit the exchange of ADP for ATP across the mitochondrial membrane (Wojtczak, 1976). Lysophospholipids may also disrupt cellular membrane structures (Weltzien, 1979).

Plasmalogenase, an enzyme that catalyzes the hydrolysis of the vinyl-ether linkage of ethanolamine or choline plasmalogens, stimulated two- to three-fold after 20 min of ligation of both carotid arteries in gerbils and may be responsible for the marked decrease in the levels of these lipids during ischemic injury (Horrocks *et al.*, 1978).

Another pathway for the release of free fatty acid that may also be activated during ischemia is the reversal of the choline and/or ethanolamine phosphotransferases (Goracci *et al.*, 1977). These enzymes normally produce phosphatidylcholine and phosphatidylethanolamine. During ischemia, however, the CMP is not removed owing to the lack of ATP production (De Medio *et al.*, 1980). Thus the reaction between phosphatidylcholine and CMP (reversal of choline phosphotransferase) produces CDP-choline and/or CDP-ethanolamine and diacylglycerol. The diacylglycerol is also produced by the action of phosphatidylinositol-specific phospholipase C. In addition, cellular diacylglycerol is generated from phosphatidylcholine (Besterman *et al.*, 1986). According to Abe *et al.* (1987), and Otani *et al.* (1988), diacylglycerol is not utilized by diacylglycerol kinase for phosphatidic acid production (owing to the lack of ATP) but is rapidly hydrolyzed to monoacylglycerol and free fatty acid by a diacylglycerol lipase. The monoacylglycerol is then hydrolyzed by monoacylglycerol lipase. It must be mentioned here that in the study by Abe *et al.* (1987), the activity of diacylglycerol lipase was not determined. Thus the relative contribution of phospholipase A_2 and the phospholipase C-diacylglycerol lipase pathway in free fatty acid release remains unknown.

Among the various membrane phospholipids, choline phosphoglycerides, phosphatidylinositol, and ethanolamine phosphoglycerides may contribute to the production of free fatty acids, in particular arachidonic acid, during ischemic injury (Sun and Foudin, 1984; Yoshida *et al.*, 1986; Abe *et al.*, 1988), and this loss of membrane phospholipids may alter the equilibrium between the membrane protein and the remaining lipid in such a way that plasma membranes become more permeable to extracellular calcium ions and the entry of high levels of this cation markedly affect the integrity and function of mitochondria (Farber *et al.*, 1981). This may result in irreversible ischemic cell damage.

4. REGULATION OF PHOSPHOLIPASE A₂ AND DIACYLGLYCEROL LIPASE ACTIVITIES

To understand the events triggering cell and tissue injury during ischemic insult, it is important to understand the regulation of phospholipase A_2 and diacylglycerol lipase activities. Phospholipase activity is regulated by calcium ions (Dennis, 1983). A calcium-binding site has been identified on phospholipase A_2 and the addition of calcium stimulates the enzymic activity whereas addition of Quin 2, a calcium chelator, inhibits this enzyme (van Scharrenburg et al., 1985; Simon et al., 1986). The ischemic insult may not only activate phospholipases but also inhibit acyltransferases (Figure 3), thus recycling the lysophospholipids (Hirashima et al., 1989). Furthermore, the diacylglycerols also stimulate the activity of phospholipase A_2 (Dawson et al., 1984). Phospholipase A_2 activity is also stimulated by platelet-activating factor (Kawaguchi and Yasuda, 1984). Several other molecular entities that are associated with transmembrane signaling may also regulate the phospholipase A_2 activity. Factors such as protein kinase C, GTP-binding proteins, diacylglycerol, and cAMP may also modulate the activities of phospholipase A_2 (Bazan, 1976; Nishizuka, 1986; Berridge, 1984). However, the effect of ischemia on GTP-binding protein and protein kinase C is not known. Finally, lipid peroxide also stimulates the activity of phospholipase A_2 (Sevanian

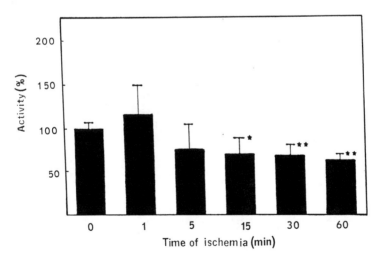

FIGURE 3. Activities of acylating enzymes after ischemic insult by decapitation. The values of enzyme activity are mean ± S.D., expressed as the percentage of 0-min ischemia ($n = 6$). * and ** denote significance at $P < 0.05$ and $P < 0.01$, respectively, compared with the control (Dunnett's test). Modified from Hirashima et al. (1989).

and Kim, 1986; Au *et al.*, 1985). It has been shown that phospholipase A_2 can be activated (in the absence of calcium ions) by peroxidized fatty acids in the phospholipids. The degree of phospholipase A_2 activation was correlated with the extent of lipid peroxidation.

Endogenous proteins called lipocortins also modulate phospholipase A_2 activity. These proteins are induced by the injection of anti-inflammatory steroids (Hirata, 1985; Dennis, 1987; Flower, 1988). The modulation of phospholipase A_2 activity by lipocortins is regulated by phosphorylation/dephosphorylation of this protein. The mechanism of phospholipase inhibition by lipocortin is not known. Initially, a direct inhibition by protein–protein interaction was implicated (Hirata, 1985). The recognition that lipocortins are able to bind to phospholipids (Schlaepfer and Haigler, 1987) suggests alternative modes of action of these proteins. Davidson *et al.* (1987) and Aarsman *et al.* (1987) have recently shown that the hydrolysis of membrane phospholipids by phospholipase A_2 is inhibited by lipocortin in a substrate-dependent manner. This suggests that lipocortins inhibit phospholipase A_2 by coating the phospholipid and thereby blocking the interaction of enzyme with its substrate. The effect of ischemic insult on lipocortins is not known.

Like phospholipase A_2, the regulation of diacylglycerol lipases is complex. The enzyme activity may be regulated by free fatty acids, which are end products of the diacylglycerol lipase reaction (Farooqui *et al.*, 1986, 1989). In vitro this inhibition can be reversed by fatty acid-free bovine serum albumin (Farooqui *et al.*, 1986). Recent studies have indicated that C-MT peptide, the C terminus of the middle-sized tumor antigen of polyomavirus, inhibits the activities of various phospholipases, including A_2, C, and D and phosphatidylinositol-specific phospholipase C (Notsu *et al.*, 1985). This peptide has an amino acid sequence similar to a portion of lipocortin I, an endogenous phospholipase-regulatory protein (Dennis, 1987; Flower, 1988). Both microsomal and plasma membrane diacylglycerol lipases are strongly inhibited by C-MT peptide (Figure 4). The degree of C-MT inhibition was several fold higher for diacylglycerol lipases than for phospholipases. The effect of lipocortin on diacylglycerol lipases is not known.

5. FREE FATTY ACIDS AND DIACYLGLYCEROLS DURING ISCHEMIC INSULT

The endogenous concentration of free fatty acid is maintained at a level approximately 1000-fold lower than that of esterified fatty acids (Bazan *et al.*, 1986). Ischemic injury causes 1.4- and 3.6-fold increase in the free fatty acid and diacylglycerol levels, respectively, over the control levels (Yoshida *et al.*, 1986). Both free fatty acids and diacylglycerols are known to have a variety of detrimental effects on brain structure and function primarily as a result of their ability to

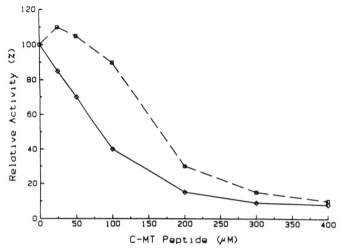

FIGURE 4. Effect of C-MT peptide on microsomal (——) and plasma membrane (– – –) diacylglycerol lipases of bovine brain. Reproduced with permssion from Farooqui et al. (1986).

disrupt cell membranes (Farber et al., 1981; Michell et al., 1976). Arachidonate, the fatty acid that is most commonly found at the sn-2 position of the glycerol moiety of membrane phospholipids, is an amphipathic molecule and is capable of forming micelles that bind either hydrophilic or hydrophobic substances (Solomonson et al., 1976). It readily intercalates into membranes and produces changes in the packing of lipid molecules (Klausner et al., 1980). Thus, arachidonate has the physical ability to modify membrane integrity. It has been reported that arachidonate inhibits Na^+,K^+-ATPase activity (Chan et al., 1983a, b). This inhibition causes a shift in cations and water (an increase in the intracellular sodium level and a concomitant decrease in the potassium level). This process may be responsible for the development of cellular edema. The disturbance in the movement of Na^+,K^+-ATPase leads to partial membrane depolarization and the opening of voltage-dependent Ca^{2+} channels (Siesjö, 1981, 1990) and the influx of Ca^{2+} (Goto et al., 1978). The influx of calcium ions may also be facilitated by Na^+-Ca^{2+} exchangers (Siesjö, 1990). The net effect of all these processes would be an increase in the concentration of cytosolic calcium ions. This increase may cause stimulation of lipolysis and proteolysis in the cell and may be responsible for brain damage (Hochachka, 1986). This may be one of the mechanisms by which arachidonate produces brain injury. Fatty acids are efficient uncouplers of oxidative phosphorylation (Harris, 1977). They markedly affect mitochondrial function (Hillered and Chan, 1988, 1990). The calcium pump that sequesters calcium in the mitochondria is activated by free fatty acids (Crompton and Heid, 1978). Free fatty acid accumulation also favors potassium loss from mitochondria, and energy is required for potassium recovery (Wojtczak, 1976).

Diacylglycerols have emerged as an important class of bioactive molecules that regulate cellular function, growth, and behavior by participating in the transfer of hormone- and growth factor-derived signals to the cell interior and by affecting the activities of a number of important enzymes. (Table 3). Increased levels of diacylglycerol have been reported to occur in ischemia, spinal cord trauma, and seizures and after electroconvulsive shock (Bazan, 1976; Demediuk et al., 1985; Bazan et al., 1986). Elevated levels of diacylglycerol disrupt cell membranes and may act as the reservoir for the massive release of free fatty acids. In vivo free fatty acids, diacylglycerols, and calcium ions may affect protein kinase C activity at very early periods of ischemic insult (because low levels of ATP are still present). However, at later periods when the cellular ATP supply is exhausted, protein kinase C may not respond to ischemic insult. However, in vitro changes in the intracellular localization of protein kinase C have been reported to occur during ischemic insult to the brain and spinal cord (Louis et al., 1988; Onodera et al., 1989; Kochhar et al., 1989). Thus the translocation of protein kinase C from the cytosol to the membrane compartment is accompanied by a marked decrease in protein kinase C activity (Louis et al., 1988; Kochhar et al., 1989). The losses in protein kinase C activity may be attributed to an increase in Ca^{2+}-dependent proteolysis during ischemic insult. The level of cAMP-dependent protein kinase is also decreased during ischemia (Kochhar et al., 1989). These findings suggest that altered protein phosphorylation may play critical roles in neuronal death during ischemic insult. Further, according to Matthys et al. (1984), diacylglycerol accumulated during ischemic insult may also increase Na^+-H^+ exchange, thus effectively slowing Na^+ exchange-based Ca^{2+} efflux.

TABLE 3. Direct Effects of Diacylglycerols
on Activities of Various Enzymes[a]

Enzyme	Effect on activity
Protein kinase C	Stimulated
Phospholipase A_2	Stimulated
Glycogen synthetase	Inhibited
Tyrosine aminotransferase	Stimulated
Ornithine decarboxylase	Stimulated
Na^+,K^+-ATPase	Inhibited
β-Glucosaminidase	Stimulated
Cytidylyltransferase	Stimulated
Lysophospholipid acyltransferase	Inhibited

[a]Modified from Farooqui et al. (1988).

The free fatty acid generated by the action of phospholipases, plasmalogenase, and lipases during ischemic insult can be metabolized to prostaglandins, prostacyclin, thromboxane, and leukotrienes by cyclooxygenases and lipoxygenases (Watson and Ginsberg, 1988; Bazan et al., 1986). Under normal conditions the above metabolites act as second messengers. However, during ischemic insult their levels are markedly increased and they may act as cytotoxic agents (Gaudet et al., 1980). For example, some prostaglandins (for example, $PGF_{2\alpha}$) are potent vasoconstrictors. $PGF_{2\alpha}$, along with the leukotrienes, may induce extravasation of material from the blood vessels into the surrounding tissue (Dahlen et al., 1981). Furthermore, the generation of free radicals in the hydrocarbon core of the cell membranes may induce cross-linking reactions with membrane phospholipids and proteins, thereby changing the microenvironment and structure of the proteins and irreversibly affecting the plasma membrane and mitochondrial functions (Demopoulos et al., 1980; Kontos et al., 1980). This may be another mechanism responsible for brain damage in hypoxic-ischemic injury.

6. LIPID PEROXIDATION AND FREE RADICALS DURING ISCHEMIC INSULT

Ischemic insult favors the formation of free radicals. The important production sites for superoxide ($\cdot O_2$) and hydroxyl ($OH\cdot$) free radicals are the mitochondrial respiratory chain and reaction sequences catalyzed by cyclooxygenase and lipoxygenase (Flamm et al., 1978; Halliwell and Gutteridge, 1985; Siesjö, 1981, 1984). These radicals are also formed during autoxidation of catecholamine and during xanthine oxidase reaction (Siesjö, 1984). As stated above, phosphatidylcholine and phosphatidylethanolamine, the most prominent cerebral phospholipids, usually have one polyunsaturated fatty acid. This is the reason why they are particularly susceptible to peroxidation (Bazan et al., 1986; Watson and Ginsberg, 1988). The most significant aspect of the peroxidative reaction is its markedly damaging effect on the polyunsaturated-acid-containing phospholipid molecules involved, leading to impaired membrane function (Demopoulos et al., 1980; Watson et al., 1984; Bazan et al., 1986; Watson and Ginsberg, 1988). This may cause inactivation of membrane-bound enzymes (such as Na^+,K^+-ATPase and adenylate cyclase). A significant rise in the lipid peroxidation, together with a rapid disappearance of free arachidonic acid, strongly indicates the occurrence of lipid peroxidation during the early recirculation periods (Siesjö, 1984; Bazan et al., 1986; Watson and Ginsberg, 1988). Thus Cooper et al. (1977) have found that cerebral polyribosomes are intact during ischemia but rapidly degrade into their subunits on recirculation, thereby losing the ability to form polypeptides. Rehncrona et al. (1979) have reported further deterioration of mitochondrial function after recirculation following incomplete ischemia. In spite of the above studies, it has not been conclusively proven that free-radical damage to unsaturated acyl chains in phospholipids and proteins constitutes a major part of the ischemic damage. At present the evidence is relatively strong for an association of free radical damage with vascular injury (Sano *et al.*, 1980; Wei *et al.*, 1981; Hall and Braughler, 1988).

7. PHARMACOLOGICAL INTERVENTION IN ISCHEMIA

Despite major advances in our understanding of biochemical events involved in the pathophysiology of cerebral ischemia, little progress has been made in our ability to arrest, prevent, or reverse ischemic insult. We know that the extent of irreversible ischemic damage is governed by both the duration of ischemic insult and the rate of blood flow within the ischemic area. A number of pharmacological agents are used in the management of stroke in humans and in experimental work on animals; these are listed in Table 4. No agent has been shown to be of unequivocal value in all cases. A few are discussed below.

7.1. Calcium-Channel Blockers

These drugs block the entry of calcium ions into the ischemic neurons. They do not themselves antagonize the effects of calcium ions; instead, they prevent the ions from gaining access to their intracellular site of action (Janis and Triggle, 1983) by blocking the entry of calcium ions. They may inhibit the essential role of this cation in the activation of lipolytic enzymes during ischemia (Chang *et al.*, 1987). Increased blood flow, dilation of cerebral vessels, decreased lactic acidosis, and decreased infarct size have been reported following treatment with calcium channel blockers (White *et al.*, 1983; Kidooka *et al.*, 1987).

7.2. Vitamin E

α-Tocopherol (vitamin E), a well-known antioxidant, has been shown (Yoshida *et al.*, 1982; Yamamoto *et al.*, 1983) to have beneficial effects on brain edema and ischemia. It inhibits the activities of phospholipase A_2 and lipoxygenase and plays a fundamental role in the stabilization of the polyunsaturated fatty acid chain in membrane phospholipids (Douglas *et al.*, 1986). Vitamin E interacts with cell membranes and prevents lipid peroxide formation by acting as a hydrogen donor (Yoshida *et al.*, 1985). The free-radical-induced damage in ischemia may also be prevented by the administration of mannitol, dimethyl sulfoxide (DMSO), and MCI-186, which possible act as specific scavengers for hydroxyl radicals (Abe *et al.*, 1988).

TABLE 4. Proposed Pharmacological Strategies for Stroke Management

Agent	Proposed mechanism of action
CDP-choline CDP-ethanolamine	Induce phospholipid synthesis, reversal of CDP-ethanolamine phosphotransferase reaction; decrease, production of free fatty acids
Ca^{2+} channel blockers (verapamil, nimodipine, flunarizine)	Decrease Ca^{2+} entry
Antioxidants/free-radical scavengers (α-tocopherol, ascorbic acid, mannitol, glutathione, catalase, superoxide dismutase)	Protect lipids from peroxidation
Opiate antagonists (naloxone)	Vasoregulation, antioxidant, anti-GABA activity
β-Adrenergic antagonists (propranolol)	Decrease edema, lactic acid production, vasodilation
Gingko biloba derivatives	Platelet-activating factor, antagonists, decrease platelet aggregation, decrease Ca^{2+} entry, free radical scavengers
Barbiturates	Membrane stabilizer, free-radical scavenger, anticonvulsant
Prostacyclin (PGI$_2$)	Vasodilation, decrease platelet aggregation
Phosphodiesterase inhibitors (aminophylline, dipyridamole, sulfinpyrazone)	Vasoconstriction of nonischemic vessels diverting blood to ischemic area
Phenothiazines (chlorpromazine, trifluoperazine)	Inhibition of Ca^{2+}-calmodulin complex
Perfluorocarbons	Hemodilution, O_2 carrier
Excitoxic amino acid blockers (2-amino-7-phosphonoheptanoic acid)	Decrease neuronal damage
Glutamate antagonist MK-801	Blockade of NMDA receptor
Cyclooxygenase inhibitors (indomethacin, aspirin)	Decrease prostaglandin synthesis
Fibrinolysins (streptokinase, urokinase, tissue plasminogen activator)	Clot dissolution
GM$_1$ ganglioside	Preservation of membrane structure, neuronal regeneration, and sprouting
S-Adenosyl-L-methionine	Improves energy metabolism, reduces brain edema

7.3. Naloxone

The use of naloxone, an opiate antagonist, for the treatment of ischemic insult is controversial (Welch and Barkley, 1986). Although endorphin levels are increased during ischemic insult, the beneficial effects of naloxone appear related to anti-inflammatory, antioxidant, vasodilatory, and membrane-stabilizing properties (Hosobuchi et al., 1982). The positive results obtained with this agent required higher doses than would be expected for opiate antagonist action alone. Therefore, further investigations are needed before this drug can be endorsed (Baskin *et al.*, 1986).

7.4. CDP-Amines

CDP-amines are key intermediates in the biosynthesis of phosphatidylcholine and phosphatidylethanolamine. The therapeutic actions of CDP-amines are thought to be due to restorative effects on phospholipid synthesis in the ischemic brain (Horrocks *et al.*, 1981; Trovarelli *et al.*, 1981). CDP-amines attenuate the fatty acid increases and restore the disruption of cerebral mitochondrial lipid metabolism induced by hypoxia (Dorman *et al.*, 1982; Horrocks and Dorman, 1985). They have been reported to inhibit the activities of phospholipases A_1 and A_2 (Freysz *et al.*, 1985; Arrigoni *et al.*, 1987). CDP-amines have also been reported to increase oxygen consumption and glucose incorporation into amino acids and phospholipids (Kakihana *et al.*, 1988). They improve cerebral blow flow and may also cause a decline in lactate production and restoration of Na^+,K^+-ATPase activity.

7.5. Glutamate Antagonist MK-801

Glutamate has been implicated in the pathophysiology of cerebral ischemia (Rothman and Olney, 1986). The glutamate antagonist MK-801 has been successfully used for the treatment of cerebral ischemia in experimental models (Ozyurt *et al.*, 1988; Park *et al.*, 1988). It has been proposed that MK-801 exerts its antagonistic effects via a site related to the ion channel (Wong *et al.*, 1986). The onset of N-methyl-D-aspartate (NMDA) receptor blockade with MK-801 is more rapid in the presence of glutamate (Wong *et al.*, 1986). These two effects may be relevant to the efficacy of MK-801 in cerebral ischemia, which putatively provokes a marked elevation in extracellular concentrations of glutamate. Westerberg *et al.* (1988) have proposed that MK-801, in addition to directing receptor blockade, protects neurons with severe, but not complete, energy failure by preserving ionic gradients across the plasma membrane and enhancing amino acid uptake.

7.6. GM_1-Ganglioside

Gangliosides have been reported to have a beneficial effect in a variety of CNS injuries by increasing CNS regeneration or sprouting (Toffano *et al.*, 1983; Carolei *et al.*, 1991). Several studies have utilized GM_1 ganglioside for the treatment of ischemic insult (Enseleit *et al.*, 1984; Bassi *et al.*, 1984; Hoffbrand *et al.*, 1988; Karpiak *et al.*, 1987). It has been proposed that GM_1 ganglioside reduces the incidence of cerebral edema and mortality by preserving the membrane structure and by preventing the deterioration of the membrane microenvironment.

7.7. Lazaroid (21-Aminosteroid U74006F)

The 21-aminosteroid U74006F, a nonglucocorticoid 21-aminosteroid, is a potential inhibitor of lipid peroxidation. It has been shown to have a beneficial effect on the recovery and survival of mice with severe head injury, posttraumatic spinal cord ischemia (Hall, 1988), and cerebral ischemia (Hall and Yonkers, 1988). The mechanism of lazaroid is not known, but Hall (1988) has proposed that lazaroid acts by inhibiting iron-dependent lipid peroxidation in the central nervous system. Furthermore, lazaroid also enhances the mean arterial blood pressure and cerebral perfusion pressure (Hall and Yonkers, 1988). Young et al. (1988) have reported that lazaroid significantly reduces Na^+ accumulation, K^+ loss, and water entry in the ischemic brain. The effect was most consistent and prominent in tissues surrounding the infarct site.

7.8. S-Adenosyl-L-Methionine

S-Adenosyl-L-methionine is the main methyl group donor in the transmethylation reaction (Hirata and Axelrod, 1980). It has been shown (Trovarelli et al., 1983; Matsui et al., 1987) that in experimental animals, S-adenosyl-L-methionine improves energy metabolism and reduces brain edema. Sato et al. (1988) have reported that this drug protects the hippocampal CA1 neurons from degeneration and necrosis in a dose-dependent manner. This compound has been successfully used in human trials in Japan (personal communication from Dr. A. Takaku, Toyama Medical and Pharmaceutical University), and beneficial results have been obtained.

8. CONCLUSION

Ischemic brain insult is accompanied by a set of complex biochemical processes that we are just beginning to understand. The ischemic damage may be caused by the influx of calcium ions from the extracellular compartment to the intracellular compartment. This disturbance in calcium ion homeostasis may activate phospholipases (A_1, A_2, and C) and proteases, resulting in liberation of free fatty acids and lysophospholipids. Both these metabolites at high levels have membrane-disrupting properties. Free fatty acids are further metabolized to prostaglandin, leukotrienes, and thromboxanes. These products at high levels have a variety of toxic effects on normal cell functions and membrane integrity. A variety of therapeutic agents such as calcium entry blockers, vitamin E, CDP-amines, MK-801, GM ganglioside, lazaroid, and S-adenosyl-L-methionine may have beneficial effects on brain ischemic insult.

REFERENCES

Aarsman, A. J., Mynbeek, G., Van Den Bosch, H., Rothhut, B., Prieur, B., Comera, C., Jordan, L., and Russo-Marie, F., 1987, Lipocortin inhibition of extracellular and intracellular phospholipases A2 is substrate concentration dependent, *FEBS Lett.* **219**:176–180.

Abe, K., Kogure, K., Yamamoto, H., Imazawa, M., and Miyamoto, K., 1987, Mechanism of arachidonic acid liberation during ischemia in gerbil cerebral cortex, *J. Neurochem.* **48**:503–509.

Abe, K., Yuki, S., and Kogure, K., 1988, Strong attenuation of ischemic and postischemic brain edema in rats by a novel free radical scavenger, *Stroke* **19**:480–485.

Alberghina, M., Biola, M., and Giuffrida, A. M., 1982, Changes in enzyme activities of glycerolipid metabolism of guinea-pig cerebral hemispheres during experimental hypoxia, *J. Neurosci. Res.* **7**:147–154.

Arrigoni, E., Averet, N., and Cohadon, F., 1987, Effects of CDP-choline on phospholipase A2 and cholinephosphotransferase activities following a cryogenic brain injury in the rabbit, *Biochem. Pharmacol.* **36**:3697–3700.

Arthur, G., Covic, L., Wientzek, M., and Choy, P. C., 1985, Plasmalogenase in hamster heart, *Biochim. Biophys. Acta* **833**:189–195.

Au, A. M., Chan, P. H., and Fishman, R. A., 1985, Stimulation of phospholipase A2 activity by oxygen-derived free radicals in isolated brain capillaries, *J. Cell. Biochem.* **27**:449–457.

Baethmann, A., and Jansen, M., 1986, Possible role of calcium entry blockers in brain protection, *Eur. Neurol.* **25**:102–114.

Baskin, D. S., Hosobuchi, Y., and Grevel, J. C., 1986, Treatment of experimental stroke with opiate antagonists, *J. Neurosurg.* **64**:99–103.

Bassi, S., Albizzati, M. G., and Sbacchi, M., 1984, Double blind evaluation of monosialoganglioside (GM) therapy in stroke, *J. Neurosci. Res.* **12**:493–498.

Bazan, N. G., 1970, Effect of ischemia and electroconvulsive shock on free fatty acid pool in the brain, *Biochim. Biophys. Acta* **218**:1–10.

Bazan, N. G., 1971, Changes in free fatty acids of brain by drug-induced convulsions, electroshock and anesthesia, *J. Neurochem.* **18**:1379–1385.

Bazan, N. G., 1976, Free arachidonic acid and other lipids in the nervous system during early ischemia and after electroshock, *Adv. Exp. Med. Biol.* **72**:317–335.

Bazan, N. G., Birkle, D. L., Tang, W., and Reddy, T. S., 1986, The accumulation of free arachidonic acid, diacylglycerols, prostaglandins, and lipoxygenase reaction products in the brain during experimental epilepsy, *Adv. Neurol.* **44**:879–902.

Becker, D. P., Verity, M. A., Povlishock, J., and Cheung, M., 1988, Brain cellular injury and recovery—horizons for improving medical therapies in stroke and trauma, *West. J. Med.* **148**: 670–684.

Bell, R. L., Kennerly, D. A., Standford, N., and Majerus, P. W., 1979, Diglyceride lipase: A pathway for arachidonic release from human platelets, *Proc. Natl. Acad. Sci. USA* **76**:3238–3241.

Benveniste, H., Brejer, J., and Schousboe, A., 1984, Elevation of the extracellular concentration of glutamate and aspartate in rat hippocampus during transient cerebral ischemia monitored by intracerebral misodialysis, *J. Neurochem.* **43**:1369–1374.

Berridge, M. J., 1984, Inositol trisphosphate and diacylglycerol as second messenger, *Biochem. J.* **220**: 345–360.

Besterman, J. M., Duronio, V., and Cuatrecasas, P., 1986, Rapid formation of diacylglycerol from phosphatidylcholine: A pathway for generation of a second messenger, *Proc. Natl. Acad. Sci. USA* **83**:6785–6789.

Carolei, A., Fieschi, C., Bruno, R., and Toffano, G., 1991, Monosialoganglioside GM1 in cerebral ischemia, *Cerebrovasc. Brain. Metab. Rev.* **3**:134–157.

Chan, P. H., Kerian R., and Fishman, R. A., 1983*a*, Reductions of GABA and glutamate uptake and (Na$^+$ + K$^+$)-ATPase activity in brain slices and synaptosomes by arachidonic acid, *J. Neurochem.* **40**:309–316.

Chan, P. H., Fishman, R. A., Caronna, J., Schmidley, J. W., and Prioleau, G., 1983*b*, Induction of brain edema following intracerebral injection of arachidonic acid, *Ann. Neurol.* **13**:625–632.

Chang, J., Blazek, E., and Carlson, R. P., 1987, Inhibition of phospholipase A2 (PLA2) activity by nifedipine and nisoldipine is independent of their calcium channel-blocking activity, *Inflammation* **11**:353–364.

Cheung, J. Y., Bonventre, J. V., Malis, C. D., and Leaf, A., 1986, Calcium and ischemic injury, *N. Engl. J. Med.* **314**:1670–1676.

Choi, D. W., 1988, Calcium-mediated neurotoxicity: Relationship to specific channel types and role in ischemic damage, *Trends Neurosci.* **11**:465–469.

Choi, D. W., 1990, Cerebral hypoxia: Some new approaches and unanswered questions, *J. Neurosci.* **10**:2493–2501.

Cooper, H. K., Zalewska, T., Kawakami, S., Hossman, K-A., and Kleihues, P., 1977, The effect of ischaemia and recirculation on protein synthesis in the rat brain, *J. Neurochem.* **28**:20–34.

Crompton, M., and Heid, I., 1978, The cycling of calcium, sodium, and protons across the inner membrane of cardiac mitochondria, *Eur. J. Biochem.* **91**:599–610.

Dahlen, S. E., Bjork, J., Hedquist, P., Arfors, K. E., Hammarstrom, S., Lindgren, J. A., and Samuelsson, B., 1981, Leukotrienes promote plasma leakage and leukocyte adhesion in postcapillary vessels: In vivo effects with relevance to the acute inflammatory response, *Proc. Natl. Acad. Sci. USA* **78**:3887–3891.

Davidson, F. F., Dennis, E. A., Powell, M., and Glenney, J. R., Jr., 1987, Inhibition of phospholipase A2 by "lipocortins" and calpactins, *J. Biol. Chem.* **262**:1698–1705.

Dawson, R. M. C., Irvine, R. F., Bray, J., and Quinn, P., 1984, Long-chain unsaturated diacylglycerols cause a perturbation in the structure of phospholipid bilayer rendering them susceptible to phospholipase attack, *Biochem. Biophys. Res. Commun.* **125**:836–842.

De Medio, G. E., Goraaci, G., Horrocks, L. A., Lazarewicz, J. W., Mazzari, S., Porcellati, G., Strosznajder, J., and Trovarelli, G., 1980, The effect of transient ischemia on fatty acid and lipid metabolism in the gerbil brain, *Ital. J. Biochem.* **29**:412–432.

Demediuk, P., Saunders, R. D., Clendenon, N. R., Means, E. D., Anderson, D. K., and Horrocks, L. A., 1985, Changes in lipid metabolism in traumatized spinal cord, *Prog. Brain Res.* **63**: 211–226.

Demopoulos, H. B., Flamm, E. E., Pietronigro, D. D., and Seligman, M. L., 1980, The free radical pathology and the microcirculation in the major central nervous system disorders, *Acta Physiol. Scand. Suppl.* **429**:91–119.

Dennis, E. A., 1983, Phospholipases, *in* "The Enzymes" (P. Boyer, ed.) pp. 307–353, Academic Press, New York.

Dennis, E. A., 1987, Regulation of eicosanoid production: Role of phospholipases and inhibitors, *Bio/Technology* **5**:1294–1300.

Dorman, R. V., Dabrowiecki, Z., De Medio, G. E., Porcellati, G., and Horrocks, L. A., 1982, Effects of cytidine nucleotides on CNS membranes during ischemia, *in* "Head Injury: Basic and Clinical Aspects" (R. G. Grossman and P. L. Gildenberg, eds.), pp. 93–101, Raven Press, New York.

Douglas, C. E., Chan, A. C., and Choy, P. C., 1986, Vitamin E inhibits platelet phospholipase A2, *Biochim. Biophys. Acta* **876**:639–645.

Edgar, A. D., Strosznajder, J., and Horrocks, L. A., 1982, Activation of ethanolamine phospholipase A2 in brain during ischemia, *J. Neurochem.* **39:**1111–1116.

Enseleit, W. H., Domer, F. R., Jarrott, D. M., and Baricos, W. H., 1984, Cerebral phospholipid content and Na, K-ATPase activity during ischemia and postischemic perfusion in the Mongolian gerbil, *J. Neurochem.* **43:**320–327.

Farber, J. L., Chien, K. R., and Mittnacht, S., Jr., 1981, The pathogenesis of irreversible cell injury in ischemia, *Am. J. Pathol.* **102:**271–281.

Farias, R. N., Blog, B., and Morero, R. D., 1975, Regulation of allosteric membrane-bound enzymes through changes in membrane lipid composition, *Biochim. Biophys. Acta* **415:**231–239.

Farooqui, A. A., and Horrocks, L. A., 1988, Methods for the determination of phospholipases, lipases and lysophospholipases, in "Neuromethods, Vol. 7, Lipids and Related Compounds" (A. A. Boulton, G. B. Baker, and L. A. Horrocks, eds.), pp. 179–209, Humana Press, Clifton, N. J.

Farooqui, A. A., Pendley, C. E., III, Taylor, W. A., and Horrocks, L. A., 1985, Studies on diacylglycerol lipases and lysophospholipases of bovine brain, in "Phospholipids in the Nervous System," 2nd ed. (L. A. Horrocks, J. N. Kanfer, and G. Porcellati, eds.), pp. 179–192, Raven Press, New York.

Farooqui, A. A., Taylor, W. A., and Horrocks, L. A., 1986, Membrane bound diacylglycerol lipases of bovine brain, in "Proceedings of Membrane Protein Symposium" (S. C. Goheen, ed.), pp. 729–746, Bio-Rad Laboratories, Richmond, Calif.

Farooqui, A. A., Farooqui, T., Yates, A. J., and Horrocks, L. A., 1988, Regulation of protein kinase C activity by various lipids, *Neurochem. Res.* **13:**499–511.

Farooqui, A. A., Rammohan, K. W., Cheng, S., Kolattukudy, P., and Horrocks, L. A., 1989, Membrane bound diacylglycerol lipase in bovine brain: Purification, regulation and cDNA cloning, *Frontiers in Chemistry Biotechnology*, pp. 75–89, compiled by R. E. Strobaugh, Chemical Abstract Service, Columbus, Ohio.

Flamm, E. S., Demopoulos, H. B., and Seligman, M. L., 1978, Free radicals in cerebral ischemia, *Stroke* **9:**445–447.

Flower, R. J., 1988, Lipocortin and the mechanism of action of the glucocorticoids, *Br. J. Pharmacol.* **94:**987–1015.

Flynn, C. J., Farooqui, A. A., and Horrocks, L. A., 1988, Ischemia, hypoxia, and edema, in "Basic Neurochemistry," 4th ed. (G. J. Siegel, R. W. Albers, B. W. Agranoff, and R. Katzman, eds.), pp. 783–795, Raven Press, New York.

Ford, D. A., Hazen, S. L., Saffitz, J. E., and Gross, R. W., 1991, The rapid and reversible activation of a calcium-independent plasmalogen-selective phospholipase A2 during myocardial ischemia, *J. Clin. Invest.* **88:**331–335.

Fourcans, B., and Jain, M. K., 1974, Role of phospholipids in transport and enzymatic reactions, *Adv. Lipid Res.* **12:**147–226.

Freysz, L., Golly, G., Avola, R., Dreyfus, H., and Massarelli, R., 1985, Metabolism of neuronal cell cultures: Modification induced by CDP-choline, in "Novel Biochemistry, Pharmacological and Clinical Aspects of Cytidinediphosphocholine" (V. Zappia, E. P. Kennedy, B. I. Nilsson, and P. Galletti, eds.), pp. 117–129, Elsevier, New York.

Gaudet, R. J., Alam, I., and Levine, L., 1980, Accumulation of cyclooxygenase products of arachidonic and metabolism in gerbil brain during reperfusion after bilateral common carotid artery occlusion, *J. Neurochem.* **35:**653–658.

Goracci, G., Horrocks, L. A., and Porcellati, G., 1977, Reversibility of ethanolamine and choline phosphotransferases (EC 2.7.8.1 and EC 2.7.8.2) in rat brain microsomes with labeled alkylacylglycerols, *FEBS Lett.* **80:**41–44.

Hagberg, H., Lehman, A., and Sandberg, M., 1985, Ischemia-induced shift of inhibitory and excitatory amino acids from intra- to extracellular compartments, *J. Cereb. Blood Flow Metab.* **5:**413–418.

Hall, E. D., 1988, Effect of the 21-aminosteroid U74006F on posttraumatic spinal cord ischemia in cats, *J. Neurosurg.* **68**:462–465.

Hall, E. D., and Braughler, J. M., 1987, The role of oxygen radical-induced lipid peroxidation in acute central nervous system-trauma, *in* "Proceedings of an Upjohn Symposium: Oxygen Radicals and Tissue Injury" (B. Halliwell, ed.), pp. 92–98, Upjohn, Kalamazoo, Mich.

Hall, E. D., and Yonkers, P. A., 1988, Attenuation of postischemic cerebral hypoperfusion by the 21-aminosteroid U74006F, *Stroke* **19**:340–344.

Halliwell, B., and Gutteridge, J. M. C., 1985, Oxygen radicals and the nervous system, *Trends Neurosci.* **8**:22–27.

Harris, E. J., 1977, The uptake and release of calcium by heart mitochondria, *Biochem. J.* **168**:447–456.

Hillered, L., and Chan, P. H., 1988, Role of arachidonic acid and other free fatty acids in mitochondrial dysfunction in brain ischemia, *J. Neurosci. Res.* **20**:451–456.

Hillered, L., and Chan, P. H., 1990, Effects of arachidonic acid on brain mitochondrial function, *in* "Lipid Mediators in Ischemic Brain Damage and Experimental Epilepsy. New Trends in Lipid Mediators Research," vol. 4 (N. G. Bazan, ed.), pp. 190–202, Karger, Basel.

Hirashima, Y., Koshu, K., Kamiyama, K., Nishijima, M., Endo, S., and Takaku, A., 1984, The activities of phospholipase A1, A2, lysophospholipase and acyl CoA: Lysophospholipid acyltransferase in ischemia dog brain, *in* "Recent Progress in the Study and Therapy of Brain Edema" (K. G. Go and A. Baethmann, eds.), pp. 213–221, Plenum Press, New York.

Hirashima, Y., Moto, A., Endo, S., and Takaku, A., 1989, Activities of enzymes metabolizing phospholipid in rat cerebral ischemia, *Mol. Chem. Neuropathol.* **10**:87–100.

Hirashima, Y. A., Takaku, A., Mills, J. S., Farooqui, A. A., and Horrocks, L. A., 1991, Purification and characterization of bovine brain cytosol phospholipase A_2, *J. Neurochem.* **57**:S115B (Abstract).

Hirata, F., 1985, Receptor mediated cascade of phospholipid metabolism, *in* "Phospholipids in the Nervous System," vol. 2 (L. A. Horrocks, J. N. Kanfer, and G. Porcellati, eds.), pp. 99–105, Raven press, New York.

Hirata, F., and Axelrod, J., 1980, Phospholipid methylation and biological signal transmission, *Science* **209**:1082–1090.

Hochachka, P. W., 1986, Defense strategies against hypoxia and hypothermia, *Science* **231**:234–241.

Hoffbrand, B. I., Bingley, P. J., Oppenheimer, S. M., and Sheldon, C. D., 1988, Trial of ganglioside GM1 in acute stroke, *J. Neurol. Neurosurg. Psychiatry* **51**:1213–1214.

Horrocks, L. A., and Dorman, R. V., 1985, Prevention by CDPcholine and CDPethanolamine of lipid changes during brain ischemia, *in* "Novel Biochemistry, Pharmacological and Clinical Aspects of Cytidinediphosphocholine" (V. Zappia, E. P. Kennedy, B. I. Nilsson, and P. Galletti, eds.), pp. 205–215, Elsevier, New York.

Horrocks, L. A., Spanner, S., Mozzi, R., Fu, S. C., D'Amato, R. A., and Krakowka, S., 1978, Plasmalogenase is elevated in early demyelinating lesions, *Adv. Exp. Med. Biol.* **100**:423–438.

Horrocks, L. A., Dorman, R. V., Dabrowiecki, Z., Goracci, G., and Porcellati, G., 1981, CDPcholine and CDPethanolamine prevent the release of free fatty acids during brain ischemia, *Prog. Lipid Res.* **20**:531–534.

Hosobuchi, Y., Baskin, D. S., and Woo, S. K., 1982, Reversal of induced ischemic neurologic deficit in gerbils by the opiate antagonist naloxone, *Science* **215**:69–71.

Hsueh, W., and Needleman, P., 1979, Cardiac and renal lipases and prostaglandin biosynthesis, *Lipids* **14**:236–240.

Janis, R. A., and Triggle, D. J., 1983, New developments in Ca^{2+} channel antagonists, *Med. Chem.* **26**:775–785.

Jenkins, L., Marmarou, A., and Lewelt, W., 1986, Increased vulnerability of the traumatized brain to early ischemia, *in* "Mechanisms of Secondary Brain Damage" (A. Baethmann, ed.), pp. 273–286, Plenum Press, New York.

Kakihana, M., Fukuda, N., Suno, M., and Nagaoka, A., 1988, Effects of CDP-choline on neurologic deficits and cerebral glucose metabolism in a rat model of cerebral ischemia, *Stroke* **19:**217–222.

Karpiak, S. E., Li, Y. S., and Mahadik, S. P., 1987, Gangliosides (GM1 and AGF2) reduce mortality due to ischemia: Protection of membrane function, *Stroke* **18:**184–187.

Kawaguchi, H., and Yasuda, H., 1984, Platelet-activating factor stimulates phospholipase in quiescent Swiss mouse 3T3 fibroblast, *FEBS Lett.* **176:**93–96.

Kidooka, M., Matsuda, M., and Handa, J., 1987, Ca^{2+} antagonist and protection of the brain against ischemia, *Surg. Neurol.* **28:**437–440.

Klausner, R. B., Kleinfeld, A. M., Hoover, R. L., Karnovsky, M. J., 1980, Lipid domains in membranes: Evidence derived from structural perturbations induced by free fatty acids and lifetime heterogeneity analysis, *J. Biol. Chem.* **255:**1286–1295.

Klee, C. B., Crouch, T. H., and Richman, P. G., 1980, Calmodulin, *Annu. Rev. Biochem.* **49:**489–515.

Kochhar, A., Saitoh, T., and Zivin, J., 1989, Reduced protein kinase C activity in ischemic spinal cord, *J. Neurochem.* **53:**946–952.

Kontos, H. A., Wei, E. P., Povlishock, J. T., Dietrich, W. D., Magiera, C. J., and Ellis, E. F., 1980, Cerebral arteriolar damage by arachidonic acid and prostaglandin G_2, *Science* **209:**1242–1244.

Louis, J.-C., Magal, E., and Yavin, E., 1988, Protein kinase C alterations in the fetal rat brain and global ischemia, *J. Biol. Chem.* **263:**19282–19285.

Matsui, Y., Kubo, Y., and Iwata, N., 1987, *S*-Adenosyl-L-methionine prevents ischemic neuronal death, *Eur. J. Pharmacol.* **144:**211–216.

Matthys, E., Patel, Y., Kreisberg, J., Stewart, J. H., and Venkatachalam, M., 1984, Lipid alterations induced by renal ischemia: Pathogenic factor in membrane damage, *Kidney Int.* **26:**153–161.

McDonald, J. W., and Johnston, M. V., 1990, Physiological and pathophysiological roles of excitatory amino acids during central nervous system development, *Brain Res. Rev.* **15:**41–70.

Michell, R. H., Allan, D., and Finean, J. B., 1976, Significance of minor glycerolipids in membrane structure and function, *Adv. Exp. Med. Biol.* **72:**3–13.

Moskowitz, N., Schook, W., and Pushkin, R., 1984, Regulation of endogenous calcium dependent synaptic membrane phospholipase A2, *Brain Res.* **290:**273–279.

Nishizuka, Y., 1986, Studies and perspectives of protein kinase C, *Science* **233:**305–312.

Notsu, Y., Namiuchi, S., Hattori, T., Matsuda, K., and Hirata, F., 1985, Inhibition of phospholipases by Met-Leu-Phe-Ile-Lys-Arg-Ser-Arg-His-Phe, C terminus of middle sized tumor antigen, *Arch. Biochem. Biophys.* **236:**195–204.

Onodera, H., Araki, T., and Kogure, K., 1989, Protein kinase C activity in the rat hippocampus after forebrain ischemia: Autoradiographic analysis by [^{3}H]phorbol 12,13-dibutyrate, *Brain Res.* **481:** 1–7.

Otani, H., Prasad, M. R., Engelman, R. M., Cordis, G. A., and Das, D. K., 1988, Enhanced phosphodiesteratic breakdown and turnover of phosphoinositides during reperfusion of ischemic rat heart, *Circ. Res.* **63:**930–936.

Ozyurt, E., Graham, D. I., Woodruff, G. N., and McCulloch, J., 1988, Protective effect of the glutamate antagonist, MK-801, in focal cerebral ischemia in the cat, *J. Cereb. Blood Flow Metab.* **8:**138–143.

Park, C. K., Nehls, D. G., Graham, D. I., Teasdale, G. M., and McCulloch, J., 1988, Focal cerebral ischaemia in the cat: Treatment with the glutamate antagonist MK-801 after induction of ischaemia, *J. Cereb. Blood Flow Metab.* **8:**757–762.

Rehncrona, S., Mela, L., and Siesjö, B. K., 1979, Recovery of brain mitochondrial function in the rat after complete and incomplete cerebral ischemia, *Stroke* **10:**437–446.

Rordorf, G., Vemura, Y., and Bonventie, J. V., 1991, Characterization of phospholipase A2 (PLA2) activity in gerbil brain: Enhanced activities of cystolic mitochondrial, and microsomal forms after ischemia and reperfusion, *J. Neurosci.* **11:**1829–1836.

Rothman, S., 1984, Synaptic release of excitatory amino acid neurotransmitter mediates anoxic neuronal death, *J. Neurosci. Res.* **4**:1884–1891.

Rothman, S. M., and Olney, J. W., 1986, Glutamate and the pathophysiology of hypoxic-ischemic brain damage, *Ann. Neurol.* **19**:105–109.

Sano, K., Asano, T., and Tanishima, T., 1980, Lipid peroxidation as a cause of cerebral vasospasm, *Neuroscience* **2**:253–261.

Sato, H., Hariyama, H., and Moriguchi, K., 1988, S-adenosyl-L-methionine protects the hippocampal CA1 neurons from the ischemic neuronal death in rat, *Biochem. Biophys. Res. Commun.* **150**: 491–496.

Schanne, F. A., Kane, A. B., Young, E. E., and Farber, J. L., 1979, Calcium dependence of toxic cell death: A common pathway, *Science* **206**:700–702.

Schlaepfer, D. D., and Haigler, H. T., 1987, Characterization of Ca^{2+} dependent phospholipid binding and phosphorylation of lipocortin-I, *J. Biol. Chem.* **262**:6931–6937.

Schlaepfer, W. W., and Zimmerman, U.-J. P., 1985, Mechanisms underlying the neuronal response to ischemic injury. Calcium-activated proteolysis of neurofilaments, *Prog. Brain Res.* **63**:1–12.

Sevanian, A., and Kim, E., 1986, Phospholipase A2 dependent release of fatty acids from peroxidized membrane, *J. Free Radicals Biol. Med.* **1**:263–271.

Siesjö, B. K., 1981, Cell damage in the brain: A speculative synthesis, *J. Cereb. Blood Flow Metab.* **1**:155–185.

Siesjö, B. K., 1984, Cerebral circulation and metabolism, *J. Neurosurg.* **60**:883–908.

Siesjö, B. K., 1986, Calcium and ischemic brain damage, *Eur. Neurol.* **25**:45–56.

Siesjö, B. K., and Wieloch, T., 1985, Cerebral metabolism in ischaemia: Neurochemical basis for therapy, *Br. J. Anaesth.* **57**:47–62.

Siesjö, B. K., 1990, Calcium in the brain under physiological and pathological conditions, *Eur. Neurol.* **30**:3–9.

Simon, M. F., Clap, H., and Douste-Blazy, L., 1986, Selective inhibition of human platelet phospholipase A2 by buffering cytoplasmic calcium with the fluorescent indicator quin-2: Evidence for different calcium sensitivities for phospholipases A2 and C, *Biochim. Biophys. Acta* **875**: 157–164.

Solomonson, L. P., Leipkalns, V. A., and Spector, A. A., 1976, Changes in ($Na^+ + K^+$)-ATPase activity of Ehrlich ascites tumor cells produced by alteration of membrane fatty acid composition, *Biochemistry* **15**:892–897.

Sun, G. Y., and Foudin, L. L., 1984, On the status of lysolecithin in rat cerebral cortex during ischemia, *J. Neurochem.* **43**:1081–1086.

Toffano, G., Savoini, G., Moroni, F., Lombardi, G., Calza, L., and Agnati, L. F., 1983, GM1 ganglioside stimulates the regeneration of dopaminergic neurons in the central nervous system, *Brain Res.* **261**:163–166.

Trovarelli, G., De Medio, G. E., Dorman, R. V., Piccinin, G. L., Horrocks, L. A., and Porcellati, G., 1981, Effect of cytidine diphosphate choline (CDP-choline) on ischemia-induced alterations of brain lipid in the gerbil, *Neurochem. Res.* **6**:821–833.

Trovarelli, G., De Medio, G. E., Porcellati, S., Stramentinoli, G., and Porcellati, G., 1983, The effect of S-adenoysl-L-methionine on ischemia-induced disturbances of brain phospholipid in the gerbil, *Neurochem. Res.* **8**:1597–1609.

van Scharrenburg, G. J. M., Slotboom, A. J., de Haas, G. H., Mulqueen, P., Breen, P. J., and Horrocks, D. W., 1985, Catalytic Ca^{2+}-binding site of pancreatic phospholipase A2: Laser- induced Eu^{3+} luminescence, *Biochemistry* **24**:334–339.

Watson, B. D., and Ginsberg, M. D., 1988, Mechanisms of lipid peroxidation potentiated by ischemia in brain, *in* "Proceedings of an Upjohn Symposium: Oxygen Radicals and Tissue Injury," (B. Halliwell, ed.), pp. 81–91, Upjohn, Kalamazoo, Mich.

Watson, B. D., Busto, R., and Goldberg, W. J., 1984, Lipid peroxidation in vivo induced by reversible global ischemia in rat brain, *J. Neurochem.* **42:**268–274.

Wei, E. P., Kontos, H. A., and Dietrich, W. D., 1981, Inhibition by free radical scavengers and by cyclooxygenase inhibitors of pial arteriolar abnormalities from concussive brain injury in cats, *Circ. Res.* **48:**95–102.

Welch, K. M. A., and Barkley, G. L., 1986, Biochemistry and pharmacology of cerebral ischemia, *in* "Stroke: Pathophysiology, Diagnosis and Management," vol. 1 (H. J. M. Barnett, B. M. Stein, J. P. Mohr, and F. M. Yatsu, eds.), pp. 75–90, Churchill Livingstone, New York.

Weltzien, H. U., 1979, Cytolytic and membrane-perturbing properties of lysophosphatidylcholine, *Biochim. Biophys. Acta* **559:**259–287.

Westerberg, E., Kehr, J., Ungerstedt, U., and Wieloch, T., 1988, The NMDA-antagonist MK-801 reduces extracellular amino acid levels during hypoglycemia and prevents striatal damage, *Neurosci. Res. Commun.* **3:**151–158.

White, B. C., Winegar, C. D., Wilson, R. F., Hoehner, P. J., and Trombley, J. H., Jr., 1983, Possible role of calcium blockers in cerebral resuscitation: A review of the literature and synthesis for future studies, *Crit. Care Med.* **11:**202–207.

Wieloch, T., 1985, Neurochemical correlates to regional selective neuronal vulnerability, *Prog. Brain Res.* **63:**69–85.

Wojtczak, L., 1976, Effect of long-chain fatty acids and acyl-CoA on mitochondrial permeability, transport and energy coupling processes, *J. Bioenerg. Ser. B.* **8:**293–301.

Wong, E. H. F., Kemp, J. A., Priestley, T., Knight, A. R., Woodruff, G. N., and Iversen, L. L., 1986, The anticonvulsant MK-801 is a potent N-methyl-D-aspartate antagonist, *Proc. Natl. Acad. Sci. USA* **83:**7104–7108.

Yamamoto, M., Shima, T., Uozumi, T., Sogabe, T., Yamada, K., and Kawasaki, T., 1983, A possible role of lipid peroxidation in cellular damages caused by cerebral ischemia and the protective effect of α-tocopherol administration, *Stroke* **14:**977–982.

Yoshida, S., Abe, K., Busto, R., Watson, B. D., Kogure, K., and Ginsberg, M. D., 1982, Influence of transient ischemia on lipid-soluble antioxidants, free fatty acids and energy metabolites in rat brain, *Brain Res.* **245:**307–316.

Yoshida, S., Busto, R., Watson, B. D., Santiso, M., and Ginsberg, M. D., 1985, Postischemic cerebral lipid peroxidation in vitro: Modification by dietary vitamin E, *J. Neurochem.* **44:**1593–1601.

Yoshida, S., Ideda, M., Busto, R., Santiso, M., Martinez, E., and Ginsberg, M. D., 1986, Cerebral phosphoinositide, triacylglycerol, and energy metabolism in reversible ischemia: Origin and fate of free fatty acids, *J. Neurochem.* **47:**744–757.

Young, W., Wojak, J. C., and DeCrescito, V., 1988, 21-Aminosteroid reduces ion shifts and edema in the rat middle cerebral artery occlusion model of regional ischemia, *Stroke* **19:**1013–1019.

ARACHIDONIC ACID LIPOXYGENASE PRODUCTS PARTICIPATE IN THE PATHOGENESIS OF DELAYED CEREBRAL ISCHEMIA

TAKASHI WATANABE, TAKAO ASANO, and TAKAO SHIMIZU

1. INTRODUCTION

It is well known that oxyhemoglobin and its breakdown products potently catalyze lipid peroxidation (Willis, 1966; Barber and Bernheim, 1967). Following sub-

TAKASHI WATANABE • Division of Neurosurgery, Institute of Neurological Sciences, Tottori University of Medicine, Yonago, Japan.   TAKAO ASANO • Department of Neurosurgery, Saitama Medical Center, Saitama Medical School, Saitama, Japan.   TAKAO SHIMIZU • Department of Biochemistry, Faculty of Medicine, University of Tokyo, Tokyo, Japan.

Neurochemical Correlates of Cerebral Ischemia, Volume 7 of *Advances in Neurochemistry*, edited by Nicolas G. Bazan, Pierre Braquet, and Myron D. Ginsberg. Plenum Press, New York, 1992.

arachnoid hemorrhage (SAH) due to aneurysmal rupture, the subarachnoid space is filled with blood clot, and subsequent erythrocyte lysis leads to the release of oxyhemoglobin. Eventually, cerebral arteries within the subarachnoid space are exposed to oxyhemoglobin and its breakdown products for a considerable length of time. Since the pathogenetic mechanism underlying cerebral vasospasm, a major complication of subarachnoid hemorrhage (SAH) due to aneurysmal rupture has remained elusive despite extensive research efforts, it seems to be a plausible hypothesis that lipid peroxidation triggered by clot lysis is involved in cerebral vasospasm (Asano *et al.*, 1981). We have already shown that the cerebrospinal fluid (CSF) level of lipid peroxides, particularly thiobarbituric acid-reactive substance (TBA-RS), was significantly higher in SAH patients who manifested symptoms of vasospasm than in those who did not (Sasaki *et al.*, 1982). Furthermore, the elevation of the CSF level of TBA-RS in SAH patients was found to be accompanied by a decrease in the CSF level of vitamin E or in the activity of CSF glutathione peroxidase and by a reciprocal activation of serum glutathione peroxidase (Watanabe *et al.*, 1988a). It seems noteworthy that the above alterations in lipid peroxides in the CSF and free-radical scavengers in the CSF or serum became prominent from 4 to 14 days after SAH, concomitant with the occurrence of delayed cerebral vasospasm.

On the other hand, autoxidation catalyzed by heme compounds is not the sole mechanism leading to lipid peroxidation. The arachidonate cascade represents the other form of lipid peroxidation, namely the enzymatic one, and the involvement of various cyclooxygenase products in the occurrence of cerebral vasospasm has been the subject of extensive research. In this regard, attention has been first directed to the vasoconstrictive prostaglandins (PGE_2, $PGF_{2\alpha}$), and then to thromboxane A_2 (TxA_2). However, the role of these vasoconstrictive PGs has remained questionable, because their levels in the CSF of SAH patients were shown to be far below the concentrations required to cause a significant constriction of the cerebral artery in vitro. TxA_2 probably synthesized and released immediately after SAH, and it has a very short half-life (Walker and Pickard, 1985). Therefore, the involvement of TxA_2 in delayed vasospasm seems unlikely unless there is a certain mechanism which permits a continuous adhesion and aggregation of platelets in the cerebral artery.

In contrast to vasoconstrictive PGs and TxA_2, prostacyclin, which is generated mainly in the vascular endothelium, inhibits the constriction of cerebral arteries that is induced by various agents (Asano *et al.*, 1982; Uski *et al.*, 1983). We showed a progressive diminution of prostacyclin synthesis in the canine basilar artery exposed to experimental SAH (Sasaki *et al.*, 1981a). This decrease in prostacyclin synthesis seems to be due to degenerative change: in the vascular endothelium, since the former occurred before the latter. Although both the increased production of TxA_2 and the decreased production of prostacyclin may play some role in symptomatic vasospasm, the administration of a TxA_2 synthetase inhibitor or a prostacyclin derivative in clinical trials did not prevent delayed vasospasm (angiographic spasm) in SAH patients (Sano *et al.*, 1986).

The whole group of lipoxygenase products are newcomers to the eicosanoid family. Arachidonic acid lipoxygenase products, such as leukotrienes (LTs), are considered possible candidates for the spasmogenic substance, because they are the chemical mediators of inflammation, possessing potent chemotactic and vasoactive properties (Goetzl, 1981; Nakao *et al.*, 1982; Larsen and Henson, 1983; Samuelsson, 1983; Lands *et al.*, 1984). However, since the data concerning the vasocontractile action of lipoxygenase products are inconsistent and the data on their synthesis following SAH are scanty (Koide *et al.*, 1982; Kamitani *et al.*, 1985; Walker and Pickard, 1985; Spallone *et al.*, 1987; Baena *et al.*, 1988), the exact role of lipoxygenase products in delayed vasospasm remains to be determined.

This paper deals with the role of lipoxygenase products in delayed cerebral vasospasm. In the first part, results of hydroxyeicosatetraenoic acid (HETE) determination in the CSF, subarachnoid clot, and the basilar artery in the canine SAH model are presented. In reference to the possible mechanism underlying the activation of 5-lipoxygenase in the cerebral artery following SAH, the effect of a lipid hydroperoxide, 15-HPETE, on the lipoxygenase activity of the canine basilar artery is also discussed. The findings that a significant amount of 12-HETE existed in the cisternal clot and that the lipoxygenase activity of the cerebral artery is stimulated by a lipid hydroperoxide, 15-HPETE, led us to suspect that its precursor, 12-HPETE, may be the culprit. Therefore, we prepared a large amount of 12-HPETE and injected it into the cisterna magna in dogs to see whether cerebral vasospasm was induced. This study is described in detail in the second part of the paper.

2. HETE DETERMINATION

2.1. Materials and Methods

2.1.1. *Operative Procedures*

Adult mongrel dogs weighing 9 to 14 kg were anesthetized by intravenous injection of pentobarbital (30 mg/kg). After endotracheal intubation each animal was left to breathe spontaneously, and the head was placed in a stereotaxic frame. In the supine position the right vertebral artery was exposed and cannulated through a small midline skin incision, and the control angiogram was taken with contrast medium. After removal of the arterial cannula and the closure of the wound, the dog was turned back and was fixed in the prone position. The cisterna magna was punctured with a no. 22 needle, and autologous arterial blood (0.2 ml/

kg) was slowly injected about 1 min after removal of the same amount of CSF. After the injection, the dog was kept in the head-down position for 20 min. On day 3, i.e., 48 hr after the first cisternal blood injection, a second injection was performed in a similar fashion. The repeat angiogram was taken via the left vertebral artery on days 2, 3, 5, 8, and 15. The diameter of the basilar artery visualized on the angiogram was measured at the midpoint between its bifurcation and the vertebrobasilar junction. The magnitude of vasospasm in each dog was expressed as the diameter ratio, calculated as the percent ratio of the basilar arterial diameter of a given angiogram to that of the control. Samples of the clot, the CSF, the serum, and the basilar artery were obtained after various time intervals following SAH. Each animal was sacrificed by exsanguination under pentobarbital anesthesia, and the brain was perfused with ice-cold saline containing heparin (5 U/ml). The clivus was removed, and the anterior surface of the pons was exposed to examine the presence of the clot in the subarachnoid space. Animals in which clot formation along the basilar artery was not sufficient were excluded from the study. The subarachnoid clot obtained from each dog ranged from 26 to 56 mg (wet weight). The basilar artery was excised and placed on an ice-cold glass plate. Under an operating microscope, the clot adhering to the artery was meticulously removed.

The magnitude of vasospasm induced in the two-hemorrhage model was compared with that in a one-hemorrhage model. In the latter model, autologous blood (0.8 ml/kg) was injected into cisterna magna only once, and angiography was carried out on days 1 and 8.

2.1.2. HPLC Measurement of HETE Content

Each sample of the subarachnoid clot, 1 ml of CSF, 1 ml of the serum, and the basilar artery segment was homogenized with 2.5 ml of methanol containing 3 nmol of 13-hydroxylinoleic acid as an internal standard for high-pressure liquid chromatography (HPLC) analysis. The solution was kept at $-20°C$ for at least 30 min and centrifuged at 2000 rpm for 15 min, and the supernatant was dried under a stream of N_2. The residue was dissolved in 0.4 ml of solvent A (acetonitrile-methanol-water-acetic acid, 350:150:250:1 by volume) and subjected to reverse-phase HPLC on a Toyo Soda TSK ODS-80TM column (5 μm, 0.46 × 15 cm), which was maintained at 35°C. The flow rate of solvent A was 0.7 ml/min, and the absorbance at 234 nm was monitored. The HETE content was determined by measuring the peak area ration with the internal standard, calculated by using a Shimadzu Chromatopac CR-3A. Each HETE was converted to a methyl ester by using an ethereal solution of diazomethane after reverse-phase HPLC isolation, and further substantiated by straight-phase HPLC with a column (Nucleosil 50-5; 0.46 × 25 cm) eluted with solvent B (hexane-isopropyl alcohol-acetic acid, 99:1:0.01 by volume; flow rate, 0.7 ml/min). Only the values measured by reverse-phase HPLC were used in this study, because the reverse-phase HPLC and the straight-phase HPLC gave almost identical values.

2.1.3. Stimulation of the Basilar Artery with A23187

To evaluate the lipoxygenase activities, basilar artery segments from normal dogs and those exposed to the two-hemorrhage procedure (day 8) were cut into small pieces with scissors and incubated for 5 min at 37°C in 0.5 ml of tris-Tyrode solution with 2 μM A23187 and 80 μM arachidonic acid. The products were analyzed by HPLC. For analysis of HETEs, the method described above was used. To determine the synthesis of leukotrienes, the evaporated sample was dissolved in 0.2 ml of solvent B (acetonitrile-methanol-water-acetic acid, 3:1:3:0.006 by volume, including 0.05% EDTA-Na$_2$, adjusted to pH 5.6 with ammonia water) and analyzed by HPLC equipped with the same Toyo Soda column at 280 nm. Prostaglandin B$_2$ (PGB$_2$) was used as an internal standard. The basilar artery obtained from dogs subjected to a sham operation without the cisternal blood injection was used as the control. The protein content in each sample of the basilar artery was measured by the method of Lowry *et al.* (1951).

2.1.4. Identification of HETEs and LTB$_4$ by GC-MS

HETEs and LTB$_4$ were further identified by gas chromatography-mass spectrometry (GC-MS) with the Shimadzu gas chromatography-mass spectrometer model QP-1000. Equipped columns contained 2% OV-1 (3 mm × 2 m) for HETEs analysis and 2% OV-1 (3.4 mm × 2 m) for LTB$_4$. The temperatures of the column and injector were 230°C for HETEs and 260°C for LTB$_4$.

2.2. Results

The diameter ratio in the two-hemorrhage SAH model was 81.1 ± 71.5% (mean ± SD, $n = 5$) on day 5, 84.6 ± 5.51% ($n = 5$) on day 3, 63.0 ± 11.0% ($n = 5$) on day 5, 41.3 ± 4.59% ($n = 19$) on day 8, and 61.2 ± 4.85% ($n = 6$) on day 15. The vasospasm in the two-hemorrhage model reached its peak on day 8. At this period, there was a significant difference in the diameter ratio between the one-hemorrhage (70.2 ± 14.8%, $n = 8$) and two-hemorrhage models (Figure 1). Results for the HETE content showed that the subarachnoid clot contained only 12-HETE (Table 1). No HETEs were detected in the watery-clear or bloody CSF (Table 2). The serum contained 5- and 12-HETEs. The serum content of 12-HETE was significantly greater on day 8 than on day 1 (Table 3). The representative HPLC charts analyzing the serum HETE content are shown in Figure 2. No HETE was found in the plasma or in the basilar artery segment sampled at various time intervals. Only the activity of 5-lipoxygenase was detected in the canine basilar

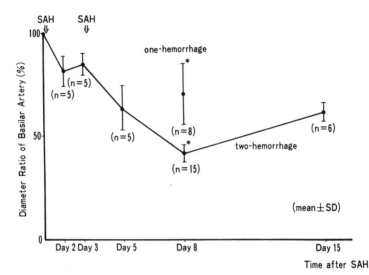

FIGURE 1. Alterations in the diameter ratio of the basilar artery in one- and two-hemorrhage models. *P < 0.001 (Student's *t* test).

artery segment. The result of HPLC analysis of products after incubation of the canine basilar artery with A23187 is shown in Figure 3. The basilar artery exposed to SAH produced a large amount of 5-HETE, whereas only a trace amount of 5-HETE was generated by the normal basilar artery (Table 4). Furthermore, the basilar artery which underwent vasospasm produced LTB_4 and LTC_4, but the normal basilar artery did not (Figure 4). In fact, considerable amounts of LTB_4 and LTC_4 were produced by the basilar artery which underwent vasospasm (Table 5). GC-MS was used for the identification of 12-HETE in the subarachnoid clot and for 5-HETE or LTB_4 in the basilar artery segment (Figures 5 and 6). LTC_4 was determined by radioimmunoassay (RIA).

TABLE 1. 12-HETE Content of Subarachnoid Clot

Day	12-HETE content (nmol/g)[a]
2	1.88 ± 2.00 (*n* = 5)
3	1.29 ± 0.60 (*n* = 5)
5	1.76 ± 2.43 (*n* = 5)
8	1.89 ± 2.16 (*n* = 6)

[a]Values are expressed as the mean ± SD.

TABLE 2. HETEs in CSF

Day 1	Day 8
Not detected ($n = 5$)	Not detected ($n = 5$)

TABLE 3. HETEs of Serum

HETE	Amount (nmol/ml)[a]	
	Day 1	Day 8
5-HETE	2.82 ± 1.86 ($n = 4$)	2.40 ± 0.70 ($n = 4$)
12-HETE	1.05 ± 0.30* ($n = 4$)	2.01 ± 0.56* ($n = 4$)

[a]Values are expressed as the mean ± SD. *$P < 0.01$ (t test).

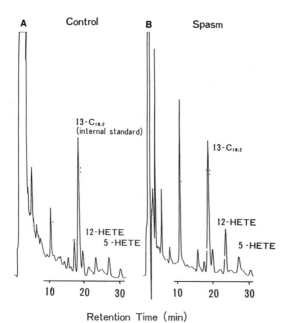

FIGURE 2. Reverse-phase HPLC analysis of serum. The absorbance at 234 nm was monitored. The serum on day 8 (B) contained more 12-HETE than did the serum on day 1 (A).

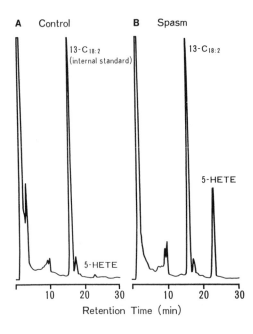

FIGURE 3. Reverse-phase HPLC analysis of HETEs produced by the basilar artery segment incubated with arachidonic acid and A23187. The absorbance at 234 nm was monitored. The artery exposed to two hemorrhages (B) produced far more 5-HETE than did the normal control (A).

2.3. Discussion

The canine two-hemorrhage model produced more pronounced vasospasm of the basilar artery than did the canine one-hemorrhage model. The severity of vasospasm in each dog as seen by angiography seemed to depend on the amount of subarachnoid clot formed along the basilar artery, and this seems to be the reason why the two-hemorrhage model induced more severe vasospasm than the one-hemorrhage models. On excising the subarachnoid clot from the basilar artery, however, it was noticed that even when a certain amount of clot was present along the artery, pronounced spasm never developed unless the clot firmly adhered to the artery, leaving no space for the CSF to dissipate between them.

TABLE 4. Formation of 5-HETE after Stimulation
of Basilar Artery with A23187

Model	Amount of 5-HETE (nmol/mg of protein)[a]
Two-hemorrhage	1.34 ± 0.52 ($n \pm 5$)
Control	0.01 ± 0.01 ($n = 5$)

[a]Values are expressed as mean $\pm$ SD. There is statistical significance ($P < 0.01$; t test).

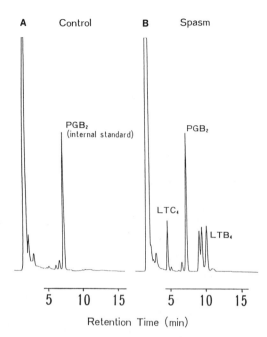

FIGURE 4. Reverse-phase HPLC analysis of products after incubation of the basilar artery with arachidonic acid and A32187. The absorbance at 280 nm was monitored. The artery exposed to SAH (B) produced LTB$_4$ and LTC$_4$, but the control artery (A) did not.

Although we had expected that various HETEs would be produced by nonenzymatic lipid peroxidation, only 12-HETE was detected in the subarachnoid clot. This indicates that the nonenzymatic reactions are not the preponderant mechanism underlying lipid peroxidation in the subarachnoid clot. It cannot be excluded, however, that very small amounts of various HETEs escaped detection by the present HPLC technique.

Whereas 5- and 12-HETEs were found in the serum from days 2 to 8 following SAH, no HETE was detected in the plasma obtained from the

TABLE 5. Formation of Leukotrienes after Stimulation of Basilar Artery with A23187

	Amount (nmol/mg of protein)[a]	
Model	LTB$_4$	LTC$_4$
Two-hemorrhage	0.085 ± 0.012 ($n = 3$)	0.072 ± 0.014 ($n = 3$)
Control	ND[b] ($n = 3$)	ND ($n = 3$)

[a]Values are expressed as the mean ± SD.
[b]ND, not detected.

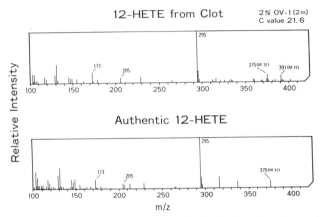

FIGURE 5. Mass-spectrometric identification of 12-HETE obtained from the subarachnoid clot. This mass spectrum, with the background subtracted, is compatible with that of authentic 12-HETE.

heparinized blood. Therefore, HETEs detected in the serum or the subarachnoid clot are believed to have been derived from platelets or leukocytes in the blood. In dogs, red blood cells reportedly have 12-lipoxygenase activity (Kobayashi and Levine, 1983); therefore, it may also have participated in the production of 12-HETE within the subarachnoid clot. The increased serum content of 12-HETE on day 8 probably is a reflection of an enhanced platelet function attributable to a reported (Denton *et al.*, 1971) increase in platelet aggregability in SAH patients.

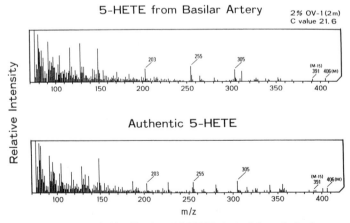

FIGURE 6. Mass-spectrometric identification of 5-HETE obtained from the basilar artery (above). This mass spectrum is identical to that of authenthic 5-HETE (below).

As the endothelial cells undergo degenerative changes concomitant with the occurrence of cerebral vasospasm (Sasaki *et al.*, 1981*b*), platelets and leukocytes adhering to the damaged intima may release their lipoxygenase products into the arterial wall.

No HETE was detected in the CSF of the present SAH model. However, we have already reported that 5-HETE was present in the CSF of SAH patients (Suzuki *et al.*, 1983) at a level which seemed to parallel the time course of cerebral vasospasm. More recently, the CSF content of LTC_4 was shown to increase following SAH (Baena *et al.*, 1988). Since the CSF level of LTs was not measured in the present study, it is not clear whether LTs were increased in the CSF of the present SAH model. The reason why 5-HETE was not detected within the CSF in this study may be that the hemorrhage and subsequent leukocytosis in the present SAH model was not so severe as in the human SAH. Nevertheless, the firm adherence of the subarachnoid clot to the cerebral artery where vasospasm developed suggests that the CSF did not serve as a vehicle for putative spasmogenic substances. It seems more likely that any spasmogenic substance produced in the subarachnoid clot is directly conveyed to the arterial wall by a diffusional process, not via the CSF. Therefore, the CSF level of any substances would be a mere reflection of their generation by the cells and tissues in and around the CSF space.

The basilar artery segment itself contained no measurable amount of HETEs. However, on incubation with arachidonic acid and A23187, the basilar artery segment exposed to SAH produced a large amount of 5-HETE, more than 100-fold that of the control. The same basilar artery segment also produced significant amounts of LTB_4 and LTC_4, whereas the unexposed basilar artery segment did not. Furthermore, we have shown by assaying enzymatic activities that 5-lipoxygenase activity of the basilar artery exposed to SAH was enhanced about 20-fold over that of the control artery whereas the activities of both LTA_4 hydrolase, which converts LTA_4 to LTB_4, and glutathione-S-transferase, i.e., LTC_4 synthetase, remained unchanged (Shimizu *et al.*, 1988). Thus, the key event leading to the enhancement of the 5-lipoxygenase pathway in the basilar artery following SAH is the increase in the activity of 5-lipoxygenase.

One possible explanation for the above phenomenon is that following SAH, the basilar artery newly acquires 5-lipoxygenase activity through the migration of leukocytes into the arterial wall. In human autopsy specimens, SAH is regularly accompanied by leukocytosis in the subarachnoid space (Hughes and Schianchi, 1978). Some cells resembling leukocytes are occasionally found within the arterial wall (Smith *et al.*, 1985), although this is not a prominent feature. In the present model, leukocyte infiltration into the arterial wall was only rarely observed. As far as the present model is concerned, therefore, it seems rather unlikely that 5-lipoxygenase is conveyed to the cerebral artery by leukocyte infiltration, although this possibility cannot be totally ruled out.

An alternative explanation is that intrinsic 5-lipoxygenase of the basilar artery was stimulated by 12-HPETE derived from the subarachnoid clot or from the platelets adhering to the intima. It has been shown that human leukocyte 5-lipoxygenase is activated by 12-HPETE released from platelets (Maclouf *et al.*, 1982). Similarly, the already increased 5-lipoxygenase activity of the basilar artery segment exposed to SAH was found to be further enhanced by 15-HPETE in a dose-dependent fashion in the concentration range of 10^{-8} to 10^{-6} M (Shimizu *et al.*, 1988). Since the subarachnoid clot contained 12-HETE in the micromolar concentration range, it seems possible that its precursor, 12-HPETE, attains a similar concentration range, particularly when blood dissipating from the ruptured aneurysm into the subarachnoid space forms a clot around cerebral arteries. The concomitant massive activation of platelets and leukocytes would lead to liberation of a large quantity of 12-HPETE, which diffuses into the arterial wall, stimulating its 5-lipoxygenase. In addition to the subarachnoid clot, platelets and leukocytes in the circulating blood would adhere to the damage intima, continuously supplying some 12-HPETE to the arterial wall.

So far, our data show that SAH is followed by activation of 12-lipoxygenase in the subarachnoid clot and of 5-lipoxygenase in the arterial wall, the former presumably triggering the latter. In this regard, it is known that a trace amount of oxygen free radicals or lipid peroxides is needed to start cyclooxygenase or lipoxygenases of the arachidonate cascade (Lands *et al.*, 1984). Therefore, it is tempting to speculate that preceding the activation of 12-lipoxygenase, there is an initial increase in the ambient level of free radicals which triggers and reinforces the subsequent activation of lipoxygenases. As stated above, the CSF space following SAH is deficient in free-radical scavenging capacity and rich in catalytic heme compounds. Whether this particular condition would lead to the initiation and propagation of lipid peroxidation due to free radical reactions remains to be clarified.

Regarding the possible actions of lipoxygenase products, it is easy to see correspondence between their known biological properties and the functional or morphological features of cerebral vasospasm, e.g., cell infiltration, increased permeability, decreased PGI_2 synthetic capacity, and smooth muscle contraction (Goetzl, 1981; Sasaki *et al.*, 1981a; Koide *et al.*, 1982). We have observed that 12-HPETE has a potent vasocontractile capacity comparable to that of 15-HPETE, whereas 12-HETE does not (unpublished data). In addition, the oxidant released from 12- or 5-HPETE in the conversion to the respective HETEs may inactivate the endothelium-derived relaxing factor (EDRF), since another species of oxygen radical, superoxide anion, reportedly does (Gryglewski *et al.*, 1986).

Putting the above pieces of evidence together, it may be conjectured that these lipoxygenase products act together to induce the complex pathological events in the cerebral artery, which culminate in cerebral vasospasm. Of prime importance among these lipoxygenase products seems to be 12-HPETE because it is presumably released at a high concentration, immediately following aneurysmal rupture and subsequent clot formation. The above speculation led us to undertake an experiment to see whether cisternal injection of 12-HPETE would provoke cerebral vasospasm. The study, which will be reported in detail elsewhere, is briefly described below.

3. EFFECT OF 12-HPETE ON CEREBRAL VASOSPASM

3.1. Materials and Methods

3.1.1. Preparation of 12-HPETE and 12-HETE

Partially purified porcine leukocyte 12-lipoxygenase was prepared by the method of Yoshimoto *et al.* (1982) and was precooled at 4°C for 5 min in 0.1 M tris-HCl buffer (pH 7.4) containing 0.03% Tween 20. Arachidonic acid was added to initiate the incubation, which was performed for 20 min at 4°C while stirring under a stream of oxygen. Ice-cold methanol was added to the reaction mixture to stop the incubation, and the resulting mixture was kept at $-20°C$ for 30 min and then subjected to centrifugation at $10,000 \times g$ for 15 min. The supernatant was acidified (to pH 2.5) with 6 M HCl, and the products were extracted with diethyl ether by the method of Borgeat and Samuelsson (1979). Products, i.e., 12-HPETE and 12-HETE, were purified on a straight-phase HPLC column (Nucleosil 50-5, 10×300 mm) with hexane-isopropanol-acetic acid (99:1:0.01 by volume; 5 ml/min flow rate, at room temperature) as the mobile phase. The details of these procedures were reported by Kitamura *et al.* (1988).

3.1.2. Cisternal Injection of 12-HPETE and 12-HETE

Adult mongrel dogs, weighing 7–12 kg, were anesthetized by intravenous injection of pentobarbital (30 mg/kg). the right vertebral artery was catheterized for angiography. The dogs were divided into three groups as follows: In group 1, nine dogs received 0.5 mg of 12-HPETE dissolved in 1 ml of 100 mM $NaHCO_3 \cdot NaOH$ (pH 9.1) intracisternally. In group 2, three dogs received 0.5 mg of 12-HETE in the same manner. In group 3, three dogs received only 1 ml of the solvent. Angiograms were obtained before and after the cisternal injection at various time intervals. The diameter of the basilar artery was measured at the midpoint, and the magnitude of vasospasm was expressed as the ratio of the diameter of the basilar artery to the control value. From one dog which received 12-HPETE, 100 μl of CSF was collected over a fixed time schedule after the cisternal injection. The samples were subjected to reverse-phase HPLC to determine the 12-HPETE and 12-HETE content, as described above.

3.2. Results

Figure 7 shows the straight-phase HPLC chart of the products of porcine leukocyte 12-lipoxygenase and demonstrates the separation of 12-HPETE, 12-HETE, and arachidonic acid. In group 1, vasoconstriction of the basilar artery was not observed during the initial 6 hr after the cisternal injection. Thereafter, prolonged constriction of the basilar artery started, lasting for 5 days (Figure 8). Representative sequential angiograms are shown in Figure 9. The angiogram on day 3 revealed the constriction of not only the basilar artery but also all the intracisternal artery. In groups 2 and 3, no definite constriction of the basilar artery was seen throughout the observation period (Figure 10). The CSF content of 12-HETE decreased very rapidly following the cisternal injection of 12-HPETE (Figure 11), and it was undetectable from day 2. Although a relatively large amount of 12-HPETE (0.5 mg) was injected into the cisterna magna, it was detected even in the CSF sampled 20 min after the injection.

3.3. Discussion

The present study revealed that prolon3ed constriction of the basilar artery and other cerebral arteries is induced by a single intracisternal injection of 12-

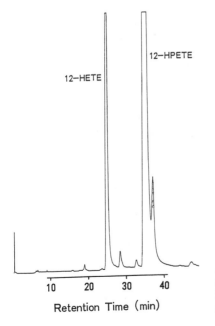

FIGURE 7. Straight-phase HPLC analysis of products after incubation of arachidonic acid with porcine leukocyte 12-lipoxygenase. The peak of 12-HPETE is clearly separate from that of 12-HETE.

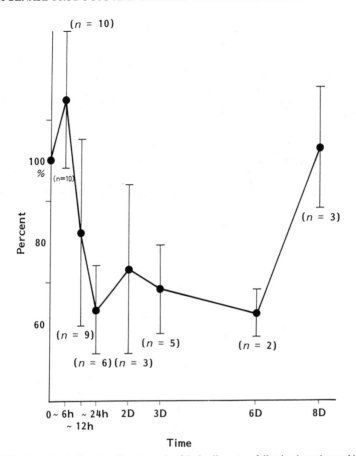

FIGURE 8. Alteration in the mean diameter ratio of the basilar artery following intracisternal injection of 12-HPETE.

HPETE. This vasoconstriction mimics cerebral vasospasm in that it has a delayed onset and a long duration once started. The magnitude and the time course of basilar artery constriction induced by 12-HPETE were comparable to those for vasospasm incurred in the one-hemorrhage model.

The above result agrees with our previous finding that the intracisternal injection of 15-HPETE in dogs causes a prolonged constriction of the basilar artery (Sasaki *et al.*, 1981*b*). The consistency between the effects of 12- and 15-HPETEs on the cerebral artery is not surprising, because these compounds share common properties as species of hydroperoxides of arachidonic acid. Rather, the importance of the present study lies in the fact that 12-HPETE, the precursor of 12-HETE, which was found to exist in the subarachnoid clot, actually induced

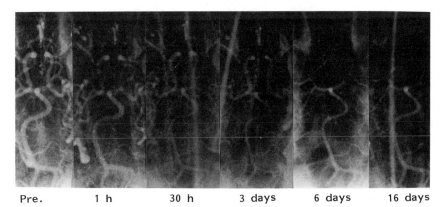

Pre.   1 h   30 h   3 days   6 days   16 days

FIGURE 9. Angiograms obtained before and after cisternal injection of 12-HPETE. In addition to the basilar artery, other intracisternal arteries were also constricted; this was particularly evident in the angiogram obtained on day 3.

prolonged constriction of cerebral arteries by a single intracisternal injection. The amount of 15-HPETE needed to elicit prolonged vasoconstriction (2 mg) was larger than that of 12-HPETE (0.5 mg). This minor discrepancy may be attributed to the difference in the pharmacological actions of the two compounds or to the difference in the vehicles used in the two studies. Nevertheless, the similarity between the effects of 12- and 15-HPETE indicates that any hydroperoxide of arachidonic acid would be capable of inducing prolonged constriction of cerebral arteries. It may be further surmised that the free radical, namely the oxygen-centered radical released from these hydroperoxides, might be the real spasmogenic substance. This is supported by the findings that 12-HETE caused no vasoconstriction and that the administration of free-radical scavengers such as 1,2-bis(nicotinamido)propane or glutathione inhibited vasospasm in the canine SAH model (Asano et al., 1984; Watanabe et al., 1988b).

The rapid disappearance of 12-HPETE from the CSF followed by the immediate appearance of 12-HETE indicates that 12-HPETE is very rapidly converted to 12-HETE in the CSF space. 12-HETE also disappears from the CSF rapidly, prior to the onset of prolonged vasoconstriction. This rapid disappearance of both 12-HPETE and 12-HETE precludes the possibility that these compounds induce prolonged vasoconstriction through their direct contractile action on the vascular smooth muscle.

Since the result of the present study is clear enough to designate 12-HPETE as the culprit responsible for SAH-induced vasospasm, the next question is why transient exposure of the cerebral artery to 12-HPETE resulted in its prolonged constriction. A possible approach to this problem would be to seek a metabolite of

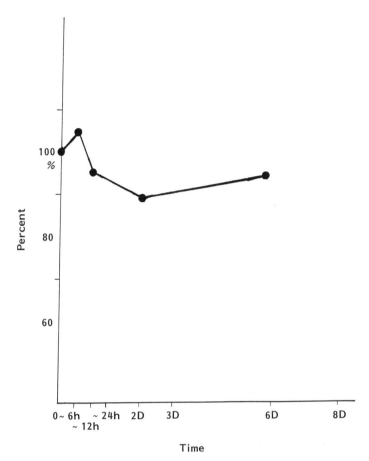

FIGURE 10. Alteration of the mean diameter ratio of the basilar artery following cisternal injection of 12-HETE.

12-HPETE that continuously existed in the subarachnoid space and exerted a contractile effect on the vascular smooth muscle. Such a substance may be found in the light of recent findings about the products of the 12-lipoxygenase pathway (Piomelli *et al.*, 1987; Setty *et al.*, 1987; Westlund, 1987; Kitamura *et al.*, 1988). Alternatively, the effect of 12-HPETE on the cerebral artery may be viewed with reference to the mechanism underlying radiation necrosis. Both 12-HPETE and irradiation cause free-radical damage to cells, the effects of which are delayed in onset. Therefore, it would not be totally absurd to postulate that 12-HPETE causes a long-lasting alteration in the cellular function which is related to the contraction

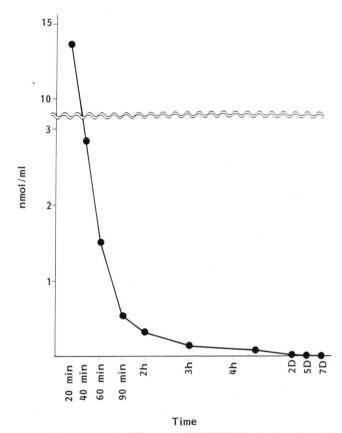

FIGURE 11. Sequential change in the CSF content of 12-HETE following intracisternal injection of 12-HPETE. Although a large amount of 12-HPETE (0.5 mg) was used, it was not detected in the CSF at 20 min after injection.

mechanism of smooth muscle cells. There has been a controversy concerning the mechanism of sustained contraction of smooth muscle. Of particular interest in this regard is the hypothesis that protein kinase C mediates sustained contraction of the smooth muscle (Rasmussen *et al.*, 1987). We have already confirmed that phorbordibutylate, an activator of protein kinase C, causes a potent and long-lasting contraction of the canine basilar artery segment in vitro (unpublished data). 12-HPETE or its metabolites may activate protein kinase C as some derivatives of arachidonic acid and other lipids do (Farooqui *et al.*, 1988). This line of investigation is in progress in our laboratory.

4. CONCLUSION

In summary, the results of our consecutive studies suggest that the activation of lipoxygenase pathways in various tissues may be the cause of cerebral vasospasm following SAH. 12-HPETE generated in the subarachnoid clot probably triggers the activation of 5-lipoxygenase in the arterial wall. Most of the organic changes accompanying cerebral vasospasm are inflammatory and therefore may well be ascribed to the phlogistic properties of lipoxygenase products. The mechanism underlying the 12-HPETE-induced prolonged constriction of the cerebral artery remains elusive. From this unknown, however, a totally new approach may evolve to reveal the mechanism underlying the sustained contraction of the vascular smooth muscle in cerebral vasospasm.

REFERENCES

Asano, T., Tanishima, T., Sasaki, T., and Sano, K., 1981, Possible participation of free radical reactions initiated by clot lysis in the pathogenesis of vasospasm after subarachnoid hemorrhage, in "Cerebral Arterial Spasm" (R. H. Wilkins, ed.), pp. 190–201, Williams & Wilkins, Baltimore.

Asano, T., Sano, K., Ochiai, C., and Takakura, K., 1982, In vitro evaluation of the inhibitory action of PGI_2 to vasoconstrictions induced by various prostaglandins, serotonin and hemoglobin using the canine basilar artery, Neurol. Med. Chir. **22**:507–512.

Asano, T., Sasaki, T., Koide, T., Takakura, K., and Sano, K., 1984, Experimental evaluation of the beneficial effect of an antioxidant on cerebral vasospasm, Neurol. Res. **6**:49–53.

Baena, R. R., Gaetani, P., and Paoletti, P., 1988, A study on cisternal CSF levels of arachidonic acid metabolites after aneurysmal subarachnoid hemorrhage, J. Neurol. Sci. **84**:329–335.

Barber, A. A., and Bernheim, F., 1967, Lipid peroxidation: Its measurement, occurrence, and significance in animal tissue, Adv. Gerontol. Res. **2**:355–403.

Borgeat, P., and Samuelsson, B., 1979, Transformation of arachidonic acid by rabbit polymorphonuclear leukocytes. Formation of a novel dihydroxyeicosatetraenoic acid, J. Biol. Chem. **254**:2643–2646.

Denton, I. C., Robertson, J. T., and Dugdale, M., 1971, An assessment of early platelet activity in experimental subarachnoid hemorrhage and middle cerebral artery thrombosis in the cat, Stroke **2**:268–272.

Farooqui, A. A., Farooqui, T., Yates, A. J., and Horrocks, L. A., 1988, Regulation of protein kinase C activity by various lipids, Neurochem. Res. **13**:499–511.

Goetzl, E. J., 1981, Oxygenation products of arachidonic acid as mediators of hypersensitivity and inflammation, Med. Clin. N. Am. **65**:809–828.

Gryglewski, R. J., Palmer, R. M. J., and Moncada, S., 1986, Superoxide anion is involved in the breakdown of endothelium-derived vascular relaxing factor, Nature **320**:454–456.

Hughes, J. T., and Schianchi, P. M., 1978, Cerebral artery spasm. A histological study at necropsy of the blood vessels in cases of subarachnoid hemorrhage, J. Neurosurg. **48**:515–525.

Kamitani, T., Little, M. H., and Ellis, E. F., 1985, Effect of leukotrienes, 12-HETE, histamine, bradykinin, and 5-hydroxytryptamine on in vitro rabbit cerebral arteriolar diameter, J. Cereb. Blood Flow Metab. **5**:554–559.

Kitamura S., Shimizu, T., Miki, I., Izumi, T., Kasama, T., Sato, A., Sano, H., and Seyama, Y., 1988, Synthesis and structural identification of four dihydroxy acids and 11,12-leukotriene C4 derived from 11,12-leukotriene A4, *Eur. J. Biochem.* **176:**725–731.

Kobayashi, T., and Levine, L., 1983, Arachidonic acid metabolism by erythrocytes, *J. Biol Chem.* **258:** 9116–9121.

Koide, T., Neichi, T., Takato, M., Matsushita, H., Sugioka, K., and Hata, S., 1982, Possible mechanisms of 15-hydroperoxyarachidonic acid-induced contraction of the canine basilar artery in vitro, *J. Pharmacol. Exp. Ther.* **221:**481–488.

Lands, W. E. M., Kulmacz, J. K., and Marshall, P. J., 1984, Lipid peroxide action in the regulation of prostaglandin biosynthesis, *in* "Free Radicals in Biology," vol. 6 (W. A. Pryor, ed.), pp. 39–63, Academic Press, London.

Larsen, G. L., and Henson, P. M., 1983, Mediators of inflammation, *Annu. Rev. Immunol.* **1:**335–359.

Lowry, O. H., Rosebrough, N. J., Farr, A. L., and Randall, R. J., 1951, Protein measurement with the Folin phenol reagent, *J. Biol. Chem.* **193:**265–275.

Maclouf, J., DeLaclos, B. F., and Borgeat, P., 1982, Stimulation of leukotriene biosynthesis in human blood leukocytes by platelet-derived 12-hydroperoxyeicosatetraenoic acid, *Proc. Natl. Acad. Sci. USA* **79:**6042–6046.

Nakao, J., Ooyama, T., Ito, H., Chang, W. C., and Murota, S., 1982, Comparative effect of lipoxygenase products of arachidonic acid on rat aortic smooth muscle cell migration, *Atherosclerosis* **44:**339–342.

Piomelli, D., Volterra, A., Dale, N., Siegelbaum, S. A., Kandell, E. R., Schwartz, J. H., and Balardetti, F., 1987, Lipoxygenase metabolites of arachidonic acid as second messengers for presynaptic inhibition of Aplysia sensory cells, *Nature* **328:**38–43.

Rasmussen, H., Takuwa, Y., and Park, S., 1987, Protein kinase C in the regulation of smooth muscle contraction, *FASEB J.* **1:**177–185.

Samuelsson, B., 1983, Leukotrienes: Mediators of immediate hypersensitivity reaction and inflammation, *Science* **220:**568–575.

Sano, K., Handa, H., Suzuki, S., Asano, T., Tamura, A., Yonekawa, Y., Ono, H., and Tachibana, N., 1986, The utility of OKY 046, a TxA$_2$ synthetase inhibitor, for angiographic and symptomatic vasospasm following subarachnoid hemorrhage due to rupture of intracranial aneurysms: Clinical assessment by a multi-institutional, double blind study, *Igaku No Ayumi (Tokyo)* **138:** 455–469.

Sasaki, T., Murota, S., Wakai, S., Asano, T., and Sano, K., 1981*a*, Evaluation of prostaglandin biosynthetic activity in canine basilar artery following subarachnoid injection of blood, *J. Neurosurg.* **55:**771–778.

Sasaki, T., Wakai, S., Asano, T., Watanabe, T., Kirino, T., and Sano, K., 1981*b*, The effect of a lipid hydroperoxide of arachidonic acid on the canine basilar artery. An experimental study on cerebral vasospasm, *J. Neurosurg.* **54:**357–365.

Sasaki, T., Asano, T., Takakura, K., Nakamura, T., Suzuki, N., Imabayashi, S., and Ishikawa, Y., 1982, Cerebral vasospasm and lipid peroxidation—lipid peroxides in the cerebrospinal fluid after subarachnoid hemorrhage, *Brain Nerve* **34:**1191–1196.

Setty, B. N. Y., Graeber, J. E., and Stuart, M. J., 1987, The mitogenic effect of 15- and 12-hydroxyeicosatetraenoic acid on endothelial cells may be mediated via diacylglycerol kinase inhibition, *J. Biol. Chem.* **262:**17613–17622.

Shimizu, T., Watanabe, T., Asano, T., Seyama, Y., and Takakura, K., 1988, Activation of the arachidonate 5-lipoxygenase pathway in the canine basilar artery after experimental subarachnoid hemorrhage, *J. Neurochem.* **51:**1126–1131.

Smith, R. R., Clower, B. R., Grotendorst, G. M., Yabuno, N., and Cruse, J. M., 1985, Arterial wall changes in early human vasospasm, *Neurosurgery* **16:**171–176.

Spallone, A., Acqui, M., Pastore, F. S., and Guidetti, B., 1987, Relationship between leukocytosis and ischemic complications following aneurysmal subarachnoid hemorrhage, *Surg. Neurol.* **27:** 253–258.

Suzuki, N., Nakamura, T., Imabayashi, S., Ishikawa, Y., Sasaki, T., and Asano, T., 1983, Identification of 5-hydroxy eicosatetraenoic acid in cerebrospinal fluid after subarachnoid hemorrhage, *J. Neurochem.* **41:**1186–1189.

Uski, T., Andersson, K. E., Brandt, L., Devinsson, L., and Ljunggren, B., 1983, Responses of isolated feline and human cerebral arteries to prostacyclin and some of its metabolites, *J. Cereb. Blood Flow Metab.* **3:**238–245.

Walker, V., and Pickard, J. D., 1985, Prostaglandins, thromboxane, leukotrienes and the cerebral circulation in health and disease, *in* "Advances and Technical Standards in Neurosurgery" (L. Symon, ed.), pp. 3–64, Springer-Verlag, Vienna.

Watanabe, T., Sasaki, T., Asano, T., Takakura, K., Sano, K., Fuchinoue, T., Watanabe, K., Yoshimura, S., and Abe, K., 1988*a*, Changes in glutathione peroxidase and lipid peroxides in cerebrospinal fluid and serum after subarachnoid hemorrhage —with special reference to the occurrence of cerebral vasospasm, *Neurol. Med. Chir.* **28:**645–649.

Watanabe, T., Asano, T., Shimizu, T., Seyama, Y., and Takakura, K., 1988*b*, Participation of lipoxygenase products from arachidonic acid in the pathogenesis of cerebral vasospasm, *J. Neurochem.* **50:**1145–1150.

Westlund, P., 1987, Formation of novel dihydroxyeicosatetraenoic acids in human platelets: Identification of 11,12-DHETEs and 5,12-DHETEs, *Adv. Prostaglandin Thromboxane Leukotriene Res.* **17:**99–104.

Willis, E. D., 1966, Mechanism of lipid peroxide formation in animal tissues, *Biochem. J.* **99:** 667–676.

Yoshimoto, T., Miyamoto, Y., Ochi, K., and Yamamoto, S., 1982, Arachidonate 12-lipoxygenase of porcine leukocyte with activity for 5-hydroxyeicosatetraenoic acid, *Biochim. Biophys. Acta* **713:**638–646.

BIOCHEMICAL CHANGES AND SECONDARY TISSUE INJURY AFTER BRAIN AND SPINAL CORD ISCHEMIA

ALAN I. FADEN, PHILLIP WEINSTEIN, ROHIT BAKSHI, SABRINA YUM, MATTHIAS LEMKE, and STEVEN H. GRAHAM

I. INTRODUCTION

Ischemia to the central nervous system (CNS) may cause tissue damage through both direct and indirect mechanisms (Siesjö, 1981; Raichle, 1983; Krause *et al.*, 1988). Direct effects occur acutely as a result of interruption of blood flow. Indirect effects are delayed and develop over a period of minutes to hours following the

ALAN I. FADEN, PHILLIP WEINSTEIN, ROHIT BAKSHI, SABRINA YUM, MATTHIAS LEMKE, and STEVEN H. GRAHAM • *Departments of Neurology and Neurosurgery, University of California, San Francisco, California.*

Neurochemical Correlates of Cerebral Ischemia, Volume 7 of *Advances in Neurochemistry*, edited by Nicolas G. Bazan, Pierre Braquet, and Myron D. Ginsberg. Plenum Press, New York, 1992.

ischemic insult; this secondary injury process results, in part, from the action of endogenous biochemical factors that are activated, synthesized, or released in response to ischemia. A partial list of such factors includes phospholipases (Edgar *et al.*, 1982; Hirashima *et al.*, 1984), membrane lipid hydrolysis products (Bazan, 1970; Bazan *et al.*, 1971; Tang and Sun, 1982, 1985; Ikeda *et al.*, 1986), eicosanoids (Moskowitz *et al.*, 1983; Chen *et al.*, 1986), oxygen radical species (Kontos, 1985), monovalent and divalent metal cations (Young *et al.*, 1987; Hoehner *et al.*, 1987), excitatory amino acids (Meldrum, 1985; Rothman and Olney, 1986), and opioid peptides (Faden, 1990). It is likely that the effects of a number of these factors are interactive, with ultimate tissue damage resulting from a complex multifactorial process.

Although it has generally been believed that even brief periods of complete ischemia (< 5 min) result in irreversible tissue damage, recent experiments indicate that it is possible to improve postischemic neurological function following much longer ischemic events (10 to 60 min) through the use of various pharmacological therapies (Hossmann, 1985; Safar, 1986; Vaagenes *et al.*, 1984; Gisvold *et al.*, 1984; Hosobuchi *et al.*, 1982; Steen *et al.*, 1985; Chen *et al.*, 1986; Faden, 1988). Using animal models of ischemia/reperfusion, we have recently tested the effects of BW755c, a mixed cyclooxygenase-lipoxygenase inhibitor, MK-801, a glutamate receptor (*N*-methyl-D-aspartate [NMDA]) antagonist, and nalmefene, an opiate receptor antagonist, in brain and/or spinal cord models of global ischemia with reperfusion. Each of the three classes of compounds resulted in significant biochemical, histological, and/or neurological improvements when compared with saline-treated controls.

2. ENDOGENOUS OPIOIDS

The primary evidence for the role of opioid peptides in ischemia has come from pharmacological experiments with opiate receptor antagonists (Faden, 1990). Although such antagonists have been shown to produce beneficial effects in a variety of models of experimental ischemic injury, there have been some discrepant findings. For example, Hosobuchi *et al.* (1982) and Avery *et al.* (1983) have reported enhancement in neurological outcome, improvement in cerebral blood flow, reductions in seizure activity, and/or enhanced survival in naloxone-treated gerbils following temporary bilateral common carotid occlusion. In contrast, several other groups failed to confirm beneficial effects of naloxone after similar common carotid occlusion in gerbils (Holaday and D'Amato, 1982; Kastin *et al.*, 1982; D. E. Levy *et al.*, 1982). However, the weight of evidence supports a therapeutic effect of naloxone, with positive results being reported in a majority of studies of focal or global CNS ischemia in various experimental animals including rats (Wexler, 1984; Capdeville *et al.*, 1985; Hariri *et al.*, 1986), rabbits (Faden *et al.*, 1984; Faden and Jacobs, 1985), cats (R. Levy *et al.*, 1982; Baskin *et al.*,

1986; Sandor et al., 1986), dogs (Faden et al., 1982; Namba et al., 1986), and primates (Baskin et al., 1982; Zabramski et al., 1984).

The mechanisms whereby endogenous opioids may contribute to secondary injury after CNS ischemia remain speculative. However, at least five classes of opiate receptors have been tentatively identified (Cox, 1982). Antagonists to these receptors can thus be used as pharmacological probes to examine the role of endogenous opioids and specific opiate receptors in ischemia tissue damage. In addition to naloxone, which is relatively nonselective, a number of other, partially receptor-selective opiate antagonists are now available (Faden, 1990). WIN44,441-3 (WIN) is a benzomorphan with apparent increased activity at κ opioid receptors. This compound significantly improved neurologic outcome following global spinal cord ischemia in rabbits, with a potency approximately 50 times greater than that of naloxone (Faden and Jacobs, 1985). Effects were stereospecific, strongly suggesting that the actions were mediated by opiate receptors. WIN also significantly improved electroencephalographic (EEG) changes, following permanent middle cerebral artery occlusion in rats, in a dose-dependent manner with an inverted U-shaped pattern (Andrews et al., 1988). Taken together, these experiments indicate that κ opiate receptors might play a role in ischemic CNS injury. Current studies with nalmefene, an exomethylene derivative of naltrexone with enhanced κ-receptor activity, in rat and rabbit models of global CNS ischemia also show marked attenuation of tissue injury as described in detail below.

3. MEMBRANE LIPIDS

One of the earliest responses of cells to ischemia appears to be an increase in the activity of lipid hydrolytic enzymes (lipases). The first studies to demonstrate increases in products of membrane lipid hydrolysis in the CNS were those of Bazan and co-workers (1970, 1971), who found that global ischemia in the rat brain was accompanied by a rapid increase in brain free fatty acid levels, with the largest relative increase being observed in arachidonic acid. Similarly, ischemia-induced increases in free fatty acid concentration have since been observed in the brain and spinal cord of a variety of experimental animals (Cenedella et al., 1975; Marion and Wolfe, 1979; Dorman et al., 1983; Tang and Sun, 1985; Abe et al., 1987; Halat et al., 1987; Bhakoo et al., 1984).

During the reperfusion period following reversible ischemia, various biologically active, oxygenated metabolites of arachidonic acid (eicosanoids) have been shown to increase in the brain and spinal cord (Chen et al., 1986; Shohami et al., 1987). Arachidonic acid is normally metabolized to eicosanoids via two different enzymatic pathways (Wolfe, 1982): the cyclooxygenase pathway, producing prostaglandins, thromboxanes, and prostacyclin; and the lipoxygenase pathway, producing leukotrienes, and hydroperoxy and hydroxy forms of arachidonic acid.

Concentrations of thromboxane, prostaglandins, and leukotrienes have all been documented to increase in brain tissue following cerebral ischemia (Dempsey *et al.*, 1986; Moskowitz *et al.*, 1983; Ment *et al.*, 1987). The hydroxy forms of arachidonate formed by 5- and 12-lipoxygenase (5-HETE and 12-HETE) (Pellerin and Wolfe, 1987) have also been found to increase in tissue after cerebral ischemia and spinal cord ischemia (Usui *et al.*, 1987; Shohami *et al.*, 1987).

The univalent reduction of molecular oxygen in living tissue produces free radicals such as superoxide anions, hydrogen peroxide, and hydroxyl radicals (Fridovich, 1978). These activated oxygen species can initiate a chain peroxidation process with polyunsaturated fatty acid side chains of membrane phospholipids (Mead, 1976). In the CNS, phospholipids are very rich in polyunsaturated fatty acids. The first step in lipid peroxidation is the abstraction of a hydrogen atom from a fatty acid side chain by an oxygen-derived free radical, resulting in a lipid radical which undergoes molecular rearrangement to form a conjugated diene. The radical diene then reacts with molecular oxygen to give a peroxy radical, which can abstract a hydrogen from an adjacent polyunsaturate, forming a hydroperoxide and a new lipid radical that propagates the chain reaction. Additional reactions of hydroperoxides lead to a variety of products, including aldehydes and radical fragments that can form cross-links between adjacent fatty acid chains. There is strong, inferential evidence that peroxidative damage to membrane lipids contributes to the progressive pathophysiology of CNS ischemia (Yoshida *et al.*, 1982, 1985; Watson *et al.*, 1984; Cooper *et al.*, 1980; Hall and Wolf, 1986). These studies have generally used indirect indicators of peroxidation such as reduction in tissue levels of the endogenous antioxidants ascorbate and α-tocopherol.

Alterations in membrane lipids following CNS ischemia may damage cells and affect physiological processes in a variety of ways. Phospholipid hydrolysis and peroxidation would be expected to alter the structure, motional dynamics (fluidity), and permeability of biomembranes (Houslay and Stanley, 1982). Because proper membrane structure is essential for cell function, perturbations of cell membranes may result in functional deficits that contribute to cell death. In addition, the eicosanoid products of arachidonate metabolism have a number of known physiological effects that may contribute to secondary CNS injury. These effects include vasoconstriction and promotion of platelet aggregation (White and Hagen, 1982; Ezra *et al.*, 1983; Rosenblum, 1985), chemoattraction of leukocytes (Wolfe, 1982), and permeabilization of vascular tissue (Woodward and Ledgard, 1985). Eicosanoid production is also directly dependent upon the presence of lipid hydroperoxides (Needleman *et al.*, 1986). In the context of CNS ischemia, a variety of compounds that can affect lipid hydrolysis, conversion of arachidonate to eicosanoids, or peroxidation have been used as potential pharmacological agents with mixed results (Yamamoto *et al.*, 1983; Yoshida *et al.*, 1985; Hall and Wolf, 1986; Norris and Hachinski, 1985; Chen *et al.*, 1986; Dorman *et al.*, 1983). We have found that BW755c, a combined cyclooxygenase-lipoxygenase inhibitor, has protective effects in a rat model of experimental spinal cord trauma (Faden *et al.*, 1988). Use of this compound has recently been extended to a rabbit model of spinal cord ischemia, the results of which will be discussed below.

4. EXCITATORY AMINO ACIDS

The neurotoxicity of excitatory neurotransmitter amino acids has long been recognized (Lucas and Newhouse, 1957; Olney *et al.*, 1971). On the basis of this and other lines of experimental evidence, it has been postulated that aspartate and glutamate may contribute to tissue damage after CNS ischemia (Rothman and Olney, 1986; Meldrum, 1985). Following cerebral ischemia, selective loss of neurons is seen in regions where glutamate is involved in neurotransmission (Jorgensen and Diemer, 1982; Ginsberg *et al.*, 1985; Pulsinelli *et al.*, 1982). Cerebral ischemia in rats and rabbits also results in rapid release of aspartate and glutamate into the extracellular space (Benveniste *et al.*, 1984; Hagberg *et al.*, 1985; Globus *et al.*, 1988; Korf *et al.*, 1988; Graham *et al.*, 1990). After ischemia and reperfusion in rat brain, rabbit brain, and dog spinal cord, there is a prolonged decrease in the total tissue levels of aspartate and glutamate (Chavko *et al.*, 1987; Erecinska *et al.*, 1984; Hagberg *et al.*, 1985).

Amino acid-induced cell death appears to be mediated through specific membrane receptors by at least two mechanisms: (1) chloride and sodium ion influx, leading to subsequent acute neuronal swelling, and (2) calcium ion influx, leading to more delayed damage (Choi, 1987). Various receptor subtypes for excitatory amino acids have been classified on the basis of their differential sensitivity to agonists such as NMDA, quisqualate, and kainate (Meldrum, 1985). Of these, the NMDA receptor is believed to play a primary role in secondary tissue death after ischemia (Simon *et al.*, 1984).

NMDA receptor antagonists have been shown to markedly reduce post-ischemic loss of cerebral neurons (Simon *et al.*, 1984; Vacanti and Ames, 1984). In our laboratories, the NMDA antagonist MK-801 [(+)-5-methyl-10,11-dihydro-5h-dibenzo[*a,d*]cyclohepten-5,10-imine maleate], which is centrally active after systemic administration (Wong *et al.*, 1986) produced beneficial effects in rabbits subjected to reversible ischemia. These studies will be discussed below.

5. EDEMA AND IONS

Although edema has long been recognized as a consequence of experimental CNS ischemia (Shibata *et al.*, 1974; Brunson *et al.*, 1973; Bartko *et al.*, 1972), the question of whether such increases in tissue water content directly contribute to secondary tissue damage remains unanswered. Concomitant with edema formation in the CNS, ischemia results in increases in the total tissue content of sodium and decreases in the tissue content of potassium (Young *et al.*, 1987; Hoehner *et al.*, 1987; Katzman and Pappius, 1973). Two recent studies involving a rat model of graded spinal cord trauma found no correlation between severity of injury and increases in tissue water content at the trauma site, suggesting that edema formation may play a lesser role in progression of secondary injury in the spinal cord than has been commonly assumed (Kwo *et al.*, 1989; Lemke and Faden, 1990).

6. BIOCHEMICAL AND PHARMACOLOGICAL STUDIES IN RAT BRAIN AND RABBIT SPINAL CORD ISCHEMIA/ REPERFUSION

Two models have been used in our laboratories to study the biochemical changes that occur as a result of global CNS ischemia and reperfusion: the seven-vessel occlusion model of global cerebral ischemia/reperfusion in the rat and a rabbit model of reversible spinal cord ischemia. The rat model of cerebral ischemia provides near-complete ischemia that is well suited for biochemical studies. The rabbit model of spinal cord ischemia reperfusion produces highly reproducible neurologic and histologic sequelae, making it ideal for pharmacologic outcome studies. We have used these models to show that several classes of drugs (an opiate antagonist, an NMDA antagonist, and a mixed cyclooxygenase-lipoxygenase inhibitor) improve outcome after CNS ischemia/reperfusion, supporting the view that multiple factors contribute to secondary injury. Furthermore, we have shown that an opiate antagonist inhibits the production of other putative secondary injury factors.

The seven-vessel occlusion model in the rat produces global cerebral ischemia by the following technique: the basilar artery and both of the pterygopalatine and external carotid arteries were occluded microsurgically to reduce collateral cerebral blood flow during ischemia. Ischemia was then induced by clip occlusion of both common carotid arteries for 60 min; this reduces blood flow in the forebrain to less than 1% of control levels. Sham-operated animals without common carotid occlusion served as controls.

Spinal cord ischemia is produced in the rabbit by transient aortic occlusion. A balloon-tipped catheter is inserted via the femoral artery into the abdominal aorta to the level of the renal arteries. The balloon is inflated, and aortic occlusion is verified by monitoring distal aortic pressure. An occlusion time of 16 min was found to produce reproducible paralysis in the rabbit. Hindlimb motor function is evaluated by a blinded observer 48 h after ischemia via a six-point neurologic score (0 = complete paralysis, 5 = normal). The animal is then perfused with formaldehyde, and the spinal cord is removed for histological examination. Alternatively, the spinal cord may be frozen in situ for chemical assays.

We used the model of spinal cord ischemia to study changes in free fatty acids, excitatory amino acids, and antioxidants after ischemia in reperfusion. Five rabbits in each group had ischemia induced for 15 min and the spinal cord removed at 15 min, 4 hr, and 24 hr. The effect of spinal cord ischemia upon fatty acids is shown in Table 1. The only significant change in free fatty acids after ischemia was an increase in the level of oleic acid (18:1) at 4 hr after ischemia. The limitation of histopathological changes to the ventral gray at this duration of ischemia (Yum and Faden, 1990) and the small sample size may explain the lack of significant changes in free fatty acids.

Figures 1 and 2 show the changes in the amino acids glutamate, glutamine, and aspartate in gray and white matter after spinal cord ischemia. In cerebral ischemia, glutamate and aspartate are released into the extracellular space (Benveniste et al., 1984), but after reperfusion extracellular levels rapidly return to normal and tissue levels of these amino acids decrease. One explanation for this is that the released excitatory amino acids are transported into the circulation during reperfusion, but metabolic effects may also play a role. The primary route for metabolism of glutamate is uptake into glia and transamination to glutamine. In contrast to previous measurements of tissue amino acid levels after cerebral ischemia reperfusion (Erecinska et al., 1984), there are no changes in either spinal cord gray or white matter glutamate levels after ischemia. The excitatory amino acid aspartate is significantly decreased in white matter 24 hr after 15 min of ischemia and 4 hr after 30 min of ischemia. There is a trend of decreasing aspartate levels in gray matter, but these changes do not reach statistical significance. In our study, the glutamine level is increased in both gray and white matter at 4 hr after 15 or 30 min of ischemia. Glutamate that is released during ischemia, taken up into cells, and transaminated may be one possible source of this increase in tissue glutamine levels.

Changes in levels of spinal cord tissue antioxidants after reperfusion are illustrated in Figure 3. There is strong inferential evidence that peroxidative damage to membrane lipids contributes to the progressive pathophysiology of CNS ischemia (Yoshida et al., 1982). Because oxidants such as superoxide and hydroxyl radicals have a short life span and usually are present at very low concentrations, it is not possible to measure the levels of these oxidants in biological samples. However, there are indirect indices that can be used to examine sequelae of radical and peroxide production, such as changes in concentrations of antioxidants. In the present study, tissue levels of ascorbate and α-tocopherol were measured following 15 min of spinal cord ischemia. Ascorbate and total ascorbic acid levels were decreased, whereas the ratio of dehydroascorbic acid to total ascorbic acid increased significantly 24 hr after reperfusion. The loss of total ascorbic acid may indicate leakage of membranes: Hillered et al. (1988) reported

TABLE 1. Changes in Fatty Acids after Spinal Cord Ischemia

Time after ischemia	Concentration (μg/mg of protein) (mean ± SEM)					
	16:0	18:0	18:1	18:2	20:4	22:6
Controls	2.6332 ± 0.9250	1.5920 ± 0.4027	2.4551 ± 0.6363	1.0759 ± 0.6627	0.1422 ± 0.0351	1.3671 ± 0.3286
15 min	2.2109 ± 0.3699	1.9095 ± 0.3168	1.9162 ± 0.3089	0.3936 ± 0.0755	0.2154 ± 0.0469	0.6535 ± 0.2542
4 hr	2.4161 ± 0.4736	2.1498 ± 0.4091	3.2823 ± 0.2827[a]	0.6722 ± 0.2307	0.1891 ± 0.0373	1.3382 ± 0.4078
24 hr	1.7961 ± 0.6443	1.6097 ± 0.6226	1.2167 ± 0.3274	0.3172 ± 0.0711	0.1565 ± 0.0390	0.1817 ± 0.0535

[a]Different from controls ($P < 0.05$).

White Matter

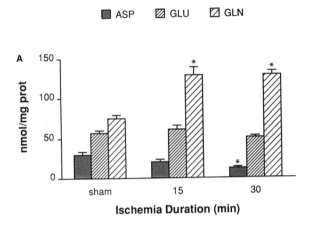

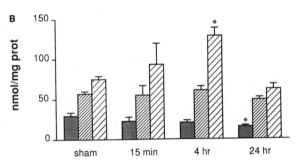

FIGURE 1. (A) Changes in the white matter spinal cord amino acids glutamate (GLU), aspartate (ASP), and glutamine (GLN) 4 hr after ischemia and reperfusion as a function of ischemia duration. *, Different from sham-operated controls ($P < 0.05$). (B) Changes in white matter spinal cord glutamate, aspartate, and glutamine after 15 min of spinal cord ischemia and reperfusion. *, Different from sham-operated controls ($P < 0.05$).

increased extracellular levels of ascorbic acid following CNS ischemia. The relative increase in dehydroascorbic acid content may indicate the actual antioxidative activity. In contrast to the changes in the level of ascorbate, a water-soluble antioxidant, levels of α-tocopherol (which is lipid soluble and membrane bound) had already declined significantly after 15 min and 4 hr of reoxygenation, but did not show significant changes after 24 hr. The different time course of these two

Gray Matter

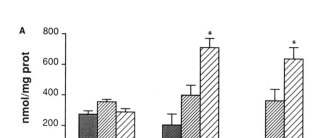

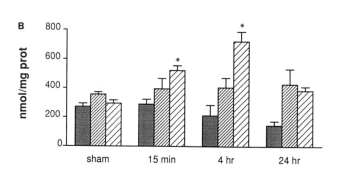

FIGURE 2. (A) Changes in the gray matter spinal cord amino acids glutamate (GLU), aspartate (ASP), and glutamine (GLN) 4 hr after ischemia and reperfusion as a function of ischemia duration. *, Different from sham-operated controls ($P < 0.05$). (B) Changes in gray matter spinal cord glutamate, aspartate, and glutamine after 15 min of spinal cord ischemia as a function of time after ischemia and reperfusion. *, Different from sham-operated controls ($P < 0.05$).

antioxidants, which are known to be closely interrelated in their antioxidative activity, may be due to their different cellular compartmentalization. Therefore, changes in antioxidants provide indirect evidence of ongoing peroxidation after CNS ischemia.

The spinal cord ischemia/reperfusion model was used to test the efficacy of

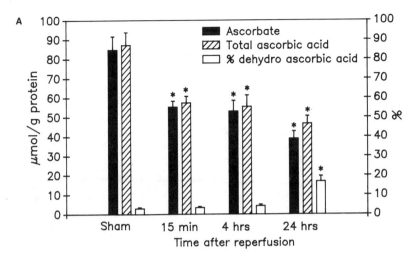

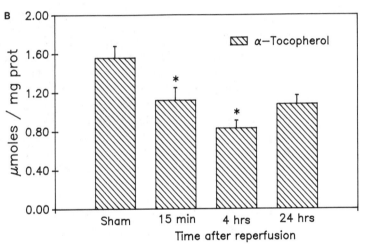

FIGURE 3. (A) Changes in ascorbate, total tissue ascorbic acid, and percent dehydroascorbic acid as a function of time after 15 min of spinal cord ischemia and reperfusion. *, Different from sham-operated controls ($P < 0.05$). (B) Changes in α-tocopherol as a function of time after 15 min of spinal cord ischemia and reperfusion. *, Different from sham-operated controls ($P < 0.05$).

three drugs in ameliorating neurological and histological damage: (1) the NMDA antagonist MK-801 (1 mg/kg); (2) the opiate antagonist nalmefene (0.1 mg/kg); and (3) the mixed cyclooxygenase-lipoxygenase inhibitor BW755c (10 mg/kg). MK-801, nalmefene, or an equal volume of saline was administered 5 min after reperfusion. Both MK-801 and nalmefene significantly ($P < 0.05$) improved neurological outcome and anterior horn cell survival (Yum and Faden, 1990). In another series of experiments, BW755c or saline was administered 15 min prior to ischemia. This dosage of BW755c significantly ($P < 0.05$) inhibited the accumulation of thromboxane B_2 (TXB_2) compared with saline controls (Faden et al., 1988). Histological and neurological outcomes were also significantly improved (Graham et al., in preparation). For purposes of comparison, the cumulative results of these experiments are illustrated in Figure 4. Figure 4A shows the neurological outcome in terms of the percentage of animals that can hop 48 hr after ischemia in the drug-treated rabbits and the grouped controls. The neurological scores of animals from each drug-treated group were significantly improved compared with those of the saline controls, but differences between various treatment groups were not significant. Figure 4B illustrates the mean number of anterior horn cells at the L4 level per section for each group. The nalmefene-treated group had the best neurological outcome, but differences among drug treatment groups did not reach statistical significance.

This illustration that three disparate pharmacological therapies are effective in ameliorating injury after CNS ischemia and reperfusion supports the view that multiple factors cause secondary injury after ischemia. The complexity of the effect of pharmacological intervention on the biochemical changes that occur after ischemia is shown by the effect of nalmefene on nonopioid injury factors. Fifteen minutes prior to the induction of global cerebral ischemia in the rat, nalmefene (100 mg/kg) or saline was given intravenously (Faden et al., 1990). Two hours after reperfusion, the brains were frozen in situ for chemical analysis of free fatty acids, amino acids, TXB_2, ascorbate and vitamin E. As shown in Table 2, brains from saline-treated rats subjected to 60 min of forebrain ischemia and 2 hr of reperfusion had higher free fatty acid levels than did sham-operated controls. Palmitate (16:0), stearate (18:0), oleate (18:1), arachidonate (20:4), adrenate (22:4), and docosahexaenoate (22:6) levels were all increased, although only the changes in stearate and arachidonate reached significance. The TXB_2 level was also significantly increased in these brain samples. Free fatty acid levels in brains from nalmefene-treated rats were indistinguishable from control values and were significantly different from levels of stearate and arachidonate in saline-treated, injured animals.

Rat brain aspartate, glutamate, glycine, γ-aminobutyrate (GABA), ascorbate, and vitamin E levels are given in Table 3. Total tissue levels of aspartate and glutamate were decreased after ischemia and reperfusion, and glycine and GABA levels were increased; however, only the changes in glutamate and glycine reached significance. Nalmefene treatment reduced the alterations in aspartate, glutamate, and GABA, but had no effect on the glycine increase. Ascorbate levels were decreased after ischemia and reperfusion, with nalmefene treatment preventing this decline. α-Tocopherol levels were unaffected in this model.

The ischemia-induced loss of neurons and/or alterations in lipid metabolism,

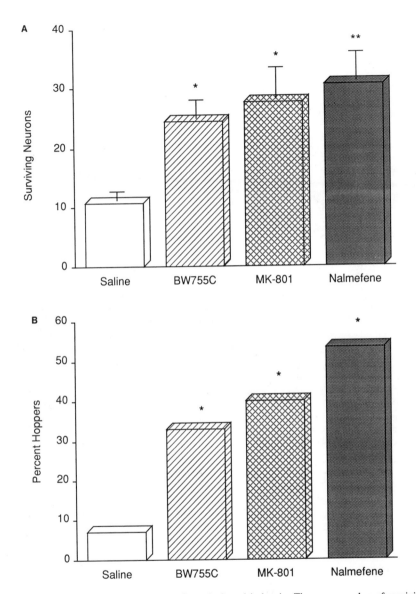

FIGURE 4. (A) Histological outcome after spinal cord ischemia. The mean number of surviving anterior horn cells 48 hr after reperfusion is shown for each treatment group and grouped controls. *, Different from group's control ($P < 0.05$). **, Different from group's control ($P < 0.01$). (B) Neurological outcome after spinal cord ischemia. The percentage of rabbits able to hop 48 hr after reperfusion is shown for each treatment group. *, Different from group's control neurological score ($P < 0.05$).

TABLE 2. Changes in Rat Brain Lipids after Ischemia and Reperfusion

| Sample | Concentration (μg/mg of protein) (mean $\pm$ SEM) | | | | | | Concentration of TXB$_2$ (pg/mg of protein) |
	16:0	18:0	18:1	18:2	20:4	22:6	
Controls	4.42 $\pm$ 0.26	3.79 $\pm$ 0.19	3.26 $\pm$ 0.18	1.13 $\pm$ 0.12	0.41 $\pm$ 0.03	0.32 $\pm$ 0.03	ND[a]
Ischemia, saline placebo	7.62 $\pm$ 0.58	9.41 $\pm$ 1.12[b,c]	5.54 $\pm$ 0.41	1.42 $\pm$ 0.07	1.16 $\pm$ 0.10[b,c]	0.60 $\pm$ 0.03	78.70 $\pm$ 18.40[b]
Ischemia, nalmefene treatment	5.00 $\pm$ 0.34	4.92 $\pm$ 0.34	4.55 $\pm$ 0.32	1.03 $\pm$ 0.05	0.48 $\pm$ 0.04	0.32 $\pm$ 0.03	35.40 $\pm$ 6.9

[a]ND, Not detectable.
[b]Different from controls ($P < 0.05$).
[c]Different from nalmefene-treated group ($P < 0.05$).

TABLE 3. Changes in Brain Amino Acids and Antioxidants after Ischemia and Reperfusion

| Sample | Concentration (μmol/mg of protein) (mean $\pm$ SEM) | | | | Concentration (μmol/g of protein) (mean $\pm$ SEM) | |
	Aspartate	Glutamate	Glycine	GABA	Ascorbate	Vitamin E
Controls	63.94 $\pm$ 6.26	246.66 $\pm$ 19.66	29.18 $\pm$ 4.59	48.93 $\pm$ 5.18	82.59 $\pm$ 4.00	1.02 $\pm$ 0.13
Ischemia, saline placebo	42.76 $\pm$ 5.89	151.17 $\pm$ 19.89[a]	49.51 $\pm$ 5.89[a]	59.20 $\pm$ 16.86	69.13 $\pm$ 3.91[a]	1.09 $\pm$ 0.17
Ischemia, nalmefene treatment	66.91 $\pm$ 10.05	207.51 $\pm$ 25.27	52.15 $\pm$ 6.33[a]	34.68 $\pm$ 4.68	82.33 $\pm$ 9.90	1.22 $\pm$ 0.19

[a]Different from controls ($P < 0.05$).

oxidant production, neurotransmitter amino acids, and neurological function reported here for rats and rabbits subjected to cerebral and spinal cord ischemia, respectively, are consistent with results of previous studies discussed in sections 1 to 6 above. These alterations and the beneficial effects observed with three different classes of pharmacological agents underscore the biochemical complexity of the secondary injury process. The present studies, in conjunction with other data from our laboratories and from the laboratories of others, suggest that some of the changes are closely related and potentially synergistic.

Although the opiate receptor antagonist nalmefene has significant beneficial biochemical effects in a rat model of cerebral ischemia/reperfusion, it is not possible to pinpoint the mechanisms whereby these effects are manifested. However, preliminary in vivo magnetic resonance spectroscopy studies with this model indicate that ATP and phosphocreatine levels recover more rapidly and to a greater degree during the reperfusion period in nalmefene-treated rats (Faden *et al.*, 1990). Thus, one important determinant of the effect of nalmefene may be improvement in the cellular bioenergetic state. For example, both reacylation of free fatty acids with lysophospholipids to re-form diacyl phosphoglycerides and de novo biosynthesis of phospholipids are energy dependent (Sun *et al.*, 1979; Stubbs and Smith, 1984). Bioenergetic improvement may therefore contribute to the postischemic reduction in free fatty acid accumulation observed in nalmefene-treated rats. Eicosanoid production, which is absolutely dependent upon the presence of free arachidonic acid, would in turn be affected. Because release and reuptake of neurotransmitter amino acids are processes that are not well understood (Nicholls, 1989), speculation regarding the potential effects of nalmefene on amino acids in the context of CNS ischemia is problematic. However, several independent studies have found CNS effects of the opioid peptide dynorphin which have been described as being "nonopiate" in nature (Faden and Jacobs, 1984; Moises and Walker, 1985; Walker *et al.*, 1982). More recently, evidence has been presented suggesting that such effects may be mediated via NMDA receptors (Caudle and Isaac, 1988). These investigators found that intrathecal injection of dynorphin in rats causes an irreversible loss of the thermally invoked tail flick reflex. Cotreatment with the NMDA receptor antagonist DL-2-amino-5-phosphonovalerate blocked this loss. In our laboratories, intrathecal administration of dynorphin in rats produces hindlimb paralysis which can be blocked by the NMDA receptor antagonist (+)-4-(3-phosphonopropyl)-2-piperazinecarboxylic acid (Bakshi and Faden, 1990). More recently, we have found that nalmefene pretreatment limits the release of glutamate and aspartate into the extracellular space after global cerebral ischemia in rats (Graham *et al.*, in preparation). Interestingly, glutamate, acting at the NMDA receptor, has been demonstrated to stimulate arachidonic acid release from mouse striatal neurons in culture, with subsequent production of eicosanoids (Dumuis *et al.*, 1988), demonstrating a potential link between action of excitatory amino acids and lipid metabolism.

7. CONCLUSIONS

Evidence has been presented here that secondary injury due to experimental ischemia/reperfusion in the brain and spinal cord may result from alterations in a number of different endogenous biochemical factors including free fatty acids, eicosanoids, oxidant production and lipid peroxidation, excitatory amino acids, and opioid peptides. The complexity of this delayed-injury process is demonstrated by the observation that three different classes of pharmacological agents have protective effects in our animal models of global ischemia reperfusion. These data, in conjunction with results of studies from other laboratories, further suggest that actions of endogenous injury factors may be interactive. Thus, the effectiveness of pharmacological therapies may be enhanced by using combinations of therapeutic agents or by using drugs that have multiple target sites.

ACKNOWLEDGMENTS

Work presented in this review was supported by Merit Review research grants from the Department of Veterans Affairs to A. I. F. and P. W. We thank Paul Demediuk for his helpful input and Carmen Warri for preparation of the manuscript.

REFERENCES

Abe, K., Kogure K., Yamamoto, H., Imazawa, M., and Miyamoto, K., 1987, Mechanisms of arachidonic acid liberation during ischemia in gerbil cerebral cortex, *J. Neurochem.* **48:** 503–509.

Andrews, B. T., McIntosh, T. K., Gonzales, M. F., Weinstein, P. R., and Faden, A. I., 1988, Levels of endogenous opioids and effects of an opiate antagonist during regional cerebral ischemia in rats, *J. Pharmacol. Exp. Ther.* 247:1248–1254.

Avery, S. F., Crockard, H., and Russel, R. W., 1983, Improved survival following severe cerebral ischemia using naloxone, *J. Cereb. Blood Flow Metab.* 3(Suppl):S331–S332.

Bakshi, R., and Faden, A. I., 1990, Competitive and non-competitive NMDA antagonists limit dynorphin A induced rat hindlimb paralysis, *Brain Res.* 507:1–5.

Bartko, D., Reulen, H. J., Koch, H., and Schuerman, K., 1972, Effect of dexamethasone on the early edema following occlusion of the middle cerebral artery in cats, *in* "Steroids and Brain Edema" (H. J. Ruelen and K. Schuerman, eds.), pp. 127–137, Springer-Verlag, Berlin.

Baskin, D. S., Kieck, C. F., and Hosobuchi, Y., 1982, Naloxone reversal of ischemic neurological deficits in baboons is not mediated by systemic effects, *Life Sci.* 31:2201–2204.

Baskin, D. S., Hosobuchi, Y., and Grevel, J. C., 1986, Treatment of experimental stroke with opiate antagonists, *J. Neurosurg.* **64:**99–103.

Bazan, N. G., 1970, Effect of ischemia and electroconvulsive shock on free fatty acid pool in the brain, *Biochim. Biophys. Acta* 218:1–10.

Bazan, N. G., Bazan, H. E. P., Kennedy, W.G., and Joel, C. D., 1971, Regional distribution and rate of production of free fatty acids in rat brain, *J. Neurochem.* 18:1387–1394.

Benveniste, H., Drejer, J., Schousboe, A., and Diemer, N. M., 1984, Elevation of the extracellular concentrations of glutamate and aspartate in rat hippocampus during transient cerebral ischemia monitored by microdialysis, *J. Neurochem.* **43**:1369–1374.

Bhakoo, K. K., Crockard, H. A., and Ascelles, P. T., 1984, Regional studies of changes in brain fatty acids following experimental ischemia and reperfusion in the gerbil, *J. Neurochem.* **43**:1025–1031.

Brunson, B., Robertson, J. T., Morgan, H., and Friedman, B. I., 1973, The measurement of cerebral infarction edema with sodium-22, *Stroke* **4**:461–464.

Capdeville, C., Pruneau, D., and Allix, M., 1985, Naloxone effect on the neurological deficit induced by forebrain ischemia in rats, *Life Sci.* **38**:437–442.

Cenedella, R. J., Galli, C., and Paoletti, R., 1975, Brain free fatty acid levels in rats sacrificed by decapitation versus focused microwave irradiation, *Lipids* **10**:290–293.

Chavko, M., Burda, J., Danielisova, V., and Marsala, J., 1987, Molecular mechanisms of ischemic damage of spinal cord, *Gerontology* **33**:220–226.

Chen, S. T., Hsu, C. Y., Hogan, E. L., Halushka, P. V., Linet, O. I., and Yatsu, F. M., 1986, Thromboxane, prostacyclin, and leukotrienes in cerebral ischemia, *Neurology* **36**:466–470.

Choi, D. W., 1987, Ionic dependence of glutamate neurotoxicity, *J. Neurosci.* **7**:369–379.

Cooper, A. J. L., Pulsinelli, W. A., and Duffy, T. E., 1980, Glutathione and ascorbate during ischemia and postischemic reperfusion in rat brain, *J. Neurochem.* **35**:1242–1245.

Cox, B. M., 1982, Endogenous opioid peptides: A guide to structures and terminology, *Life Sci.* **31**:1645–1658.

Dempsey, R. J., Roy, M. W., Meyer, K., Cowen, D. E., and Tai, H., 1986, Development of cyclooxygenase and lipoxygenase metabolites of arachidonic acid after transient cerebral ischemia, *J. Neurosurg.* **64**:118–124.

Dorman, R. V., Dabrowiecki, Z., and Horrocks, L. A., 1983, Effects of CDPcholine and CDPethanolamine on the alterations in rat brain lipid metabolism induced by global ischemia, *J. Neurochem.* **40**:276–279.

Dumuis, A., Haynes, S. L., Pin, J. P., and Bockaert, J., 1988, NMDA receptors activate the arachidonic acid cascade system in striatal neurons, *Nature* **336**:68–70.

Edgar, A. D., Stroznajder, J., and Horrocks, L. A., 1982, Activation of ethanolamine phospholipase A_2 in brain during ischemia, *J. Neurochem.* **39**:1111–1116.

Erecinska, M., Nelson, D., Wilson, D. F., and Silver, I. A., 1984, Neurotransmitter amino acids in the CNS. I. Regional changes in amino acid levels in rat brain during ischemia and reperfusion, *Brain Res.* **304**:9–22.

Ezra, D., Boyd, L. M., Feuerstein, G., and Goldstein, R. E., 1983, Coronary constriction by leukotriene C_4, D_4 and E_4 in the intact pig heart, *Am. J. Cardiol.* **51**:1451–1454.

Faden, A. I., 1988, Role of thyrotropin-releasing hormone and opiate receptor antagonists in limiting central nervous system injury, *Adv. Neurol.* **47**:531–546.

Faden, A. I., 1990, Role of opiate antagonists in the treatment of stroke, *in* "Current Neurosurgical Practice, vol. III. Protection of the Brain from Ischemia" (P. R. Weinstein and A. I. Faden, eds.), pp. 265–271, Williams & Wilkins, Baltimore.

Faden, A. I., and Jacobs, T. P., 1984, Dynorphin-related peptides cause motor dysfunction in the rat through a non-opiate action, *Br. J. Pharmacol.* **81**:271–276.

Faden, A. I., and Jacobs, T. P., 1985, Opiate antagonist WIN44,441-3 stereospecifically improves neurological recovery after ischemic spinal injury, *Neurology* **35**:1311–1315.

Faden, A. I., Hallenbeck, J. M., and Brown, C. Q., 1982, Treatment of experimental stroke: Comparison of naloxone and thyrotropin-releasing hormone, *Neurology* **32**:1083–1087.

Faden, A. I., Jacobs, T. P., Smith, M. T., and Zivin, J. A., 1984, Naloxone in experimental spinal cord ischemia: Dose response studies, *Eur. J. Pharmacol.* **103**:115–120.

Faden, A. I., Lemke, M., and Demediuk, P., 1988, Effects of BW755c, a mixed cyclooxygenase-lipoxygenase inhibitor, following traumatic spinal cord injury in rats, *Brain Res.* **463**:63–68.

Faden, A. I., Shirane, R., Chang, L. H., James, T. L., Lemke, M., and Weinstein, P. R., 1990, Opiate receptor antagonist reduces metabolic and neurochemical alterations associated with reperfusion after global brain ischemia in rats, *J. Pharmacol. Exp. Ther.* **255:**451–458.

Fridovich, I., 1978, The biology of oxygen radicals, *Science* **201:**875–888.

Ginsberg, M. D., Graham, D. I., and Busto, R., 1985, Regional glucose utilization and blood flow following graded forebrain ischemia in the rat: Correlation with neuropathology, *Ann. Neurol.* **18:**470–481.

Gisvold, S. E., Safar, P., and Rao, G., 1984, Multifaceted therapy after global brain ischemia in monkeys, *Stroke* **15:**803–812.

Globus, M. Y. T., Buston, R., Dietrich, W. D., Martinez, E., Valdes, I., and Ginsberg, M. D., 1988, Effect of ischemia on the in vivo release of striatal dopamine, glutamate, and gamma-aminobutyric acid studied by intracerebral microdialysis, *J. Neurochem.* **51:**1455–1464.

Graham, S. H., Shiraishi, K., Panter, S. S., Simon, R. P., and Faden, A. I., 1990, Changes in extracellular amino acid neurotransmitter produced by focal cerebral ischemia, *Neurosci. Lett.* **110:**124–130.

Hagberg, H., Lehmann, A., Sandberg, M., Nystrom, B., Jacobson, I., and Hamberger, A., 1985, Ischemia-induced shift of inhibitory and excitatory amino acids from intra- to extracellular compartments, *J. Cereb. Blood Flow Metab.* **5:**413–419.

Halat, H., Lukacova, N., Chavko, M., and Marsala, J., 1987, Effects of incomplete ischemia and subsequent recirculation on free palmitate, stearate, oleate, and arachidonate levels in lumbar and cervical spinal cord of rabbit, *Gen. Physiol. Biophys.* **6:**387–399.

Hall, E. D., and Wolf, D. F., 1986, A pharmacological analysis of the pathophysiological mechanisms of posttraumatic spinal cord ischemia, *J. Neurosurg.* **64:**951–961.

Hariri, R. J., Supra, E. L., and Roberts, J. P., 1986, Effect of naloxone on cerebral perfusion and cardiac performance during experimental cerebral ischemia, *J. Neurosurg.* **64:**780–786.

Hillered, L., Persson, L., Bolander, H. G., Hallstrom, A., and Ungerstedt, U., 1988, Increased extracellular levels of ascorbate in the striatum after middle cerebral artery occlusion in the rat monitored by intracerebral microdialysis, *Neurosci. Lett.* **95:**286–290.

Hirashima, Y., Koshu, K., Kamiyama, K., Nishijima, M., Endo, S., and Takaku, A., 1984, Activities of phospholipase A_1, A_2, lysophospholipase, and acylCoA: Lysophospholipid acyltransferase, *in* "Recent Progress in the Study and Therapy of Brain Edema," (K. G. Go and A. Baethman, eds.), pp. 213–221, Plenum Press, New York.

Hoehner, T. J., Garritano, A. M., DiLorenzo, R. A., O'Neill, B. J., Kumar, K., Koehler, J., Nayini, R., Huang, R. R., Krause, G. S., Aust, S. D., and White, B. C., 1987, Brain cortex tissue Ca, Mg, Fe, Na, and K following resuscitation from cardiac arrest in dogs, *Am. J. Emerg. Med.* **5:**19–23.

Holaday, J. W., and D'Amato, R. J., 1982, Naloxone or TRH fails to improve neurological deficits in gerbil models of stroke, *Life Sci.* **31:**385–392.

Hosobuchi, Y., Baskin, D. S., and Woo, S. K., 1982, Reversal of induced ischemic neurological deficit in gerbils by the opiate antagonist naloxone, *Science* **215:**69–71.

Hossmann, K., 1985, Post-ischemic resuscitation of the brain: Selective vulnerability versus global resistance, *Prog. Brain Res.* **63:**3–17.

Houslay, M. D., and Stanley, K. K., 1982, "Dynamics of Biological Membranes. Influence on Synthesis, Structure, and Function," John Wiley, New York.

Ikeda, M., Yoshida, S., Busto, R., Santiso, M., and Ginsberg, M. D., 1986, Polyphosphoinositides as a probable source of brain free fatty acids accumulated at the onset of ischemia, *J. Neurochem.* **47:**123–132.

Jorgensen, M. B., and Diemer, N-H., 1982, Selective neuron loss after cerebral ischemia in the rat: Possible role of transmitter glutamate, *Acta Neurol. Scand.* **66:**536–546.

Kastin, A. J., Nissen, C., and Olson, R. D., 1982, Failure of MIF or naloxone to reverse ischemic-induced neurological deficits in gerbils, *Pharmacol. Biochem. Behav.* **17:**1083–1085.

Katzman, R., and Pappius, H. M., 1973. "Brain Electrolytes and Fluid Metabolism," Williams & Wilkins, Baltimore.

Kontos, H. A., 1985, Oxygen radicals in cerebral vascular injury, *Circ. Res.* **157**:508–516.

Korf, J., Klein, H. C., Venema, K., and Postema, F., 1988, Increases in striatal and hippocampal impedance and extracellular levels of amino acids by cardiac arrest in freely moving rats, *J. Neurochem.* **50**:1087–1096.

Krause, G. S., White, B. C., Aust, S. D., Nayini, N. R., and Kumar, K., 1988, Brain cell death following ischemia and reperfusion: A proposed biochemical sequence, *Crit. Care Med.* **16**: 714–726.

Kwo, S., Young, W., and DeCrescito, V., 1989, Spinal cord sodium, potassium, calcium, and water concentration changes in rats after graded contusion injury, *J. Neurotrauma* **6**:13–24.

Lemke, M., and Faden, A. I., 1990, Edema development and ion changes in rat spinal cord after impact trauma: Injury dose-response studies, *J. Neurotrauma* **7**:41–54.

Levy, D. E., Pike, C. L., and Rawlinson, D. G., 1982, Failure of naloxone to limit clinical or morphological brain damage in gerbils with unilateral carotid artery occlusion, *Soc. Neurosci. Abstr.* **8**:248.

Levy, R., Feustel, P., Severinghaus, J., and Hosobuchi, Y., 1982, Effect of naloxone on neurologic deficit and cortical blood flow during focal cerebral ischemia in cats, *Life Sci.* **31**:2205–2208.

Lucas, D. R., and Newhouse, J. P., 1957, The toxic effect of sodium L-glutamate on the inner layers of the retina, *Arch. Ophthalmol.* **58**:193–201.

Marion, J., and Wolfe, L. S., 1979, Origin of the arachidonic acid released post-mortem in rat forebrain, *Biochim. Biophys. Acta* **574**:25–32.

Mead, J. F., 1976, Free radical mechanisms of lipid damage and consequences for cellular membranes, *in* "Free Radicals in Biology," vol. 1 (W. A. Pryor, ed.), pp. 51–68, Academic Press, New York.

Meldrum, B., 1985, Possible therapeutic applications of antagonists of excitatory amino acid neurotransmitters, *Clin. Sci.* **68**:113–122.

Ment, L. R., Stewart, W. B., Duncan, C. C., Pitt, B. R., and Cole, J., 1987, Beagle pup model of brain injury: Regional cerebral blood flow and cerebral prostaglandins, *J. Neurosurg.* **67**:278–283.

Moises, H. C., and Walker, J. M., 1985, Electrophysiological effects of dynorphin peptides on hippocampal pyramidal cells in rat, *Eur. J. Pharmacol.* **108**:85–98.

Moskowitz, M. A., Kiwak, K. J., Hekemian, K., and Levine, L., 1983, Synthesis of compounds with properties of leukotrienes C_4 and D_4 in gerbil brains after ischemia and reperfusion, *Science* **224**: 886–889.

Namba, S., Nishigaki, S., and Fujiwara, N., 1986, Opiate-antagonist reversal of neurological deficits—experimental and clinical studies, *Jpn. J. Psych. Neurol.* **40**:61–79.

Needleman, P., Turk, J., Jakschik, B. A., Morrison, A. R., and Lefkowith, J. B., 1986, Arachidonic acid metabolism, *Annu. Rev. Biochem.* **55**:69–102.

Nicholls, D. G., 1989, Release of glutamate, aspartate, and gamma-aminobutyric acid from isolated nerve terminals, *J. Neurochem.* **52**:331–341.

Norris, J. W., and Hachinski, V. C., 1985, Megadose steroid therapy in ischemic stroke, *Stroke* **16**: 150–157.

Olney, J. W., Ho, O. L., and Rhee, V., 1971, Cytotoxic effects of acidic and sulphur containing amino acids on the infant mouse central nervous system, *Exp. Brain Res.* **14**:61–76.

Pellerin, L., and Wolfe, L. S., 1987, New findings on the biosynthesis of lipoxygenase products by intact pieces of rat cerebral cortex, *J. Neurochem.* **48**:S84.

Pulsinelli, W. A., Brierly, J. B., and Plum, F., 1982, Temporal profile of neuronal damage in a model of transient forebrain ischemia, *Ann. Neurol.* **11**:491–498.

Raichle, M. E., 1983, The pathophysiology of brain ischemia, *Ann. Neurol.* **13**:2–10.

Roseblum, W. I., 1985, Constricting effect of leukotrienes on cerebral arterioles of mice, *Stroke* **16**: 262–263.

Rothman, S. M., and Olney, J. W., 1986, Glutamate and the pathophysiology of hypoxic-ischemic brain damage, *Ann. Neurol.* **19**:105–111.

Safar, P., 1986, Cerebral resuscitation after cardiac arrest: A review, *Circulation* **74**(Suppl. IV):138–153.

Sandor, P., Gotoh, F., and Tomita, M., 1986, Effects of a stable enkephalin analogue, (D-Met2,Pro5)-enkephalinamide, and naloxone on cortical blood flow and cerebral blood volume in experimental brain ischemia in anesthetized cats, *J. Cereb. Blood Flow Metab.* **6**:553–558.

Shibata, S., Hodge, C. P., and Pappius, H. M., 1974, Effect of experimental ischemia on cerebral water and electrolytes, *J. Neurosurg.* **41**:146–159.

Shohami, E., Jacobs, T. P., Hallenbeck, J. M., and Feuerstein, G., 1987, Increased thromboxane A_2 and 5-HETE production following spinal cord ischemia in the rabbit, *Prostaglandins Leukotrienes Med.* **28**:169–181.

Siesjö, B. K., 1981, Cell damage in the brain: A speculative synthesis, *J. Cereb. Blood Flow metab.* **1**: 155–185.

Simon, R. P., Swan, J. H., Griffiths, T., and Meldrum, B. S., 1984, Blockade of N-methyl-D-aspartate receptors may protect against ischemic damage in the brain, *Science* **226**:850–852.

Steen, P. A., Gisvold, S. E., and Milde, J. H., 1985, Nimodipine improves outcome when given after complete ischemia in primates, *Anesthesiology* **62**:406–414.

Stubbs, C. D., and Smith, A. D., 1984, The modification of mammalian membrane polyunsaturated fatty acid composition in relation to membrane fluidity and function, *Biochim. Biophys. Acta* **779**:89–137.

Sun, G. Y., Su, K. L., Der, O. M., and Tang, W., 1979, Enzymic regulation of arachidonate metabolism in brain membrane phospholipids, *Lipids* **14**:229–235.

Tang, W., and Sun, G. Y., 1982, Factors affecting the free fatty acids in rat brain cortex, *Neurochem. Int.* **4**:269–273.

Tang, W., and Sun, G. Y., 1985, Effects of ischemia on free fatty acids and diacylglycerols in developing rat brain, *Int. J. Dev. Neurosci.* **3**:51–56.

Usui, M., Asano, T., and Takakura, K., 1987, Identification and quantitative analysis of hydroxyeicosatetraenoic acids in rat brains exposed to regional ischemia, *Stroke* **18**:490–494.

Vaagenes, P., Cantadore, R., and Safar, P., 1984, Amelioration of brain damage by lidoflazine after prolonged ventricular fibrillation cardiac arrest in dogs, *Crit. Care Med.* **12**:846–855.

Vacanti, F. X., and Ames, A., 1984, Mold hypothermia and Mg^{++} protect against irreversible damage during CNS ischemia, *Stroke* **15**:695–698.

Walker, J. M., Moises, H. C., Coy, D. H., Baldrighi, G., and Akil, H., 1982, Nonopiate effects of dynorphin and des-tyr-dynorphin, *Science* **218**:1136–1138.

Watson, B. D., Busto, R., Goldberg, W. J., Santiso, M., Yoshida, S., and Ginsberg, M. D., 1984, Lipid peroxidation in vivo induced by reversible global ischemia in rat brain, *J. Neurochem.* **42**: 268–274.

Wexler, B. C., 1984, Naloxone ameliorates the pathophysiologic changes which lead to and attend an acute stroke in stroke-prone/SHR, *Stroke* **15**:630–634.

White, R. P., and Hagan, A. A., 1982, Cerebrovascular actions of prostaglandins, *Pharmacol. Ther.* **18**:313–331.

Wolfe, L. S., 1982, Eicosanoids: Prostaglandins, thromboxane, leukotrienes, and other derivatives of carbon-20 unsaturated fatty acids, *J. Neurochem.* **38**:1–14.

Wong, E. H. F., Kemp, J. A., and Priestly, T., 1986, The novel anticonvulsant MK-801 is a potent N-methyl-D-aspartate antagonist, *Proc. Natl. Acad. Sci. USA* **83**:7104–7108.

Woodward, D. F., and Ledgard, S. E., 1985, Effect of LTD_4 on conjunctival vasopermeability and blood-aqueous barrier integrity, *Invest. Ophthalmol. Visual Sci.* **26**:481–485.

Yamamoto, M., Shima, T., Uozumi, T., Sogabe, T., Yamada, K., and Kawasaki, T., 1983, A possible role of lipid peroxidation in cellular damage caused by cerebral ischemia and the protective effect of vitamin E, *Stroke* **14**:977–982.

Yoshida, S., Abe, K., Busto, R., Watson, B. D., Kogure, K., and Ginsberg, M. D., 1982, Influence of transient ischemia on lipid-soluble antioxidants, free fatty acids, and energy metabolites in rat brains, *Brain Res.* **245:**307–316.

Yoshida, S., Busto, R., Watson, B. D., and Ginsberg, M. D., 1985, Postischemic cerebral lipid peroxidation in vitro: Modification by dietary vitamin E, *J. Neurochem.* **44:**1593–1601.

Young, W., Rapaport, Z. H., Chalif, D. J., and Flamm, E. S., 1987, Regional brain sodium, potassium, and water changes in the rat middle cerebral artery occlusion model, *Stroke* **18:**751–759.

Yum, S. W., and Faden, A. I., 1990, Comparison of the protective effects of the *N*-methyl-D-aspartate receptor antagonist, MK-801, and the opiate receptor antagonist, nalmefene, in spinal cord ischemia in rabbits, *Arch. Neurol.* **47:**277–281.

Zambramski, J. M., Spetzler, R. F., Selman, W. R., Hershey, L. A., and Roessman, U., 1984, Naloxone improves neurological function during and outcome after temporary focal cerebral ischemia, *Stroke* **15:**621–627.

CHAPTER 10

FREE FATTY ACID LIBERATION IN THE PATHOGENESIS AND THERAPY OF ISCHEMIC BRAIN DAMAGE

EDWIN M. NEMOTO, RHOBERT W. EVANS, and PATRICK M. KOCHANEK

1. INTRODUCTION

Unraveling the mechanisms of neuronal membrane degradation and failure after ischemic anoxia stands as one of our greatest and most exciting challenges today. By gaining an understanding of the mechanisms of irreversible membrane degra-

EDWIN M. NEMOTO, RHOBERT W. EVANS, and PATRICK M. KOCHANEK • *Department of Anesthesiology and Critical Care Medicine, University of Pittsburgh, School of Medicine, Pittsburgh, Pennsylvania.*

Neurochemical Correlates of Cerebral Ischemia, Volume 7 of *Advances in Neurochemistry*, edited by Nicolas G. Bazan, Pierre Braquet, and Myron D. Ginsberg. Plenum Press, New York, 1992.

dation and dysfunction after ischemic anoxia, we may be able to understand the basis for not only irreversible neuronal injury but also the apparent differential susceptibility of synaptic transmission, mitochondrial oxidative phosphorylation, protein synthesis, and perhaps other subcellular organelles or processes to ischemic anoxia. There is little doubt that the inability of the plasma membrane to maintain transmembrane ionic gradients with the help of various membrane ion pumps such as the Na^+,K^+- and Ca^{2+}-ATPase pumps is tantamount to irreversible cellular injury. But where exactly are we in understanding the mechanisms of membrane degradation and failure, and how did we get to this point? We present a brief historical perspective of past investigations on the pathogenesis of ischemic anoxic brain damage and how appreciation of the role of free fatty acids (FFA) evolved. Then, our current understanding of the origins and mechanisms of FFA accumulation will be discussed. Finally, we will suggest potentially fruitful directions for future research.

2. HISTORICAL PERSPECTIVES

2.1. Tolerance of the Brain to Global Ischemia

An important question addressed since the mid-1900s (Grenell, 1946; Boyd and Connolly, 1962; Hirsch et al., 1957; Wright and Ames, 1964) and again more recently (Miller and Myers, 1970; Nemoto et al., 1977; Wolin et al., 1971; Hossmann and Zimmerman, 1974) is what exactly is the tolerance of the brain to global brain ischemia as occurs during cardiac arrest? Earlier studies seeking to answer these questions in long-term-recovery animal models were generally crude (Boyd and Connolly, 1962; Hirsch et al., 1957). Postinsult recovery of the animals was largely left to chance, without life support. Nevertheless, it was generally accepted that the tolerance of the brain to complete cerebral ischemic anoxia exceeded the clinically accepted limit of 5 min and was believed to lie somewhere between 10 and 15 min (Miller and Myers, 1970; Nemoto et al., 1977; Wolin et al., 1971). Studies by Hossmann and colleagues showed that the brain could tolerate periods of ischemia of even up to 1 hr (Hossmann and Zimmerman, 1974). The hypothetical relationship between the duration of ischemia and the degree of neurologic deficit, partly based on data obtained in monkeys, could explain the difficulty in determining the threshold of ischemic brian damage (Figure 1). The steep increase in neurologic deficit at the threshold would explain the variability and high sensitivity of the model to small differences in physiological variables which could markedly influence the brain damage sustained. The severity of the injury is also critical for the successful demonstration of the efficacy of therapy. Too severe an insult precludes any demonstration of efficacy, whereas too mild an insult would result in a difference too small to detect. It is clear, however, that the

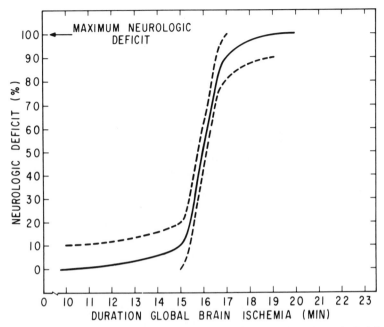

FIGURE 1. Relationship between duration of complete global brain ischemia and neurologic deficit in Rhesus monkeys. (From Nemoto *et al.*, 1977.)

severity of brain damage and neurologic dysfunction sustained increases as the duration of ischemia is prolonged beyond 5 min.

2.2. Biochemical Correlates of Ischemic Brain Damage

To put our current interest in FFA accumulation and membrane lipid degradation as it relates to ischemic brain damage in proper perspective, we briefly review the major recent concepts on the pathogenesis of ischemic brain damage. The "vascular lesion" hypothesis of Spielmeyer (1922) and the "pathoclisis" or selective neuronal vulnerability hypothesis of Vogt (1925) attempt to relate the distribution of ischemic brain damage directly to the vascular bed and neurons, respectively. They mark the beginning of 60 years of intensive research into the pathogenesis of ischemic anoxic brain damage. These hypotheses were still being debated nearly 50 years later by Ames and Brierley (Plum, 1973). The intervening years of research provided information critical to the development of concepts elaborated upon in the subsequent 10 years. The question of the tolerance of the brain to complete global brain ischemia was addressed, and changes in brain high-energy metabolites and glycolytic intermediates and their relationship to the duration of ischemia were investigated as a means of assessing the severity of brain damage sustained (Ljunggren *et al.*, 1974; Lowry *et al.*, 1964; Nemoto, 1978). The protective effects of hypothermia (Kopf *et al.*, 1975; Thorn and Heimann, 1958) and drugs such as the barbiturates (Michenfelder and Theye, 1970; Smith *et al.*, 1974; Yatsu *et al.*, 1972) were reported. Finally, the potential detrimental role of neurotransmitter (NT) hyperactivity and the contribution of failure of synaptic transmission to the neurologic deficit sustained were hypothesized along with the notion that synaptic transmission mechanisms were more susceptible to ischemic damage than was mitochondrial function.

The last 10 years of research have been marked by the development of new insights gained from an interdisciplinary focus on the pathogenesis of ischemic anoxic brain damage at the level of the cell membrane. Membrane metabolism in general and membrane lipid metabolism in particular, with respect to membrane degradation, membrane function (permeability, ionic conductance, receptor function, etc.), and the role of lipid mediators, are now topics of intensive investigation in the pathogenesis of ischemic brain damage.

2.2.1. Brain High-Energy Metabolites

A biochemical or metabolic correlate of the degree of brain damage sustained after ischemic anoxia could provide considerable insight into the mechanisms of ischemic brain damage. However, studies of the changes in brain high-energy phosphates, energy charge potential, lactate, glucose, various Krebs cycle intermediates, etc., were disappointing. Neither brain high-energy phosphates nor adenylate charge potential correlated with dysfunction of brain electrical activity at the onset of ischemia (Duffy *et al.*, 1972; Kaasik *et al.*, 1970) or recovery postischemia (Hinzen *et al.*, 1972; Hossmann and Kleihues, 1973). However, it is difficult to relate biochemical data to neurologic function. Whereas brain high-energy phosphates may recover to 80% or even 95% of normal, the relevance of a 20% or a 5% decrease in ATP levels or energy charge potential to neurologic dysfunction is unknown. Is a 30% decrease in brain ATP levels the result of 30% neuronal necrosis or of 30% decrease in ATP levels in all cells? Ueki *et al.* (1988) suggested that while normal or near-normal levels of brain high-energy phosphate levels postischemia may not necessarily reflect complete recovery of neurologic function, a dramatic fall in the level of brain high-energy phosphates is a prerequisite for severe neurologic dysfunction.

Within 2 min after the onset of complete global brain ischemia, brain high-energy phosphates, glucose, and lactate plateau to minimum or maximum levels and therefore cannot be correlated with the duration of ischemia (Figure 2). It is generally accepted that the longer the duration of ischemia, the greater the neurologic deficit sustained. That 20 min of ischemia results in greater brain

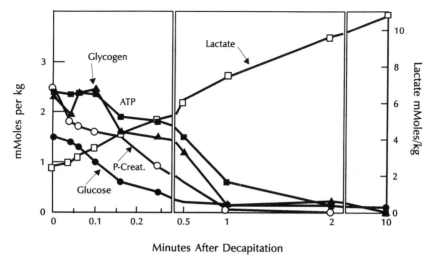

FIGURE 2. Changes in levels of brain high-energy phosphates and other metabolites during decapitation ischemia in adult, unanesthetized mice. (From Lowry *et al.*, 1964.)

damage than 10 min and that 10 min results in greater damage than 5 min is well known. However, the metabolic changes occurring during ischemia reveal nothing that would indicate evolving damage as the duration of ischemia is prolonged. Indeed, it was partly on this basis, along with their observations that cats would occasionally survive 30 and even up to 60 min of complete global brain ischemia with almost complete recovery (Hossmann and Sato, 1970; Ueki *et al.*, 1988) under optimal circumstances, that Hossmann and associates suggested that during complete global brain ischemia, the brain may be in metabolic arrest (Hossmann *et al.*, 1973).

2.2.2. Synaptic Transmission Dysfunction

Following reperfusion after complete global brain ischemia in dogs, Hinzen *et al.* (1972) reported full recovery of brain high-energy phosphates but with severely abnormal brain electrical activity. Thus, it was noted that failure of synaptic transmission could occur without neuronal death, which would add to the neurologic dysfunction attributable to neuronal necrosis and infarction (Figure 3). Neurologic dysfunction, the ultimate measure of brain damage, could be related to histological, biochemical (high-energy phosphates), and electrophysiological

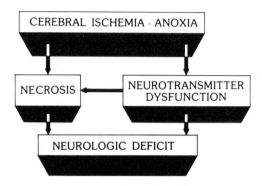

FIGURE 3. Hypothesized components of neurologic deficit after cerebral ischemia-anoxia. Neurologic deficit is due to a combination of neuronal necrosis (irreversible) and neurotransmission dysfunction (reversible or irreversible). (From Nemoto, 1978.)

(i.e., electroencephalography [EEG], evoked potential) changes, but discussion of how well each relates to neurologic dysfunction is beyond the scope of this chapter. It is likely that neurons would either go on to die or recover with or without function, the latter as "quiescent" or "silent" neurons (Nemoto, 1978).

Investigations into the role of synaptic processes in the pathogenesis of ischemic/traumatic brain damage initially focused on their exacerbation of the damage sustained. Osterholm and associates (Osterholm and Mathews, 1972*a,b*) suggested that NT released during ischemia or after traumatic injury in the spinal cord exacerbated the injury sustained. This was demonstrated by measuring the release of NT (Osterholm and Mathews, 1972*a*), the effect of inhibition of catecholamine synthesis (Osterholm and Mathews, 1972*b*), and the effects of the direct application of serotonin onto the cortex (Osterholm and Bell, 1969).

It was subsequently shown that receptor blockade with α-adrenergic receptor blockers such as phenoxybenzamine or depletion of catecholamines prior to ischemia resulted in improved biochemical and physiological recovery (Busto *et al.*, 1985; Clemens and Phebus, 1988; Kogure *et al.*, 1976; Welch *et al.*, 1976). NT release during cerebral ischemia-anoxia could exacerbate the injury sustained through either the excessive stimulation of cerebral metabolism, when perfusion is unable to meet excessive metabolic demands (i.e., postischemic hypoperfusion), or their cerebrovascular effects, promoting development of vasospasm or vasoparalysis. Indeed, increased turnover and release of NT (Kogure *et al.*, 1975; Lavyne *et al.*, 1975; Moskowitz and Wurtman, 1976) into the brain parenchyma does occur, as shown by brain microdialysis (Brannan *et al.*, 1987; Busto *et al.*, 1989; Globus *et al.*, 1988; Slivka *et al.*, 1988; Yao *et al.*, 1988). The complete suppression of striatal glutamate release during ischemia at 33°C compared with 36°C indicates that glutamate release plays a prominent role in the pathogenesis of striatal damage during ischemia (Figure 4). The role of the excitatory amino acids such as glutamate, aspartate, and glycine and the *N*-methyl-D-aspartate (NMDA) and non-NMDA receptors has recently spawned a flurry of research in this area which is of special interest in delayed neuronal death (Choi, 1990; Kirino, 1982; Pulsinelli *et al.*, 1982). The delayed recovery of brain electrical activity correlates with continued altered dysfunction in brain NT even after recovery of brain high-energy phosphates (Busto *et al.*, 1989; Globus *et al.*, 1988), again suggesting that brain mitochondrial function is less sensitive to ischemic damage than are processes of synaptic transmission. However, there was still no biochemical correlate that could be associated with the evolution of ischemic brain injury during complete global brain ischemia.

2.2.3. Brain Free Fatty Acid Accumulation

Initial investigations into the effects of ischemia on brain FFA levels were prompted not by an interest in ischemia but, rather, to determine the level of FFA found in the normal brain and hence to try to explain the markedly divergent values of brain FFA levels reported by different investigators. Galli and ReCecconi (1966) first reported unbelievably high brain FFA levels of 2 to 3 mg/brain. Lunt and Rowe (1968) reported that the quantity and composition of brain FFA varied with the method of tissue preparation. Finally, Bazan and associates (Bazan, 1970; Bazan *et al.*, 1971) subjected rats to decapitation ischemia of various durations and found that the rate of increase in brain FFA was rapid in the first 4 to 5 min, slowed

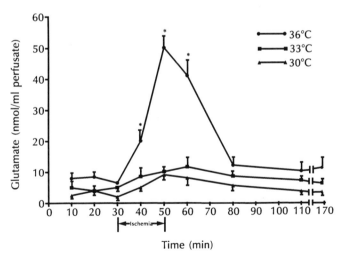

FIGURE 4. Rat brain striatal glutamate levels during and after four-vessel occlusion ischemia and arterial hypotension at brain temperatures of 36°C ($n = 10$), 33°C ($n = 4$), and 30°C ($n = 8$). *, $P < 0.01$ compared with control values. (From Busto *et al.*, 1989.)

considerably between 5 and 10 min, and achieved a plateau after 10 min (Figure 5). Later, they suggested that the FFA released during ischemia achieved levels that could be detrimental to mitochondrial oxidative metabolism and other processes such as excitable membrane function (Aveldano and Bazan, 1975*a*; Bazan, 1975).

3. FREE FATTY ACID AS AN INDICATOR FOR SEVERITY OF ISCHEMIC BRAIN DAMAGE DURING COMPLETE GLOBAL BRAIN ISCHEMIA

3.1. Time Course and Magnitude of Free Fatty Acid Accumulation

Perplexed by the fact that changes in brain high-energy phosphates, glucose, lactate, etc., during complete global brain ischemia failed to reflect the fact that longer durations of ischemia caused increasingly greater brain damage, we searched for biochemical variables that might show a progressive change as the duration of ischemia was prolonged. The FFA data obtained by Bazan and associates (Bazan, 1970; Bazan *et al.*, 1971) appeared to be such an indicator except for a relative plateau in FFA accumulation beyond 10 min of ischemia, which we attributed to a rapid postdecapitation fall in brain temperature (Figure 6). Therefore, we repeated the studies done by Bazan and associates, except that after

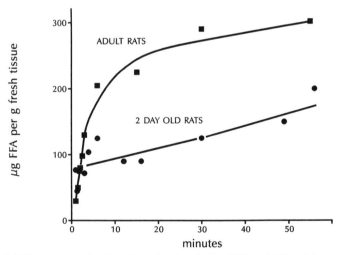

FIGURE 5. FFA content as a function of time after decapitation of 130- and 170-g adult rats and 2-day-old rats. Curves were fitted by eye. (From Bazan *et al.*, 1971.)

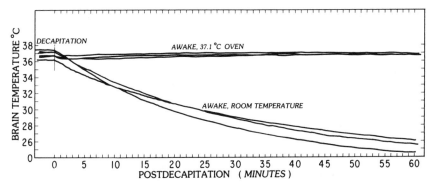

FIGURE 6. Changes in brain temperature after decapitation of awake rats. Brain temperatures were measured by using subdural thermistors sealed with methylmethacrylate. Rats were allowed to recover from anesthesia after insertion of the thermistors and decapitated at time 0. The brains were sealed in plastic bags with water-soaked sponges; three were kept in an incubator at 37.1°C, and three were left at room temperature (25°C). (From Shiu and Nemoto, 1981.)

decapitation, the brains were kept at 37°C in plastic bags humidified with water-soaked sponges (Shiu *et al.*, 1983*a*; Shiu and Nemoto, 1981). Under these conditions, brain FFA levels continued to rise at an impressive rate even after 60 min of ischemia, although there was a definite decrease in the rate of increase after the first 5 min (Figures 7 and 8). Arachidonic acid levels increased 10-fold. The accumulations of stearic (18:0) and arachidonic (20:4) acids appeared to parallel each other with a larger and more rapid rate of increase, whereas oleic and palmitic acid showed a smaller and less rapid rate.

3.2. Evidence That Free Fatty Acid Accumulation Reflects the Evolution of Ischemic Brain Damage

The evidence indicating that brain FFA accumulation during ischemia reflects the evolution of ischemic brain damage is circumstantial and indirect. First, as discussed above, the basic premise in our work on the relationship between brain FFA accumulation and ischemic brain damage is that the longer the duration of complete global brain ischemia, the greater the brain damage sustained. The continued accumulation of FFA in the absence of changes in other known metabolites further supports the notion that FFA accumulation reflects the evolution of ischemic brain damage.

Second, the enzymes primarily responsible for the hydrolysis of membrane phospholipids are heterogeneously distributed at the cellular level. Phospholipase

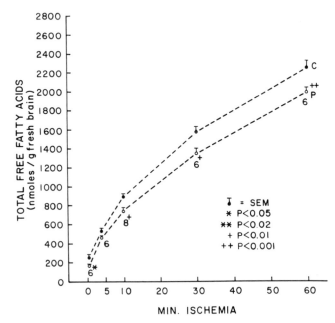

FIGURE 7. Whole rat brain total FFA levels during decapitation ischemia in unanesthetized control (C) and pentobarbital-anesthetized (P) rats. Numbers below the curves indicate the number of rats studied at each point. (From Shiu *et al.*, 1983*a*.)

A_1 and A_2 activity is eight- and fivefold higher in neurons than in glia, respectively (Woelk *et al.*, 1978), and neurons are more sensitive to ischemic injury than are glia.

Third, the rate and magnitude of FFA production in gray matter far exceed those in white matter after complete ischemia in monkeys (Bazan, 1971*a*) and rats (Bazan *et al.*, 1971), which is consistent with the greater damage sustained in the gray matter than in the white matter.

Fourth, it is clear that NT are involved in the activation of phospholipases and tri- and diglyceride lipases. Norepinephrine and 5-hydroxytryptamine (5-HT) increased the concentration of FFA in synaptosomes and synaptic membrane (Price and Rowe, 1972), whereas monoamine oxidase inhibition by iproniazid phosphate increases FFA levels in synaptosomes, indicating that endogenous biogenic amines elicit a similar effect to that previously hypothesized by Bazan (1971*b*, 1975). Aveldano and Bazan (1979) showed that inhibition of catecholamine synthesis by α-methyl-*p*-tyrosine pretreatment reduced brain arachidonic acid levels by 42% and almost completely inhibited a 48% increase in brain arachidonic

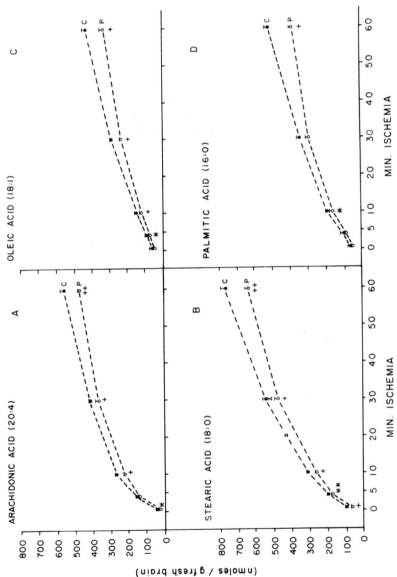

FIGURE 8. Changes in whole rat brain arachidonic (A), stearic (B), oleic (C), and palmitic (D) acid levels during decapitation ischemia at 37°C in unanesthetized control (C) and pentobarbital-anesthetized (P) rats. (From Shiu et al., 1983a).

acid levels caused by electroconvulsive shock. The rise in brain FFA levels after 3 min of ischemia, however, was unaffected. The hydrolysis of phosphatidylinositol (PI) and the polyphosphoinositides by phospholipase C appears to be particularly linked to receptor activation (Smith *et al.*, 1986) by K^+-induced depolarization of synaptosomes (Majewska and Sun, 1982), noradrenaline (Kemp and Downs, 1986); muscarinic agonists (Larocca *et al.*, 1987), and glutamate (Ninomiya *et al.*, 1990). Therefore, it is apparent that the liberation of FFA is associated with synaptic events.

Fifth, there is substantial evidence that newborns and poikilotherms have a greater tolerance to ischemic anoxic brain damage and that the rate of increase of FFA during decapitation ischemia is also substantially lower (Aveldano and Bazan, 1975*a*).

Sixth, neurons in the CA1 region of the hippocampus are selectively vulnerable to ischemia compared with neurons in the CA3 region in rats and gerbils (Kogure *et al.*, 1975, 1976). Accordingly, rats subjected to decapitation ischemia of up to 12 min showed a larger increase in brain arachidonic acid accumulation in the CA1 than in the CA3 region of the hippocampus (Westerberg *et al.*, 1987).

Finally, the importance of FFA liberation and phospholipid hydrolysis in the normal mechanisms of membrane transduction in processes of membrane receptor activation (Hokin, 1985; Sekar and Hokin, 1986; Smith *et al.*, 1986) and membrane ion channel opening (Berridge, 1982; Majewska and Sun, 1982) supports the notion that the accumulation of FFA in ischemia may be related to the damage sustained during ischemia.

Despite the foregoing evidence that the accumulation of FFA during complete global brain ischemia reflects the evolution of ischemic brain damage, the following suggests that this may not be the case. It has long been known that the rate of increase of brain FFA levels during seizures is much higher than even that caused by cerebral ischemia (Bazan and Rakowski, 1970; Bazan, 1970, 1971*b*) although the absolute levels are lower during seizures than during ischemia. Therefore, the increase in brain FFA levels per se does not indicate brain damage. It has also been reported (Busto *et al.*, 1989) that moderate hypothermia (i.e., 33°C), which effectively attenuates the severity of ischemic brain damage, completely blocked glutamate release during ischemia but failed to attenuate FFA accumulation in the striatum. Curiously, the FFA level in the striatum was higher after ischemia at 33°C than at 36°C, but this was not the case in the cortex, where there was some attenuation in the amount of FFA accumulated. The reason for these results is unknown but could be attributable to the process of freezing the brain in situ. The striatum is deeper in the brain than the cortex and may have suffered hypoxia or anoxia before freezing by surface cooling. Nevertheless, definitive proof of a relationship between FFA accumulation and brain damage has yet to be obtained.

3.3. Efficacy of Various Drugs in Attenuating Free Fatty Acid Accumulation during Ischemia

If FFA liberation during cerebral ischemia-anoxia is related to processes of brain injury, as we suggest, then therapies proven effective in ameliorating ischemic anoxic damage should attenuate FFA accumulation. Also, the degree of the attenuation of FFA accumulation by a particular drug should be related to its therapeutic efficacy. Therefore, the effects of FFA accumulation of various drugs of proven, suspected, or no efficacy in ameliorating ischemic brain damage were studied (Nemoto *et al.*, 1982) (Figure 9).

Of the anesthetics, the barbiturates are the most extensively tested and are, in our opinion, most consistently effective in attenuating ischemic brain damage (Aldrete *et al.*, 1979; Bleyaert *et al.*, 1978; Hoff *et al.*, 1975; Moseley *et al.*, 1975; Smith *et al.*, 1974; Yatsu *et al.*, 1972). They were among the most effective in

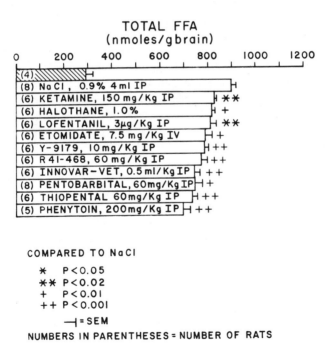

FIGURE 9. Whole-brain total FFA levels (nanomoles/gram of brain) in rats after 10 min of normothermic decapitation ischemia following treatment with various drugs. (From Nemoto *et al.*, 1982.)

attenuating the increase in brain FFA levels during 10 min decapitation ischemia in the rat. Diphenylhydantoin, an anticonvulsant, also effectively attenuated FFA accumulation with similar effectiveness to thiopental and is also reportedly effective in attenuating ischemic damage in animals (Aldrete *et al.*, 1979). The other drugs tested are essentially unproven in their effectiveness, and ketamine and halothane have no protective effects, at least relative to barbiturates (Moseley *et al.*, 1975). However, ketamine has recently been shown to be effective in ameliorating ischemic brain damage in gerbils (Marcoux *et al.*, 1988) and rats (Church *et al.*, 1988).

In the therapeutic application of these potent drugs, determination of the minimum dose resulting in maximal protective effects is important because many of these drugs, such as the barbiturates, are potent cardiovascular and respiratory depressants. To determine the minimum dose resulting in maximal protective effects as judged by the attenuation of FFA accumulation, we studied the dose-related effects of thiopental, pentobarbital, dilantin, and ketamine on FFA accumulation during ischemia of 10 min duration (Shiu *et al.*, 1983*b*). The point at which an increase in dose no longer results in further attenuation of FFA accumulation is of interest. Pentobarbital (Figure 10) and thiopental (Figure 11) maximally reduced FFA accumulation at subanesthetic intraperitoneal (i.p.) doses of 30 mg/kg, whereas phenytoin (Figure 12) maximally attenuated FFA accumulation at the anticonvulsant dose in the rat of 150 mg/kg i.p. These results suggest that it is unnecessary to achieve an isoelectric EEG for maximal protective effects. This is also supported by the observation that the cerebral metabolic rate for glucose is depressed by 90% at subanesthetic doses of barbiturates (Crane *et al.*, 1978). High barbiturate doses could easily exacerbate the severity of brain damage sustained as a consequence of cardiovascular and respiratory depression.

The opiate antagonist naloxone is also effective in attenuating focal ischemic brain damage. Naloxone is effective in reversing the neurologic deficit resulting from stroke in animals (Baskin *et al.*, 1986; Faden *et al.*, 1982; Hosobuchi *et al.*, 1982; Zambramski *et al.*, 1984), and there is even some indication of usefulness in improving recovery in human patients (Jabaily and Davis, 1984) or for use as a diagnostic tool (Estanol *et al.*, 1985). There are, however, conflicting reports in animals (Hubbard and Sundt, 1983) and patients (Fallis *et al.*, 1984), which leaves the question open. The effect of naloxone in attenuating FFA accumulation during ischemia was not particularly impressive compared with that of pentobarbital (Figure 13). Similarly, xylocaine (lidocaine) was a poor inhibitor of FFA accumulation.

The changing proportions of the major FFA accumulating with increasing duration of ischemia suggests that either the origins or the mechanisms of FFA liberation change as ischemia is prolonged. This notion is also supported by studies on the effects of various calcium channel blockers and antagonists on FFA

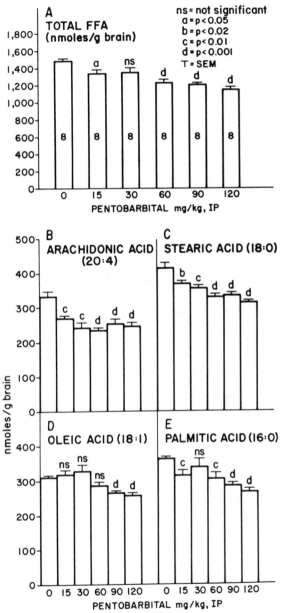

FIGURE 10. Dose-related effects of pentobarbital on whole-brain FFA accumulation after 10 min of decapitation ischemia at 37°C. Numbers in the columns indicate the number of rats studied. (From Shiu *et al.*, 1983*b*.)

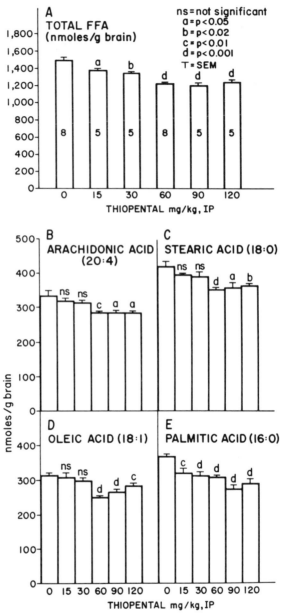

FIGURE 11. Dose-related effects of thiopental on whole-brain FFA accumulation after 10 min of decapitation ischemia at 37°C. Numbers in the columns indicate the number of rats studied. (From Shiu et al., 1983b.)

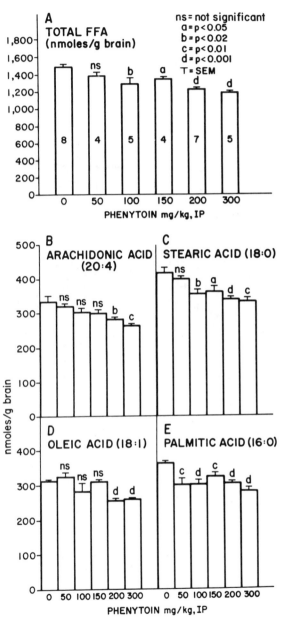

FIGURE 12. Dose-related effects of phenytoin on whole-brain FFA accumulation after 10 min of decapitation ischemia at 37°C. Numbers in the columns indicate the number of rats studied. (From Shiu *et al.*, 1983*b*.)

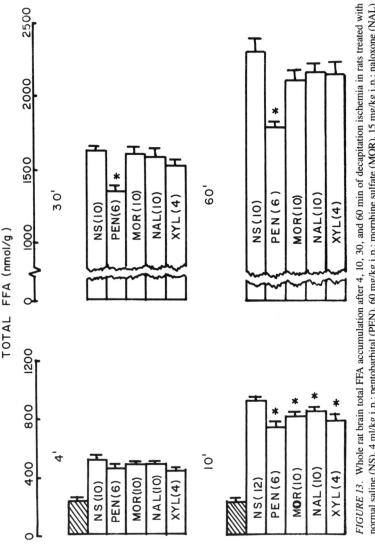

FIGURE 13. Whole rat brain total FFA accumulation after 4, 10, 30, and 60 min of decapitation ischemia in rats treated with normal saline (NS), 4 ml/kg i.p.; pentobarbital (PEN), 60 mg/kg i.p.; morphine sulfate (MOR), 15 mg/kg i.p.; naloxone (NAL) 10 mg/kg i.p.; and xylocaine (XYL; lidocaine), 40 mg/kg i.p. The rats were all decapitated at 10 min after drug administration, except for morphine sulfate-treated rats, which were decapitated 30 min after treatment. *, $P < 0.05$ compared with NS. Numbers in parentheses indicate the number of animals studied. Hatched bars represent total FFA levels after 0.5 min ischemia.

accumulation during decapitation global brain ischemia in rats (Shiu *et al.*, 1983*c*). The Ca^{2+} antagonists differed in their effects on attenuation of FFA accumulation. Whereas nifedipine, like pentobarbital, attenuated the rate of FFA accumulation throughout 60 min of ischemia, cinnarazine, lidoflazine, D-600, and flunarizine were effective only in the first 10 to 30 min (Table 1). It is likely that calcium antagonists and blockers differ in their efficacy in attenuating FFA depending upon their mode and site of action. Reports on the therapeutic effects of Ca^{2+} antagonists vary, and although some studies report a lack of efficacy with flunarizine (Newberg *et al.*, 1984), the majority indicate a beneficial effect (Deshpande and Wieloch, 1985; Steen *et al.*, 1983, 1985; Vaagenes *et al.*, 1984).

4. RELEVANCE OF MEMBRANE PHOSPHOLIPID HYDROLYSIS AND FREE FATTY ACID ACCUMULATION TO THE PATHOGENESIS OF ISCHEMIC BRAIN DAMAGE

The liberation and accumulation of FFA during ischemia are important for three primary reasons (Figure 14). First, they arise primarily from the differential hydrolysis of membrane phospholipids (Begin, 1987), which alters membrane

TABLE 1. Effect of Various Drugs on Whole Rat Brain Total FFA Accumulation after Decapitation Ischemia in Rats[a]

Drug	FFA accumulation (nmoles/g wet brain) after ischemia duration (min)[b]				
	0.5	4	10	30	60
Saline (4 ml/kg, i.p.)	253 ± 33	534 ± 32	899 ± 19	1578 ± 44	2255 ± 80
Pentobarbital (60 mg/kg, i.p.)	167 ± 15*	461 ± 19	745 ± 35*	1353 ± 51*	1794 ± 40*
Nifedipine (20 mg/kg, p.o.)	117 ± 13*	437 ± 5*	685 ± 28*	1288 ± 108*	1837 ± 106*
Cinnarizine (10 mg/kg, p.o.)	114 ± 11*	445 ± 28	717 ± 29*	1438 ± 52	2163 ± 34
Lidoflazine (10 mg/kg, p.o.)	149 ± 3	575 ± 84	765 ± 32	1427 ± 14*	2121 ± 58
D-600 (20 mg/kg, i.p.)	213 ± 33	513 ± 42	787 ± 33*	1423 ± 14*	2021 ± 143
Flunarizine (20 mg/kg, p.o.)	196 ± 6	460 ± 16	806 ± 33	1370 ± 17*	2061 ± 65

[a]Reproduced with permission from Shiu *et al.* (1983*c*).
[b]Asterisks indicate $P < 0.05$ compared with rats treated with 0.9% NaCl, i.p.

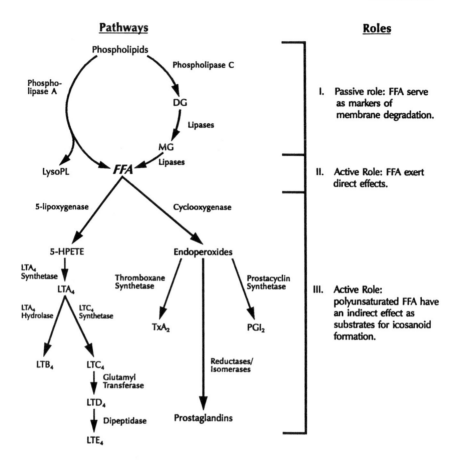

Pathways   **Roles**

FIGURE 14. Diagrammatic illustration of the potential roles of FFA in influencing the pathogenesis of ischemic brain damage. Abbreviations: DG, diglyceride; MG, monoglyceride; Lyso PL, lysophospholipid; FFA, free fatty acid; 5-HPETE, 5-hydroperoxyeicosatetraenoic acid; LT, leukotriene; TxA$_2$, thromboxane A$_2$; PGI$_2$, prostacyclin.

phospholipid composition and thereby impacts on membrane function (Chester *et al.*, 1986; North and Fleischer, 1983; Yeagle, 1983). Second, the accumulated FFA and other degradation products such as the lysophospholipids and diacylglycerols exert a direct perturbing effect on membranes, disrupting their integrity and affecting their function and processes. Third, the polyunsaturated fatty acids (PUFA) serve as substrates for the formation of eicosanoids: a diverse group of oxygenated fatty acids with potent pharmacological effects.

4.1. Relevance of the Mechanisms and Origins of Free Fatty Acid Liberation and Accumulation to the Pathogenesis of Ischemic Brain Damage

The mechanisms and origins of FFA liberation during ischemia are topics of great interest to investigators in that their delineation could shed light on the specific membrane processes that fail and lead to neuronal necrosis. The potential insight provided by such studies is considerable and will be discussed in detail in section 5.

4.2. Direct Detrimental Effects of Hydrolysis Products of Membrane Phospholipid Degradation during Ischemia

The liberation of the degradation products of phospholipid hydrolysis such as lysophospholipids and the polyunsaturated fatty acids, which are normally present in very low concentrations (Bazan, 1971b), is highly toxic to the cell because of detergent like effects of these products on the cell membrane (Bazan, 1971b, 1975; Begin, 1987; Chan and Fishman, 1978; Chan et al., 1983a; Das and Rand, 1984; Hillered and Chan, 1988; Wojtczak, 1976). These metabolites are potent membrane disrupters and have been shown to cause membrane disruption and brain edema (Begin, 1987; Chan and Fishman, 1978; Chan et al., 1983a,b). The polyunsaturated FFAs arachidonate, linoleate, and docosahexanoate induce edema in rat brain cortical slices in vitro (Chan and Fishman, 1978). Arachidonic, linoleic, oleic, and docosahexaenoic acids, at concentrations of 6×10^{-5} M and higher, uncouple mitochondrial oxidative phosphorylation, reduce ATP formation (Das and Rand, 1984; Wojtczak, 1976), and induce superoxide radical formation (Chan et al., 1988). These processes are closely linked to the development of cellular edema in rat brain (Chan et al., 1982, 1983b). Attenuation of brain edema by superoxide dismutase after brain trauma (Chan et al., 1987) and activation of phospholipase A_2 activity by oxygen-derived free radicals (Au et al., 1985) implicate free radical generation in the process. Arachidonic acid also inhibits choline uptake and depletes the acetylcholine content in rat synaptosomes (Boksa et al., 1988), suggesting that PUFA could also have profound effects on membrane transport processes.

Table 2 reminds us of the FFA levels attained during global ischemia. The data are taken from Shiu et al. (1983a) and are given in micromoles per gram. However, assuming that 1 g of brain has a volume of about 1 ml, then the values are also approximate measures of millimolar concentration.

FFA uncouple oxidative phosphorylation (Hillered and Chan, 1988; Van den Bosch and Van den Vesselaar, 1978). Kuwashima et al. (1978) measured the P/O ratio in mitochondria isolated from the cerebrum of normal rats. Addition of

TABLE 2. Concentrations of FFA
in Brain during Global Ischemia

Ischemia duration (min)	Brain concentration (μmol/g wet brain)				
	16:0	18:0	18:1	20:4	Total
0.5	0.05	0.10	0.05	0.04	0.25
5	0.11	0.20	0.09	0.16	0.53
10	0.20	0.31	0.15	0.27	0.87
30	0.34	0.54	0.29	0.42	1.60
60	0.50	0.80	0.50	0.54	2.26

saturated fatty acids (16:0 and 18:0) had little effect. However, the unsaturated fatty acids (16:1, 18:1, 18:2, and 20:4) inhibited oxidative phosphorylation. At concentrations of 20 and 100 μM arachidonic acid, the most potent fatty acid studied, reduced the P/O ratio by 15 and 80%, respectively. Thus the effect of ischemia on oxidative phosphorylation observed in vivo was mimicked in vitro by FFA.

FFA also modify enzymatic activity. Ballou and Cheung (1985) studied their effects on phospholipase A_2 activity, and again saturated FFA had little effect whereas unsaturated FFA inhibited the enzyme. The concentrations required for 50% inhibition of enzyme activity (I_{50}s) for 18:1 and 20:4 (the weakest and most potent inhibitors, respectively) were 2.0 and 0.2 μM. Thus, the FFA exhibit product inhibition, reducing their own formation by phospholipase A_2. In contrast, diglyceride (DG) initially promotes phospholipase A_2 activity, including that of phospholipase C, which results in DG formation. However, the effects were observed only at high concentrations, > 5 mol% (Dawson et al., 1983).

All the FFA effects described above occur at FFA concentrations observed during ischemia. Indeed, the 0.5-min "control" values noted in Table 1 are at concentrations such that the FFA would be expected to exert significant detrimental effects. This raises the question of the authenticity of the 0.5-min value. The FFA values may be elevated as a result of the delay in freezing the brain tissue. Biochemical activity may continue for about 1 min, with considerable degradation. The data, however, also raises the question of protein binding and the extent to which it may nullify or neutralize the detrimental effect of FFA. Do saturated fatty acids fail to cross the aqueous barrier to reach their target, or are they incorporated into membranes with little deleterious effect?

The membrane perturbation caused by the degradation products of phospholipid hydrolysis, namely FFA, strongly perturbs the bilayer structure of membranes, and the in vivo concentration is presumably kept low. However, disruption of the bilayer membrane may be necessary during cell division, exocytosis, and fertilization. Lysophosphatidylcholine (lysoPC) enhances fusion between liposomes, but FFA (14:0) may have a greater tendency to promote molecular mixing between liposomes via exchange diffusion (Papahadajopoulos *et al.*, 1972). Meizel and Turner (1983) studied the effect of FFA on the fusion/vesiculation of the plasma membrane with the outer acrosomal membrane of spermatozoa (acrosome reaction), a prerequisite for fertilization. Saturated fatty acids (16:0 and 18:0) had no effect, whereas *cis* fatty acids at concentrations of 0.18 or 0.09 mM greatly stimulated the acrosome reaction. LysoPC, another product of phospholipid degradation, via phospholipase A, was shown to have a similar effect.

4.3. Free Fatty Acid Precursors of the Eicosanoids and Their Secondary Effects

The FFA liberated most rapidly during ischemia, arachidonic acid, is the major precursor of the eicosanoids (Figure 14). Prostaglandin I_2 (PGI_2) is a vasodilator with platelet-antiaggregatory effects, and thromboxane A_2 (TXA_2) has the opposite effect. PGI_2 and TXA_2 may be involved in the development of delayed postischemic hypoperfusion since inhibition of cyclooxygenase by indomethacin and indomethacin plus PGI_2 attenuate the postischemic hypoperfusion observed (Hallenbeck, 1977; Hallenbeck *et al.*, 1982; Kochanek *et al.*, 1987).

Ischemia promotes eicosanoid synthesis by increasing the concentration of the precursor fatty acids including the main substrate, arachidonic acid. It is the availability of substrate that is normally considered to be the limiting step in the synthesis of eicosanoids (Lands and Samuelsson, 1968).

Studies have focused on the synthesis of eicosanoids during reperfusion, when oxygen is available for fatty acid oxidation. However, it should be noted that synthesizing 0.01 nmol of TxB_2, a large amount per gram of tissue, requires only 0.02 nmol of O_2. This may be satisfied at very low cerebral blood flow rates since at a normal brain blood flow rate of 0.60 ml/g/min and an arterial oxygen content of 20 vol% or 9 μmol/ml, oxygen delivery to the brain is 5,400 nmol of O_2/g of brain/min. The situation is complicated by the large number of reactions that will compete for the available oxygen. However, cyclooxygenase is known to have a very low K_m for oxygen (Siesjö, 1981). Incomplete ischemia may cause more severe brain damage than complete ischemia, since the conditions permit continual release of FFA and influx of oxygen. However, even during complete ischemia, synthesis of some eicosanoids is promoted (Crockard *et al.*, 1982; Dorman, 1988).

During reperfusion, eicosanoid concentrations are considerably elevated. The responses are complex, and Kempski *et al.* (1982) report that the patterns vary with the eicosanoid, brain region, and time. However, it may be that the level of 5-lipoxygenase products increases more slowly than that of the cyclooxygenase eicosanoids but remains elevated for longer (Minamisawa *et al.*, 1988). These authors also suggested that the time course of leukotriene formation, but not that of TXB_2 or 6-*keto*-PGF_1, correlates with the upward trend in brain water content observed during reperfusion.

Considerable work has been done with inhibitors of eicosanoid synthesis, particularly indomethacin, but the therapeutic effects are conflicting, and several explanations may apply. Indomethacin blocks eicosanoid formation at the level of cyclooxygenase. Therefore, synthesis of all prostaglandins is inhibited. Thus, formation of eicosanoids with opposing effects, PGF_2 and TXB_2 versus PGE_2 and PGI_2 is blocked, yielding questionable results. The effects are further complicated by a shunting effect: inhibition of cyclooxygenase provides more arachidonic acid for the lipoxygenase pathways and hence may increase leukotriene levels. Ideally, in studies such as this, all eicosanoid metabolites should be measured during treatment with indomethacin but this is extremely difficult, expensive, and time-consuming. Nevertheless, at least two eicosanoids should be monitored to evaluate whether the inhibitor is effective in vivo. Shohami *et al.* (1982) reported that the use of indomethacin lowered the levels of PGF_2, TXB_2 and 6-*keto*-PGF_1 but that none of these decreases was significant. Dempsey *et al.* (1986) reported that although treatment with indomethacin lowered brain TXB_2, PGF_2, B_4 and 6-*keto*-PGF_1 concentrations in gerbils, the level of leukotriene (LTB_4) was elevated, presumably as a result of a shunting effect.

In a similar approach, Dorman (1988) studied pentobarbital as a potential inhibitor of eicosanoid synthesis. Pentobarbital has beneficial effects during treatment of ischemia, and Nemoto and associates (Shiu *et al.*, 1983a; Shiu and Nemoto, 1981) showed that pentobarbital reduces the accumulation of the precursor fatty acids. Surprisingly, not only was the pentobarbital ineffective in lowering the levels of eicosanoids but also PGF_2 and 6-*keto*-PGF_1 formation was stimulated.

A fundamental unresolved question on the synthesis of eicosanoids in the ischemic/reperfused brain is the site of formation. Although brain cells are known to synthesize eicosanoids, considerable attention has been devoted to the role of blood elements, in particular platelets and leukocytes. Saito *et al.* (1988) used a common carotid artery occlusion model of cerebral ischemia followed by recirculation with saline or pretreatment with busulfan, which decreases leukocyte and platelet numbers by greater than 99%. Both saline and busulfan pretreatment reduced the level of LTD_4 but not of PGD_2, indicating that blood elements, probably leukocytes, were the source of LTD_4.

Brain microvessels manifest enhanced eicosanoid synthesis after exposure to ischemia in vivo followed by in vitro incubation (Asano *et al.*, 1985). They were more efficient at converting exogenous [^{14}C]arachidonic acid into eicosanoids, particularly hydroxy fatty acids, independent of substrate concentration. The increase in eicosanoid formation was therefore due to an actual change in enzyme activity that occurred during ischemia and that was retained during isolation.

Although it is difficult to ascertain to what extent increased eicosanoid formation in vivo is controlled by substrate concentration or increased enzyme activity, it is clear that considerably more arachidonic acid is available than can be accounted for by the amount of eicosanoids formed. The arachidonic acid content can be more than 100 $\mu g/g$ of brain, whereas eicosanoid levels are in the range of picograms to nanograms per g of brain. What limits the oxidation of arachidonic acid when both fatty acid substrate and oxygen are present in abundance? Since cyclooxygenase is a suicide enzyme, it may be rendered inactive after a brief burst of eicosanoid production. Eicosanoids are considerably more water soluble than FFA and hence would be more susceptible to washout during reperfusion. Similarly, washout of the FFA may lead to enhanced eicosanoid formation in peripheral tissue. Future analyses of FFA and eicosanoids during ischemia/reperfusion should include not only brain tissue but also blood.

5. ORIGINS AND MECHANISMS OF FREE FATTY ACID LIBERATION AND ACCUMULATION DURING ISCHEMIA

Two lipid-based membrane transduction mechanisms have been described, namely, the PI response (Downes and Mitchell, 1985; Hawthorne and Prickard, 1979; Hokin-Neaverson, 1977; Michell, 1975) and the methylation response (Hirata and Axelrod, 1980), both of which are activated by various agonists and appear to be involved in controlling intracellular Ca^{2+} concentration by controlling membrane Ca^{2+} permeability. The methylation response is elicited by the stimulation of cellular metabolism by a variety of agonists such as catecholamines, peptide hormones, and antigens, resulting in the conversion of phosphatidylethanolamine (PE) to phosphatidylcholine (PC) in a series of methylation reactions and, in the process, redistributing PC to the outer layer of the membrane, which is believed to alter the generation of second messengers (Hirata and Axelrod, 1980). The PI response involves the hydrolysis of phosphatidylinositol 4,5 diphosphate (PIP_2), which represents a minor component of membrane phospholipids, by phospholipase C, resulting in inositol triphosphate (IP_3) and diacylglycerol formation. The importance of IP_3 has been clearly associated with intracellular second messengers involved with calcium-mediated events (Dempsey *et al.*, 1986). Thus, membrane phospholipid hydrolysis by phospholipases is associated with normal physiological and biochemical events in membrane transduction, and it appears that in pathological states such as cerebral ischemic anoxia, the exaggeration of these events as a result of either the hydrolysis of membrane phospholipids or the marked accumulation of FFA has a detrimental effect on membrane function, as hypothesized by Bazan (1975).

Although the first paper by Bazan (Bazan, 1970) to explore the source of the FFA reported that 20% could result from breakdown of triglycerides, subsequent work has focused on the phospholipids. Two major pathways of phospholipid degradation are considered: (1) phospholipase A hydrolysis producing FFA and lysophospholipids; and (2) phospholipase C activity yielding water-soluble head groups and diglycerides, which are then hydrolyzed by lipases to give FFA (Figure

14). Although both phospholipases C, A_1, and A_2 are reportedly activated after ischemia (Edgar *et al.*, 1982) and head injury (Wei *et al.*, 1982), the necessity of assaying the activities of these enzymes in vitro in an artificial medium raises questions about the relevance of these estimates to the enzyme activities in situ. In addition, studies have tended to concentrate on the relative contributions of polyphosphoinositides (poly-PI), minor but functionally important components of membranes, or the major membrane phospholipids, PC and PE. It is suggested that phospholipase C activity favors poly-PI, whereas PC and PE are the primary substrates for phospholipase A. The activation of phospholipase C and the hydrolysis of PI and poly-PI appear to be the primary mechanisms involved in the early, receptor-coupled hydrolysis of phospholipids and accumulation of FFA via the actions of phospholipase C and diglyceride lipase (Aveldano and Bazan, 1975*b*; Huang and Sun, 1986; Abe *et al.*, 1989; Yoshida *et al.*, 1986). These observations are supported by the previously cited reports on the activation of phosphoinositide hydrolysis by a variety of neurotransmitters including noradrenalin, K^+, glutamate, and muscarinic agonists. The observations on the effects of calcium antagonists attenuating primarily the early rise in brain FFA soon after the onset of ischemia also suggest that the early accumulation of FFA is attributable to the activation of phospholipase C. This topic is discussed in greater detail in Chapter 11. The activation of phospholipase A_1 and A_2 may predominate after longer durations of ischemia and in concert with phospholipase C activation.

During periods of ischemia extending for more than 10 min, hydrolysis of lipids involves all the major classes of phospholipids except possibly sphingomyelin (Bralet *et al.*, 1987). Some selectivity must still occur during the hydrolytic process, however, since the composition of the FFA pool even after 60 min of ischemia differs from that of the source: the total bound fatty acid (unpublished observations). These analyses were made after complete global ischemia, conditions under which the FFA pool would not be expected to be modified by posthydrolytic events (oxidation, reacylation, or washout).

During brain ischemia, the poly-PIs are extensively hydrolyzed in the first 3 min (Huang and Sun, 1986; Ikeda *et al.*, 1986) and the level of poly-PI reached a minimum of one-third of the initial concentration within 10 min (Ikeda *et al.*, 1986). In the first 3 min, the loss of poly-PI completely accounted for arachidonic and stearic acid levels in the diglyceride and FFA fraction. However, the accumulation of additional acids, 16:0 and 18:1, in both the diglyceride and FFA fractions indicated that hydrolysis of other lipids also occurs during the initial 3 min of ischemia (see below), as also suggested by the findings of Huang and Sun (1986).

Although the levels of poly-PI do not plateau until 10 min of ischemia, the greatest rate of hydrolysis occurs within the first 3 to 5 min and thus resembles other biochemical parameters (glucose, high-energy phosphates, lactate, and pH) in proving to be a poor marker of severity of ischemic damage and eventual neurologic outcome at least during the ischemic insult.

The loss of poly-PI is reversible. Yoshida *et al.* (1986) reported that initial levels of poly-PI were reestablished during reperfusion (30 to 180 min) after 15 or 45 min of ischemia. However, Abe *et al.* (1988) commented that the poly-PI content did not return to normal during 3 hr of reperfusion after 3 hr of ischemia. To further complicate the interpretation of poly-PI degradation, Yoshida *et al.* (1986) noted that although the levels of poly-PI recovered during reperfusion, normal function did not. EEG activity was still abnormal after 45 min of ischemia and 180 min of reperfusion, although the poly-PI content had returned to pre-ischemic concentrations.

Direct measurements of poly-PI by the above investigators were necessary and have much improved our attempts to use the composition of the FFA pool as an indicator of the lipid source. Much has been made of the apparent link in the appearance of 20:4 and 18:0. These two acids account for more than 90% of the acyl moieties found in poly-PI, and the similar time course taken for their release is suggested as proof that poly-PI are specifically degraded. However, the evidence that 20:4 and 18:0 do follow a similar pattern of release is not compelling (Yoshida *et al.*, 1986). In any case, since PC and PE include major components containing both 20:4 and 18:0, these moieties could be the source of the released acids, as shown by Goto *et al.* (1988). These authors reported that 18:0 to 20:4 PE was reduced by 60% during the first 5 min of ischemia.

The detailed lipid analysis of Goto *et al.* (1988) indicated that the level of diacyl-PE decreased sharply within 5 min of ischemia but showed little additional loss. The diacyl-PC level, however, had a tendency to decrease throughout the 60 min of ischemia without a significant change in the total PC level. For both diacyl-PE and diacyl-PC the reduction was greatest for the polyunsaturated moieties. Levels of saturated and monounsaturated species of PE did decrease, but no significant loss of these moieties was observed for PC. In no case was there a significant difference between the 5- and 60-min ischemia samples, although there was a tendency to further hydrolysis. It is therefore not clear whether any of these changes can be related to the extent of ischemic damage and neurologic outcome. Interpretation is complicated by the large variation in the data on neurologic outcome and the time-consuming and difficult nature of the lipid analyses. Nevertheless, it would be much more informative to take analyses even further and analyze the ether moieties of PC and PE at the molecular species level.

Since the level of FFA does bear some relationship to the extent of ischemic damage and neurologic outcome, investigators have attempted to inhibit the release of fatty acids. Nemoto *et al.* (1982) studied a series of agents known to have a beneficial effect during ischemia. These agents inhibited the rise in FFA after 10 min of decapitation ischemia in the rat, and the degree of inhibition correlated with their therapeutic efficacy. However, the extent of the inhibition was disappointing: the most effective group was that containing phenytoin, thiopental, pentobarbital, and Innovar-vet (a combination of droperidol and fentanyl), all of which attenuated the rise in FFA by about 23%. This result may not be surprising, since many enzymes with different specificities may have to be targeted by inhibitors.

A puzzling feature of lipid analyses of ischemic tissue is that the extent of phospholipid breakdown is considerably greater than that indicated by the accumulated FFA and DG. Levels of FFA tend to plateau at about 2 μmol of total FFA/g of tissue (Table 1), whereas concentrations of diglyceride tend to plateau at much lower levels (about 0.2 μmol/g of brain tissue) (Goto *et al.*, 1988; Ikeda *et al.*, 1986; Yoshida *et al.*, 1986). Since the brain contains about 60 μmol of phospholipid/g, these levels of FFA and DG could be obtained by hydrolysis of about 1% of the total phospholipid (Cuzner and Davison, 1967). However, there are reports documenting extensive breakdown of phospholipids. Bralet *et al.* (1987) reported a 40% loss of PC and PE and a 25% loss of PI and phosphatidylserine (PS) after 24 hr of ischemia in an embolization model. In this model of incomplete ischemia, the residual flow may wash out most of the FFA. There may also be sufficient oxygen and energy available to oxidize the fatty acids. This interpretation is supported by the observation that PUFA accumulation is greatly moderated during incomplete versus complete ischemia, and this is assumed to result from preferential washout and/or metabolism of the PUFA. However, it is surprising that even in the complete global ischemia used by Goto *et al.* (1988) their data indicate that during 60 min of ischemia, 40 and 60% of the diacyl-phospholipid and diacyl-PE were hydrolyzed respectively. The disparity between FFA levels and phospholipid degradation thus makes FFA concentration a poor quantitative marker of membrane degradation. Nevertheless, a relationship of unknown quantitative significance between FFA content and membrane breakdown may exist. It is questionable, however, whether the reported correlation between FFA levels and ischemic damage and neurologic outcome results from the passive marker role of the FFA or from their active roles as membrane perturbers and as substrates for icosanoid biosynthesis.

6. FUTURE DIRECTIONS OF RESEARCH

Aside from elucidating in detail the mechanisms leading to the degradation of membrane lipids and the accumulation of FFA, the effects of these alterations in membrane lipid composition on membrane function will have to be determined. The changes in the composition of these membrane lipids must cause dramatic changes in the biophysical characteristics of biological membranes, which would ultimately affect membrane permeability and membrane function in terms of receptor/effector coupling. Thus, the elucidation of the major changes in membrane lipid composition and the evaluation of the impact on the biophysical characteristics of the membrane will have to be addressed in the near future. Our recent preliminary studies indicate that changes in lipid composition profoundly

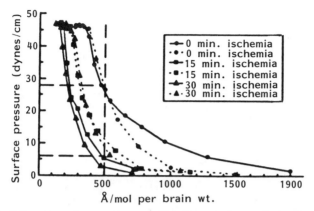

FIGURE 15. Shift in the surface pressure–area phase diagrams of rat cerebral cortex phospholipid mixtures obtained from rats subjected to 0, 15, or 30 min of complete global brain ischemia without recirculation. The units for the x axis correct for differences in phospholipid concentrations in rats.

influence membrane biophysical characteristics, namely monolayer/membrane surface pressure, which could alter membrane function (Goodman et al., 1989) (Figure 15). Changes of such magnitude on the pressure-area phase diagrams of the membrane phospholipids indicate a substantial change in monolayer surface pressure, which may profoundly affect membrane-associated enzyme and perhaps receptor activities and affinities.

REFERENCES

Abe, K., Yuki, S., and Kogure, K., 1988, Strong attenuation of ischemic and postischemic brain edema in rats by a novel free radical scavenger, Stroke 19:480–485.

Abe, K., Kogure, K., Yamamoto, H., Imazawa, M., and Miyamoto, K., 1989, Mechanism of arachidonic acid liberation during ischemia in gerbil cerebral cortex, J. Neurochem. 48: 503–509.

Aldrete, J. A., Romo-Salas, F., Jankovsky, L., and Franatovic, Y., 1979, Effect of pretreatment with thiopental and phenytoin on postischemic brain damage in rabbits, Crit. Care Med. 7:466–470.

Asano, T. A., Gotoh, O., Koide, T., and Takakura, K., 1985, Ischemic brain edema following occlusion of the middle cerebral artery in the rat. II. Alteration of the eicosanoid synthesis profile of brain microvessels, Stroke 16:110–113.

Au, A. M., Chan, P. H., and Fishman, R. A., 1985, Stimulation of phospholipase A_2 activity by oxygen-derived free radicals in isolated brain capillaries, J. Cell. Biochem. 27:449–453.

Aveldano, M. I., and Bazan, N. G., 1975a, Differential lipid deacylation during brain ischemia in homeotherm and poikilotherm, content and composition of free fatty acids and tracylglycerol, Brain Res. 100:99–100.

Aveldano, M. I., and Bazan, N. G., 1975b, Rapid production of diacylglycerols enriched in arachidonate and stearate during early brain ischemia, J. Neurochem. 25:919–920.

Aveldano, M. I., and Bazan, N. G., 1979, Alpha-methyl-p-tyrosine inhibits the production of free arachidonic acid and diacylglycerols in brain after a single electroconvulsive shock, *Neurochem. Res.* **4:**213–221.

Ballou, L. R., and Cheung, W. Y., 1985, Inhibition of human platelet phospolipane A₂ activity by unsaturated fatty acids, *Proc. Natl. Acad. Sci.* **82:**371–375.

Baskin, D. S., Hosobuchi, Y., and Grevel, J. C., 1986, Treatment of experimental stroke with opiate antagonists. Effects of neurological function, infarct size, and survival, *J. Neurosurg.* **64:**99–103.

Bazan, N. G., 1970, Effects of ischemia and electroconvulsive shock on free fatty acid pool in the brain, *Biochim. Biophys. Acta* **218:**1–10.

Bazan, N. G., 1971*a*, Free fatty acid production in cerebral white and grey matter of the squirrel monkey, *Lipids* **6:**211–212.

Bazan, N. G., 1971*b*, Changes in free fatty acids of brain by drug-induced convulsions, electroshock and anaesthesia, *J. Neurochem.* **18:**1379–1385.

Bazan, N. G., 1975, Free arachidonic acid and other lipids in the nervous system during early ischemia and after electroshock, *in* "Functional and Metabolism of Phospholipids in the Central and Peripheral Nervous Systems" (G. Procellati, L. Amaducci, and C. Galli, eds.), pp. 317–335, Plenum Publishing Corp., New York.

Bazan, N. G., and Rakowski, H., 1970, Increased levels of brain free fatty acids after electroconvulsive shock, *Life Sci.* **9:**501–507.

Bazan, N. G., De Bazan, H. E. P., Kennedy, W. G., and Joel, C. D., 1971, Regional distribution and rate of production of free fatty acids in rat brain, *J. Neurochem.* **18:**1387–1393.

Begin, M. E., 1987, Effects of polyunsaturated fatty acids and of their oxidation products on cell survival, *Chem. Phys. Lipids.* **45:**269–313.

Berridge, M. J., 1982, A novel cellular signaling system based on the interaction of phospholipid and calcium metabolism, *in* "Calcium and Cell Function," vol. III (W. Y. Cheung, ed.), pp. 1–36, Academic Press, New York.

Bleyaert, A. L., Nemoto, E. M., Safar, P., Stezoski, S. W., Mickell, J. J., Moossy, J., and Rao, G. R., 1978, Thiopental amelioration of brain damage after global ischemia in monkeys, *Anesthesiology* **49:**390–398.

Boksa, P., Mykita, S., and Collier, B., 1988, Arachidonic acid inhibits choline uptake and depletes acetylcholine content in rat cerebral cortical synaptosomes, *J. Neurochem.* **50:**1309–1317.

Boyd, R. J., and Connolly, J. E., 1962, Total cerebral ischemia in the dog, *Arch. Surg.* **34:**72–76.

Bralet, J., Beley, P., Jemaa, R., Bralet, A. M., and Beley, A., 1987, Lipid metabolism, cerebral metabolic rate, and some related enzyme activities after brain infarction in rats, *Stroke* **18:**418–425.

Brannan, T., Weinberger, J., Knott, P., Taff, I., Kaufmann, H., Togasaki, D., Nieves-Rosa, J., and Maker, H., 1987, Direct evidence of acute massive striatal dopamine release in gerbils with unilateral strokes, *Stroke* **18:**108–110.

Busto, R., Harik, S. I., Yoshida, S., Scheinberg, P., and Ginsberg, M. D., 1985, Cerebral nor-epinephrine depletion enhances recovery after brain ischemia, *Ann. Neurol.* **18:**329–336.

Busto, R., Globus, M., Dietrich, W. D., Martinez, E., Valdez, I., and Ginsberg, M. D., 1989, Ischemia induced release of neurotransmitters and free fatty acids in the rat brain: Effect of mild intraischemic hypothermia, *Stroke* **20:**904–910.

Chan, P. H., and Fishman, R. A., 1978, Brain edema: Induction in cortical slices by polyunsaturated fatty acids, *Science* **28:**358–360.

Chan, P. H., Yurko, M., and Fishman, R. A., 1982, Phospholipid degradation and cellular edema induced by free radicals in brain cortical slices, *J. Neurochem.* **38:**525–531.

Chan, P. H., Fishman, R. A., Caronna, J., Wchmidley, J. W., Prioleau, G., and Lee, J., 1983*a*, Induction of brain edema following intracerebral injection of arachidonic acid, *Ann. Neurol.* **13:**625–632.

Chan, P. H., Fishman, R. A., Chen, S. F., and Chew, S., 1983*b*, Effects of temperature on arachidonic acid-induced cellular edema and membrane perturbation in rat brian cortical slices, *J. Neurochem.* **41**:1550–1557.

Chan, P. H., Longar, S., and Fishman, R. A., 1987, Protective effects of liposome-entrapped superoxide dismutase on posttraumatic brain edema, *Ann. Neurol.* **21**:540–547.

Chan, P. H., Chen, S. F., and Yu, A. C. H., 1988, Induction of intracellular superoxide radical formation by arachidonic acid and by polyunsaturated fatty acids in primary astrocytic cultures, *J. Neurochem.* **50**:1185–1193.

Chester, D. W., Tourtellotte, M. E., Melchior, D. L., and Romano, A. H., 1986, The influence of saturated fatty acid modulation of bilayer physical state on cellular membrane structure and function, *Biochim. Biophys. Acta* **860**:383–398.

Choi, D., 1990, Possible mechanisms limiting N-methyl-*D*-aspartate receptor overactivation and the therapeutic efficacy of N-methyl-*D*-aspartate antagonists, *Stroke* **21**(Suppl. III):III-20–III-22.

Church, J., Zeman, S., and Lodge, D., 1988, The neuroprotective action of ketamine and MK-801 after transient cerebral ischemia in rats, *Anesthesiology* **69**:702–709.

Clemens, J. A., and Phebus, L. A., 1988, Dopamine depletion protects striatal neurons from ischemia-induced cell death, *Life Sci.* **42**:707–713.

Crane, P. D., Brau, L. D., Cornford, E. M., Cremer, J. E., Glass, J. M., and Odendorf, W. H., 1978, Dose-dependent reduction of glucose utilization by pentobarbital in rat brian, *Stroke* **9**:12–18.

Crockard, H. A., Bhakoo, K. K., and Larcelles, P. T., 1982, Regional prostaglandin levels in cerebral ischemia, *J. Neurochem.* **38**:1311–1314.

Cuzner, M. L., and Davison, A. N., 1967, Quantitative thin layer chromatography of lipids, *J. Chromatogr.* **27**:388–397.

Das, S., and Rand, R. P., 1984, Diacylglycerol causes major structural transitions in phospholipid bilayer membranes, *Biochem. Biophys. Res. Commun.* **124**:491–496.

Dawson, R. M. C., Hemington, N. L., and Irvine, R. F., 1983, Diacylglycerol potentiates phospholipase attack upon phospholipid bilayers: Possible connection with cell stimulation, *Biochem. Biophys. Res. Commun.* **117**:196–201.

Dempsey, R. J., Roy, M. W., Meyer, K., Cowen, D. E., and Tai, H. H., 1986, Development of cyclooxygenase and lipoxygenase metabolites of arachidonic acid after transient cerebral ischemia, *J. Neurosurg.* **64**:118–124.

Deshpande, J. K., and Wieloch, T., 1985, Amelioration of ischemic brain damage following post-ischemic treatment with flunarizine, *Neurol. Res.* **7**:27–29.

Dorman, R. V., 1988, Effects of cerebral ischemia and reperfusion on prostanoid accumulation in unanesthetized and pentobarbital-treated gerbils, *J. Cereb. Blood Flow Metab.* **8**:609–612.

Downes, C. P., and Mitchell, R. H., 1985, Inositol phospholipid breakdown as a receptor-controlled generator of second messenger, in "Molecular Mechanisms of Transmembrane Signalling" (P. Cohen and M. D. Houslay, eds.), pp. 3–56, Elsevier, New York.

Duffy, T. E., Nelson, S. R., and Lowry, O. H., 1972, Cerebral carbohydrate metabolism during acute hypoxia and recovery, *J. Neurochem.* **19**:959–977.

Edgar, A. D., Strosznajder, J., and Horrocks, L. A., 1982, Activation of ethanolamine phospholipase A$_2$ in brain during ischemia, *J. Neurochem.* **39**:1111–1116.

Estanol, B., Aguilar, F., Corona, T., 1985, Diagnosis of reversible versus irreversible cerebral ischemia by the intravenous administration of naloxone, *Stroke* **16**:1006–1009.

Faden, A. I., Hallenbeck, J. M., and Brown, C. Q., 1982, Treatment of experimental stroke: Comparison of naloxone and thyrotropin releasing hormone, *Neurology* **32**:1083–1087.

Fallis, R. J., Fisher, M., and Lobo, R., 1984, A double blind trial of naloxone in the treatment of acute stroke, *Stroke* **15**:627–629.

Galli, C., and ReCecconi, D., 1966, Lipid changes in rat brain during maturation, *Lipid* **2**:76–82.

Globus, M. Y. T., Busto, R., Dietrich, W. D., Martinez, E., Valdes, I., and Ginsberg, M. D., 1988, Intra-ischemia extracellular release of dopamine and glutamate is associated with striatal vulnerability to ischemia, *Neurosci. Lett.* **91**:36–40.

Goodman, D. M., Nemoto, E. M., Evans, R. W., and Winter, P. M., 1989, Cerebral phospholipid (PL) monolayer surface (SP) pressure after decapitation ischemia in rats, *J. Neurosurg. Anesthesiol.* **1**:162.

Goto, Y., Okamoto, S., Yonekawa, Y., Taki, W., Kikuchi, H., Handa, H., and Dito, M., 1988, Degradation of phospholipid molecular species during experimental cerebral ischemia in rats, *Stroke* **19**:728–735.

Grenell, R. G., 1946, Central nervous system resistance. I. The effect of temporary arrest of cerebral circulation for periods of two to ten minutes, *J. Neuropathol. Exp. Neurol.* **5**:131–154.

Hallenbeck, J. M., 1977, Prevention of post-ischemic impairment of microvascular perfusion, *Neurology* **27**:3–10.

Hallenbeck, J. M., Leitch, D. R., Dutka, A. J., Greenbaum, L. J., and McKee, A. E., 1982, Prostaglandin I2, indomethacin, and heparin promote postischemic neuronal recovery in dogs, *Ann. Neurol.* **12**:145–156.

Hawthorne, J. N., and Prickard, M. R., 1979, Phospholipids in synaptic function, *J. Neurochem.* **32**:5–15.

Hillered, L., and Chan, P. H., 1988, Effects of arachidonic acid on respiratory activities in isolated brain mitochondria, *J. Neurosci. Res.* **19**:94–100.

Hinzen, D. H., Muller, U., Sobotka, P., Gebert, E., Lang, R., and Hirsch, H., 1972, Metabolism and function of dog's brain recovering from longtime ischemia, *Am. J. Physiol.* **223**:1158–1164.

Hirata, F., and Axelrod, J., 1980, Phospholipid methylation and biological signal transmission, *Science* **209**:1082–1090.

Hirsch, H., Euler, K. H., and Schneider, M., 1957, Uber die Erholung und Wiederbelebung des Gehirns nach Ischamie bei Normothermie, *Pfluegers Arch.* **265**:281–313.

Hoff, J. T., Smith, A. L., Hankinson, H. L., and Neilsen, S. L., 1975, Barbiturate protection from cerebral infarction in primates, *Stroke* **6**:28–33.

Hokin, L. E., 1985, Receptors and phosphoinositide-generated second messengers, *Annu. Rev. Biochem.* **54**:205–235.

Hokin-Neaverson, M., 1977, Metabolism and role of phosphatidylinositol in acetylcholine stimulated membrane function, *Adv. Exp. Biol. Med.* **83**:429–446.

Hosobuchi, Y., Baskin, D. S., and Woo, S. K., 1982, Reversal of induced ischemic neurologic deficit in gerbils by the opiate antagonist naloxone, *Science* **215**:69–71.

Hossmann, K.-A., and Kleihues, P., 1973, Reversibility of ischemic brain damage, *Arch. Neurol.* **29**:375–384.

Hossmann, K.-A., and Sato, K., 1970, Recovery of neuronal function after prolonged cerebral ischemia, *Science* **168**:375–376.

Hossmann, K.-A., and Zimmerman, V., 1974, Resuscitation of the monkey brain after 1 h complete ischemia. I. Physiological and morphological observations, *Brain Res.* **81**:59–74.

Hossmann, K.-A., Lechtape-Gruter, H., and Hossmann, V., 1973, The role of cerebral blood flow for the recovery of the brain after prolonged ischemia, *Z. Neurol.* **204**:281–299.

Huang, S. F. L., and Sun, G. Y., 1986, Cerebral ischemia induced quantitative changes in rat brain membrane lipids involved in phosphoninositide metabolism, *Neurochem. Int.* **9**:185–190.

Hubbard, J. L., and Sundt, T. M., 1983, Failure of naloxone to affect focal incomplete cerebral ischemia and collateral blood flow in cats, *J. Neurosurg.* **59**:237–244.

Ikeda, M., Yoshida, S., Busto, R., Santiso, M., and Ginsberg, M. D., 1986, Polyphosphoinositides a probable source of brain free fatty acids accumulated at the onset of ischemia, *J. Neurochem.* **47**:123–132.

Jabaily, J., and Davis, J. N., 1984, Naloxone administration to patients with acute stroke, *Stroke* **15**:36–39.

Kaasik, A. E., Nilsson, L., and Siesjö, B. K., 1970, The effects of asphyxia upon the lactate, pyruvate and bicarbonate concentrations of brain tissue and cisternal CSF and upon the tissue concentrations of phosphocreatine and adenine nucleotides in anesthetized rats, *Acta Physiol. Scand.* **78:** 433–447.

Kemp, J. A., and Downes, C. P., 1986, Noradrenaline-stimulated inositol phospholipid breakdown in rat dorsal lateral geniculate nucleus neurons, *Brain Res.* **371:**314–318.

Kempski, O., Shohami, E., Von Lubitz, D., Hallenbeck, J. M., and Feuerstein, G., 1982, Postischemic production of eicosanoids in gerbil brain, *Stroke* **18:**111–119.

Kirino, T., 1982, Delayed neuronal death in the gerbil hippocampus following ischemia, *Brain Res.* **239:**57–69.

Kochanek, P. M., Dutka, A. J., Kumaroo, K. K., Tanishima, T., and Hallenbeck, J. M., 1987, Leukotrienes, prostaglandins and granulocyte accumulation in cerebral ischemia, *in* "Cerebral Ischemia and Hemorheology" (A. Hartmann and W. Kuschinsky, eds.), pp. 257–265, Springer Verlag, Berlin.

Kogure, K., Scheinberg, P., Matsumoto, A., Busto, R., and Reinmuth, O. M., 1975, Catecholamines in experimental brain ischemia, *Arch. Neurol.* **32:**21–24.

Kogure, K., Scheinberg, P., Kishikawa, H., and Busto, R., 1976, The role of monoamines and cyclic-AMP in ischemic brain edema, *in* "Dynamics of Brain Edema" (H. M. Pappius and W. H. Feindel, eds.), pp. 203–214, Springer Verlag, New York.

Kopf, G. S., Mirvis, D. M., and Myers, R. E., 1975, Central nervous system tolerance to cardiac arrest during profound hypothermia, *J. Surg. Res.* **18:**29–34.

Kuwashima, J., Nakamura, K., Fujitani, B., Dadokawa, T., Yoshida, K., and Shimizu, M., 1978, Relationship between cerebral energy failure and free fatty acid accumulation following prolonged brain ischemia, *Jpn. J. Pharmacol.* **28:**277–287.

Lands, W. E. M., and Samuelsson, B., 1968, Phospholipid precursors of prostaglandins, *Biochim. Biophys. Acta* **164:**426–429.

Larocca, J. N., Cervone, A., and Ledeen, R., 1987, Stimulation of phosphoinositide hydrolysis in myelin by muscarinic agonist and potassium, *Brain Res.* **436:**357–362.

Lavyne, M., Moskowitz, M. A., Larin, F., Zervas, N., and Wurtman, R. J., 1975, Brain ^{3}H-catecholamine metabolism in experimental cerebral ischemia, *Neurology* **25:**483–485.

Ljunggren, B., Norberg, K., and Siesjö, B. K., 1974, Influence of tissue acidosis upon restitution of brain energy metabolism following total ischemia, 1974, *Brain Res.* **77:**173–183.

Lowry, O. H., Passoneau, J. V., Hasselberger, F. X., and Schulz, D. W., 1964, Effect of ischemia on known substrates and cofactors of the glycolytic pathway in brain, *J. Biol. Chem.* **239:**18–30.

Lunt, G. G., and Rowe, C. E., 1968, The production of unesterified fatty acid in brain, *Biochim. Biophys. Acta* **152:**681–693.

Majewska, M. D., and Sun, G. Y., 1982, Activation of arachidonyl-phosphatidylcholine formation by K^+-evoked stimulation of brain synaptosomes, *Neurochem. Int.* **4:**427–433.

Marcoux, F. W., Goodrich, J. E., and Dominick, M. A., 1988, Ketamine prevents ischemic neuronal injury, *Brain Res.* **452:**329–335.

Meizel, S., and Turner, K. O., 1983, Stimulation of an exocytotic event, sperm acrosome reaction, by cis-unsaturated fatty acids, *FEBS Lett.* **161:**315–318.

Michell, R. H., 1975, Inositol phospholipids and cell surface receptor function, *Biochim. Biophys. Acta* **415:**81–147.

Michenfelder, J. D., and Theye, R. A., 1970, Cerebral protection by thiopental during hypoxia, *Anesthesiology* **33:**430–439.

Miller, J. R., and Myers, R. E., 1970, Neurological effects of systemic circulatory arrest in the monkey, *Neurology* **20:**715–724.

Minamisawa, H., Terashi, A., Katayama, Y., Kanda, Y., Shimizu, J., Shiratori, T., Inamwa, K., Kaseki, H., and Yoshino, Y., 1988, Brain eicosanoid levels in spontaneously hypertensive rats after ischemia with reperfusion: Leukotriene C4 as a possible cause of cerebral edema, *Stroke* **19:** 372–377.

Moseley, J. I., Laurent, J. P., and Molinari, G. F., 1975, Barbiturate attenuation of the clinical course and pathologic lesions in a primate stroke model, *Neurology* **25:**870–874.

Moskowitz, M., and Wurtman, R. J., 1976, Acute stroke and brain monoamines, *in* "Cerebrovascular Disease" (P. Scheinberg, ed.), pp. 153–166, Raven Press, New York.

Nemoto, E. M., 1978, Pathogenesis of cerebral ischemia-anoxia, *Crit. Care Med.* **6:**203–214.

Nemoto, E. M., Bleyaert, A. L., Stezoski, S. W., Moossy, J., Gutti, R. R., and Safar, P., 1977, Global brain ischemia: A reproducible monkey model, *Stroke* **8:**558–564.

Nemoto, E. M., Shiu, G. K., Nemmer, J. P., and Bleyaert, A. L., 1982, Attenuation of brain free fatty acid liberation during global ischemia: A model for screening potential therapies of efficacy? *J. Cereb. Blood Flow Metab.* **2:**475–480.

Newberg, L. A., Steen, P. A., Milde, J. H., and Michenfelder, J. D., 1984, Failure of flunarizine to improve cerebral blood flow or neurological recovery in a canine model of complete cerebral ischemia, *Stroke* **15:**666–671.

Ninomiya, H., Taniguchi, T., and Fujiwara, M., 1990, Phosphoinositide breakdown in rat hippocampal slices: Sensitivity to glutamate induced by in vitro anoxia, *J. Neurochem.* **55:**1001–1007.

North, P., and Fleischer, S., 1983, Alterations of synaptic membrane cholesterol/phospholipid ratio using a lipid transfer protein, *J. Biol. Chem.* **258:**1242–1253.

Osterholm, J. L., and Bell, J., 1969. Experimental effects of free serotonin on the brain and its relation to brain injury. 1. The neurological consequences of intracerebral serotonin injections. 2. Trauma-induced alterations in spinal fluid and brain. 3. Serotonin-induced cerebral edema, *J. Neurosurg.* **31:**408–421.

Osterholm, J. L., and Mathews, G. J., 1972*a*, Altered norepinephrine metabolism following experimental spinal cord injury. 1. Relationship to hemorrhagic necrosis and post-wounding neurological deficits, *J. Neurosurg.* **36:**386–394.

Osterholm, J. L., and Mathews, G. J., 1972*b*, Altered norepinephrine metabolism following experimental spinal cord injury. 2. Protection against traumatic spinal cord hemorrhagic necrosis blockade with alpha-methyl-p-tyrosine, *J. Neurosurg.* **36:**395–401.

Papahadajopoulos, D., Hui, S., Shiu, G. K., Vail, W. J., Poste, G., 1976, Studies on membrane fusion interactions of pure phospholipid membranes and the effects of myristic acid, lysolecithin, proteins and dimethylsulfoxide, *Biochim. Biophys. Acta* **448:**245–264.

Plum, F., 1973, The clinical problem: How much anoxia damages the brain? Symposium held at New York Hospital—Cornell Medical Center: The Threshold and Mechanisms of Anoxic-Ischemic Brain Injury, New York, June 10, 1973, *Arch. Neurol.* **29:**359–360.

Price, C. J., and Rowe, C. E., 1972, Stimulation of the production of unesterified fatty acids in nerve endings of guinea pig brain in vitro by noradrenalin and 5-hydroxy tryptamine, *Biochem. J.* **126:** 575–585.

Pulsinelli, W. A., Brierley, J. B., and Plum, F., 1982, Temporal profile of neuronal damage in a model of transient forebrain ischemia, *Ann. Neurol.* **11:**491–498.

Saito, K., Levine, L., and Moskowitz, M. A., 1988, Blood components contribute to rise in gerbil brain levels of leukotriene-like immunoreactivity after ischemia and reperfusion, *Stroke* **19:** 1395–1398.

Sekar, M. C., and Hokin, L. E., 1986, The role of phosphoinositides in signal transduction, *J. Membr. Biol.* **89:**193–210.

Shiu, G. K., and Nemoto, E. M., 1981, Barbiturate attenuation of brain free fatty acid liberation during global ischemia, *J. Neurochem.* **37:**1448–1456.

Shiu, G. K., Nemmer, J. P., and Nemoto, E. M., 1983*a*, Reassessment of brain free fatty acid liberation during global ischemia and its attenuation by barbiturate anesthesia, *J. Neurochem.* **40:**880–884.

Shiu, G. K., Nemoto, E. M., and Nemmer, J. P., 1983*b*, Dose of thiopental, pentobarbital and phenytoin for maximal therapeutic effects in cerebral ischemic anoxia, *Crit. Care Med.* **11:** 452–459.

Shiu, G. K., Nemoto, E. M., Nemmer, J. P., and Winter, P. M., 1982c, Comparative evaluation of barbiturate and Ca^{++} antagonist attenuation of brain free fatty acid liberation during global brain ischemia, *in* "Brain Protection—Morphological and Clinical Aspects" (K. Wiedemann and S. Hoyer, eds.), pp. 45–54, Springer, Verlag, Berlin.

Shohami, E., Rosenthal, J., and Lavy, S., 1982, The effect of incomplete cerebral ischemia on prostaglandin levels in rat brain, *Stroke* **13:**494–499.

Siesjö, B. K., 1981, Cell damage in the brain: A speculative synthesis, *J. Cereb. Blood Flow Metab.* **1:** 155–185.

Slivka, A., Brannan, T. S., Weinberger, J., Kott, P. J., and Cohen, G., 1988, Increase in extracellular dopamine in the striatum during cerebral ischemia: A study utilizing cerebral microdialysis, *J. Neurochem.* **50:**1714–1718.

Smith, A. L., Hoff, J. T., Nielsen, S. L., and Larson, C. P., 1974, Barbiturate protection in acute focal cerebral ischemia, *Stroke* **5:**1–7.

Smith, C. D., Cox, C., and Snyderman, R., 1986, Receptor-coupled activation of phosphoinositides-specific phospholipase C by an N protein, *Science* **232:**97–100.

Spielmeyer, W., 1922, "Histopathologie des Nervensystems," Springer Verlag, Berlin.

Steen, P. A., Newberg, L. A., Milde, J. H., and Michenfelder, J. D., 1983, Nimodipine improves cerebral blood flow and neurological recovery after complete cerebral ischemia in the dog, *J. Cereb. Blood Flow Metab.* **3:**38–43.

Steen, P. A., Gisvold, S. E., Milde, H. J., Newberg, L. A., Scheithauser, B. W., Lanier, W. L., and Michenfelder, J. D., 1985, Nimodipine improves outcome when given after complete cerebral ischemia in primates, *Anesthesiology* **62:**406–414.

Thorn, W., and Heimann, J., 1958, Beeinflussung der Ammoniak-konzentration in Hypothermie, *J. Neurochem.* **2:**166–177.

Ueki, M., Linn, F., and Hossmann, K.-A., 1988, Functional activation of cerebral blood flow and metabolism before and after global ischemia of rat brain, *J. Cereb. Blood Flow Metab.* **8:** 486–494.

Vaagenes, P., Cantadore, R., Safar, P., Moossy, J., Rao, G., and Diven, W., 1984, Amelioration of brain damage by lidoflazine after ten minutes ventricular fibrillation in dogs, *Crit. Care Med.* **12:** 846–855.

Van den Bosch, H., and van den Vesselaar, A. M. H. P., 1978, Intracellular formation and removal of lysophospholipids, *Adv. Prostaglandin Thromboxane Res.* **3:**69–75.

Vogt, O., 1925, Der Begriff der Pathoklise, *J. Psychol. Neurol.* **31:**245–260.

Wei, E. P., Lamb, R. G., Kontos, H. A., 1982, Increased phospholipase C activity after experimental brain injury, *J. Neurosurg.* **56:**695–698.

Welch, K. M. A., Chabi, E., Dodson, R. F., Wang, T. P. F., Nell, J., and Bergin, B., 1976, The role of biogenic amines in the progression of cerebral ischemia and edema: Modification by p-chlorophenyl-alanine, methysergide and pentoxyfilline, *in* "Dynamics of Brain Edema" (H. M. Pappius and W. A. Feindel, eds.), pp. 193–202, Springer Verlag, New York.

Westerberg, E., Deshpande, J. K., and Wieloch, T., 1987, Regional differences in arachidonic acid release in rat hippocampal CA1 and CA3 regions during cerebral ischemia, *J. Cereb. Blood Flow Metab.* **7:**189–192.

Woelk, H., Goracci, G., Areinti, G., and Porcellati, G., 1978, On the activity of phospholipases A1 and A2 in glial and neuronal cells, *Adv. Prostaglandin Thromboxane Res.* **3:**77–83.

Wojtczak, L., 1976, Effect of long-chain fatty acids and acyl-CoA on mitochondrial permeability, transport and energy-coupling processes, *J. Bioenerg. Biomembr.* **8:**293–311.

Wolin, L. R., Massopust, L. C., and Traslitz, N., 1971, Tolerance to arrest of cerebral circulation in the Rhesus monkey, *Exp. Neurol.* **30:**103–115.

Wright, R. L., and Ames, A., III, 1964, Measurement of maximal permissible cerebral ischemia and a study of its pharmacologic prolongation, *J. Neurosurg.* **21:**567–574.

Yao, H., Sadoshima, S., Ishitsuka, T., Nagao, T., Fujishima, M., Tsutsumi, T., and Uchimura, H., 1988, Massive striatal dopamine release in acute cerebral ischemia in rats, *Experientia* **44:** 506–508.

Yatsu, F. M., Diamond, I., Graziano, C., and Lindquist, P., 1972, Experimental brain ischemia: Protection from irreversible damage with a rapid-acting barbiturate (methohexital), *Stroke* **3:** 726–732.

Yeagle, P., 1983, Cholesterol modulation of (Na^+ + K^+) ATPAse ATP hydrolyzing activity in the human erythrocyte, *Biochim. Biophys. Acta* **727:**39–44.

Yoshida, S., Ikeda, M., Busto, R., Santiso, M., Martinez, E., and Ginsberg, M. D., 1986, Cerebral phosphoinositide, triacylglycerol, and energy metabolism in reversible ischemia: Origin and fate of free fatty acids, *J. Neurochem.* **47:**744–757.

Zambramski, J. M., Spetzler, R. F., Selman, W. R., Roessmann, U. R., Hershey, L. A., Crumrine, R. C., and Macko, R., 1984, Naloxone therapy during focal cerebral ischemia evaluation in a primate model, *Stroke* **15:**621–627.

CHAPTER 11

CEREBRAL ISCHEMIA AND POLYPHOSPHOINOSITIDE METABOLISM

GRACE Y. SUN

1. INTRODUCTION

Cerebral ischemia due to cerebrovascular occlusion is one of the most devastating diseases confronting mankind. The brain is critically dependent on a balanced supply of oxygen and glucose from blood, and cessation of blood flow even for a short time may result in severe neuronal damages and eventually neuronal cell death. In many ways, the initial phase of ischemic insult is like an acute neuronal stimulation which is accompanied by synaptic membrane depolarization, calcium influx and neurotransmitter release (see the review by Nemoto [1985]). However, unlike electroconvulsive shock or drug-induced seizures, neuronal events associated with ischemia are further complicated by cellular deprivation of glucose and high-energy metabolites, and this, in turn, may lead to an increase in the levels of lactate and other metabolic end products (Lowry *et al.*, 1964; Kobayashi *et al.*,

GRACE Y. SUN • *Biochemistry Department, University of Missouri, Columbia, Missouri.*

Neurochemical Correlates of Cerebral Ischemia, Volume 7 of *Advances in Neurochemistry*, edited by Nicolas G. Bazan, Pierre Braquet, and Myron D. Ginsberg. Plenum Press, New York, 1992.

1977; Levy and Duffy, 1977, 1985; Nowak *et al.*, 1985). There are also changes in membrane phospholipids as a result of the ischemic insult; some of these have been described previously (Sun, 1988).

It has been well demonstrated that many neurotransmitters in the brain are able to transduce their signals postsynaptically through a receptor-mediated mechanism associated with generation of intracellular second messengers (Berridge, 1984). Our interest here is directed mainly to examining the signal transduction system involving the hydrolysis of polyphosphoinositides (poly-PI) by phospholipase C (see reviews by Downes [1986], Abdel-Latif [1986], Fisher and Agranoff [1987]). This signal transduction system is known to produce two types of second messengers, namely, diacylglycerols (DG) for activation of protein kinase C (Nishizuka, 1984, 1986) and inositol triphosphate (IP_3) for mobilization of intracellular Ca^{2+} stores (Berridge, 1984; Williamson *et al.*, 1986). During the past few years, the significance of this signal transduction in the nervous system has been probed by using brain slices as well as cultured cells of neural origin (Berridge, 1983; Brown *et al.*, 1984; Gonzales and Crews, 1984, 1985). Nevertheless, little information is available with regard to the response of poly-PI in the brain. This is due mainly to the functional heterogeneity of the neural tissue and the complex organization of the subcellular organelles in the brain.

2. BIOCHEMICAL REACTIONS ASSOCIATED WITH THE POLY-PI CYCLE

Compared with other peripheral tissues, the brain is considered a rich source of poly-PI. Not only are poly-PI in the brain associated with the nerve ending particles, but also they are found in several other subcellular fractions such as in the somal plasma membranes (Sun *et al.*, 1988a) and in myelin (Eichberg and Hauser, 1973). Therefore, experiments to assess the extent of poly-PI degradation due to stimulation of agonists should consider the presence of metabolically active and inactive poly-PI pools in the tissue (Gonzalez-Sastre *et al.*, 1971).

Since poly-PI are known to play an important role in the signal transduction process, it is not surprising to find these compounds metabolically very active and that the metabolic events are stringently controlled. As shown in the metabolic scheme depicted in Figure 1, phosphatidylinositol 4,5-bisphosphate (PIP_2) is synthesized from its precursor molecule, phosphatidylinositol (PI), through two stepwise ATP-dependent kinase reactions. Our earlier studies have indicated that these two kinases (PI and PIP kinases) in the brain exhibit different properties and subcellular localizations (Stubbs *et al.*, 1988). Microsomes and somal plasma membranes (Sun *et al.*, 1988a) from rat brain cortex were shown to have higher PI kinase activity than PIP kinase activity, whereas the synaptic membranes showed

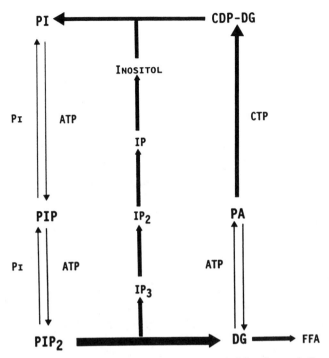

FIGURE 1. Scheme depicting various enzymatic pathways underlying the metabolic turnover of phosphoinositides.

higher PIP kinase activity than the PI kinase. Although the key function of these two kinases is to synthesize PIP_2 for phospholipase C, it is not clear whether phosphatidylinositol 4-phosphate (PIP) in cells or tissue has any physiological role other than acting as an intermediate for the biosynthesis of PIP_2. A number of calcium-mobilizing receptor agonists are known to stimulate the hydrolysis of PIP_2 (Abdel-Latif, 1986). Recent studies have given strong evidence that this signal transduction mechanism is mediated by a GTP-binding protein similar to that mediating the adenylate cyclase system (Litosch, 1987; Chiu *et al.*, 1988; Li *et al.*, 1989).

Phospholipase C in the brain is present in both soluble and membrane-bound forms (Abdel-Latif, 1986), and its catalytic activity is dependent on the presence of Ca^{2+} (Manning and Sun, 1983). Because PIP_2 shows a high affinity for binding Ca^{2+} (Sun, unpublished observation), the Ca^{2+} bound to poly-PI (presumably in the inner leaflet of the membrane surface) may be important for regulating the activity of phospholipase C. Hydrolysis of PIP_2 by phospholipase C results in the generation of $Ins(1,4,5)P_3$, a water-soluble product, and DG, which is expected to remain bound to the membrane. Owing to the second-messenger role of these two products (Berridge, 1984; Williamson et al., 1985), several enzymic mechanisms have been identified for catabolic removal of these compounds. The removal of Ins(1,4,5)P$_3$ can bring about either through hydrolysis to Ins(1,4)P$_2$ by a phosphatase or conversion to Ins(1,3,4,5)P$_4$ by a kinase (Inhorn et al., 1987). The Ins(1,3,4,5)P$_4$ is then sequentially hydrolyzed to Ins(1,3,4)P$_3$, inositol bisphosphates (IP$_2$), inositol monophosphates (IP$_1$) and free inositol. The exact pathway for hydrolysis of Ins(1,3,4,5)P$_4$ and the properties of the phosphatases responsible for hydrolysis of inositol phosphates have not been clearly defined. The sequential hydrolysis of Ins(1,4,5)P$_3$ in brain can be best demonstrated by observing the accumulation of IP$_1$ after pretreating animals with lithium, a compound known to inhibit the IP$_1$ phosphatase activity (Hallcher and Sherman, 1980; Sherman et al., 1981).

The DG generated from hydrolysis of PIP$_2$ by phospholipase C may be further catabolized by DG lipase to monoacylglyceride (MG) and free fatty acids (FFA) (Farooqui et al., 1986) or converted to phosphatidic acid (PA) by the ATP-dependent DG kinase. The MG formed may be further hydrolyzed to release more FFA by the MG lipase (Farooqui et al., 1986). Although DG and MG lipases have been purified from brain microsomes and somal plasma membranes in the brain, they are relatively insensitive to Ca^{2+} (Farooqui et al., 1986). At this point, it is not clear whether other cellular factors regulate these enzymes. DG kinase in the brain is present in both cytosolic and membrane-bound forms (Strosznajder et al., 1986; Stubbs et al., 1988). Results from a more recent study have further indicated that activity of the membrane-bound DG kinase can be stimulated severalfold by oleic acid whereas the cytosolic enzyme can be translocated to the membrane by oleoyl-Coenzyme A (Kelleher and Sun, 1989). To date, there is no direct indication that DG or MG lipase activities are elevated during ischemia, although it is reasonable to assume that the DG kinase activity would be impaired under ischemic conditions due to ATP depletion.

Cerebral ischemia may alter key enzymes involved in the turnover of poly-PI in the brain (Figure 1). In most instances, alterations are due to either a change in cellular Ca^{2+} homeostasis or ATP availability. If the initial onset of an ischemic insult is marked by neuronal stimulation and subsequent neurotransmitter release, this event would have led to a stimulation of phospholipase C in the postsynaptic membranes (Figure 1). However, it is not clear whether the increase in synaptic Ca^{2+} due to opening of the voltage-dependent Ca^{2+} channel also has a role in the activation of phospholipase C in presynaptic membranes. In nonischemic brain tissue where there is an abundant supply of ATP, the agonist-stimulated poly-PI breakdown can be readily replenished. In ischemic tissue, however, the rapid depletion of ATP would have inevitably limited the activity of the PI and PIP kinases as well as other kinases involved in the poly-PI cycle (such as DG kinase and IP$_3$ kinase). On the other hand, these conditions may favor the activation of phosphatases, thus allowing PA to be converted to DG, poly-PI to PI, and IP_3 to IP (Figure 1).

3. LABELING OF PHOSPHOINOSITIDES AND INOSITOL PHOSPHATES IN THE BRAIN

Poly-PI are known to make up around 1% of the total phospholipids in the brain (Sun et al., 1988a). Therefore, to examine the metabolism of these compounds, it is necessary to be able to label them. Proper procedures are also needed to extract and separate these highly charged lipid compounds. Recently, our laboratory has devoted considerable time and effort to establishing procedures for labeling as well as extraction and separation of these phospholipids in the brain (Sun et al., 1988b; Sun and Lin, 1989). Using brain membranes prelabeled with ^{32}Pi, we were able to monitor the recovery of poly-PI during procedures such as subcellular fractionation, lipid extraction, and separation. It was subsequently realized that the instability of these compounds was due mainly to activation of phospholipase C in the presence of Ca^{2+}, and this activity can be inhibited by either microwave fixation of the tissue (Soukup et al., 1978) or by homogenization of brain tissue in ice-cold sucrose medium containing EDTA or EGTA if subcellular membranes were to be isolated.

Intracerebral injection of [^{32}P]ATP into rat brain results in labeling of all the membrane phospholipids. Different labeling patterns could be observed among different subcellular fractions (Sun and Lin, 1989). For example, a high proportion of the radioactivity in the myelin fraction was attributed to labeling of the PIP_2 and PA, whereas the poly-PI in the microsomal fraction were only sparingly labeled (Figure 2). After injection of [^{32}P]ATP into rat brain, labeling of the phosphoinositides in the synaptosomal fraction reached a plateau by 2 to 4 hr and then started to decline after this time (Figure 3). On the other hand, labeling of other phospholipids, such as phosphatidylcholine (PC), phosphatidylserine (PS), phosphatidylethanolamine (PE), and ethanolamine plasmalogen (PEpl) in the same fraction continued to show a steady increase in radioactivity between 1 and 16 hours. These results revealed the presence of two distinct modes for the uptake of the ^{32}P label by the phospholipids in the brain. By using the improved high-performance thin-layer chromatography (HPTLC) procedure described by Sun and Lin (1989), it is possible to separate PIP and PIP_2 together with all other phospholipids within the same TLC plate. This two-dimensional HPTLC system involves the use of three types of solvents and an intermittent exposure of the plate to HCl fumes in order to separate the PEpl from the diacyl species. An example of the separation, as well as an autoradiogram depicting the labeling of phospholipids, is shown in Figure 4.

With [^3H]inositol as the precursor, the same injection procedure can be used

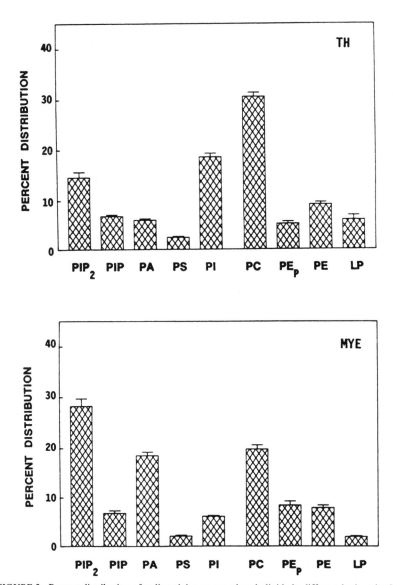

FIGURE 2. Percent distribution of radioactivity among phospholipids in different brain subcellular fractions 4 hr after intracerebral injection of [^{32}P]ATP. Results are mean ± S.D. from subcellular fractions obtained from four rats. Procedures for subcellular fractionation are the same as described by Sun *et al.* (1988*a*), and procedures for extraction and separation of phospholipids are same as described by Sun and Lin (1989). Abbreviations for fractions: TH, total brain homogenate; MYE, myelin; MIC, microsomes; PM, somal plasma membranes; P$_2$, crude mitochondria-synaptosomes; SYN, purified synaptosomes; SV, synaptic vesicles; SPM, synaptic plasma membranes.

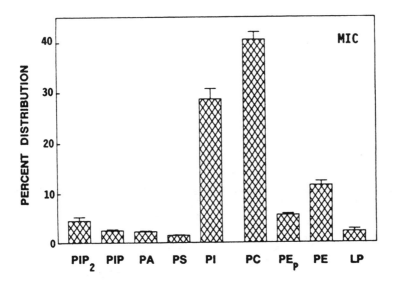

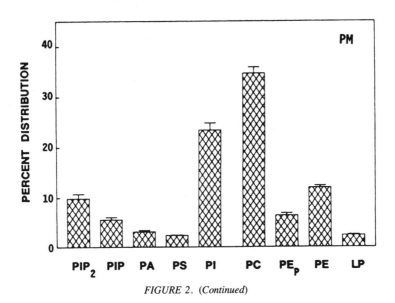

FIGURE 2. (Continued)

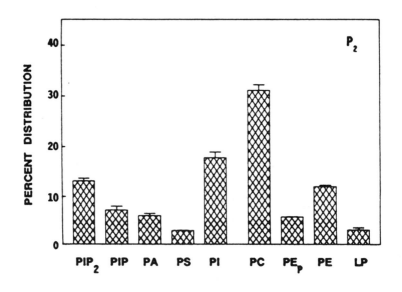

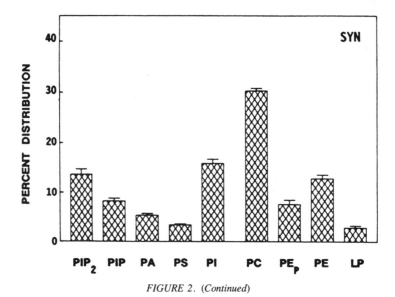

FIGURE 2. (*Continued*)

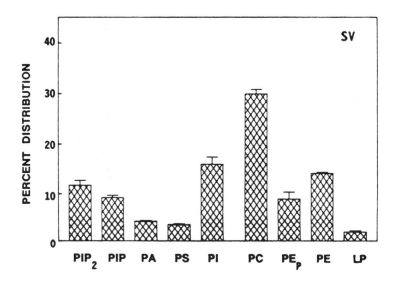

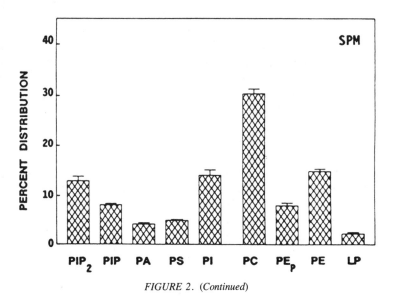

FIGURE 2. (Continued)

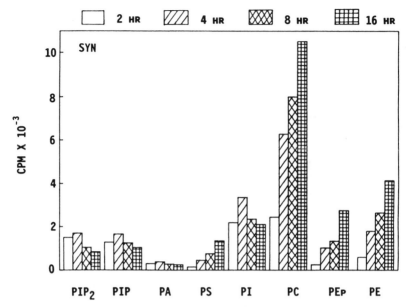

FIGURE 3. Labeling of phospholipids in rat brain synaptosomes with respect to time after intracerebral injection of [^{32}P]ATP. Prior to calculation of data, radioactivity in the brain homogenate of each sample was normalized. Results for each time point represent mean results for three to four brains.

to label the phosphoinositides and inositol phosphates in the brain. With this precursor, incorporation of labeled inositol into the inositol phospholipids (PI, PIP, and PIP$_2$) was less rapid than the ^{32}P-labeling procedure and showed a steady increase with time between 1 and 16 hr (Sun *et al.*, 1988*b*). The water-soluble inositol phosphates (IP, IP$_2$, and IP$_3$), however, seem to be able to attain maximum labeling within a shorter time (4 hr) as compared to the inositol phospholipids (Figure 5). It is important to realize that a relatively large amount of [^{3}H]inositol is needed to sufficiently label the poly-PI and the inositol phosphates in the brain, especially if reliable counts for IP$_3$ are to be obtained. Labeled inositol phosphates extracted into the aqueous fraction can be separated by a Dowex AG 1-X8 ion exchange column (formate form; Bio-Rad Laboratories, Richmond, Calif.) by the elution procedure described by Berridge *et al.* (1983). However, owing to the lack of strong chromophore, this column procedure cannot be used to quantitate the amount of inositol phosphates present in the samples. Our laboratory has recently tested the ion chromatography procedures for analysis of inositol phosphates isomers and mass determination (Dionex Corp., Sunnyvale, Calif.) (Smith *et al.*, 1988). The procedure was found suitable for analysis of the IP$_1$ and IP$_2$ in the brain, but the level of IP_3 was too low for detection by the conductivity detector (Sun et al., 1990).

4. ISCHEMIA INDUCES AN INCREASE IN DIACYLGLYCEROLS IN THE BRAIN

Before the discovery that DG may have a second-messenger role for the activation of protein kinase C, it was already recognized that ischemic insult could result in a rapid increase in the level of DG in the brain (Aveldano and Bazan, 1975; Banschbach and Geison, 1974; Tang and Sun, 1985). The DG released during the ischemic insult showed a high level of stearic and arachidonic acids, a profile similar to that in the phosphoinositides (Figure 6). On the basis of the similarity in the acyl groups, Keough et al. (1972) had suggested a metabolic link between DG and PI. In general, DG increase as a result of post-decapitation ischemic insult is rapid and reaches a plateau after 2 min (Figure 7). This mode of DG increase is different from that indicated by the FFA, which is slower and continues for a much longer period (Figure 5). Using the in situ freezing technique to inactivate brain tissue, Abe and Kogure (1986) reported a value of 80 nmol/g (wet weight) for the DG in the gerbil forebrain, and this level increased 83% after 5 min of ischemia induced by bilateral carotid ligation.

Rat pups up to two weeks of age did not elicit an obvious increase in the level of DG or FFA in the brain due to the decapitation ischemic insult (Figure 6) (Tang and Sun, 1985; Bazan, 1971a). These results suggest a postnatal development of the ischemia-induced event. Because most of the ischemia-induced lipid changes can be found in the synaptosomal fraction but not in the myelin (Huang and Sun, 1986), it is reasonable to conclude that this event is more closely associated with synaptogenesis than myelination.

5. ISCHEMIA INDUCES BREAKDOWN OF POLY-PI IN THE BRAIN

The observation that there is a transient and rapid increase in the level of DG with a fatty acid profile resembling that of phosphoinositides has prompted us to further investigate the biochemical mechanism underlying this event. Determination of the phosphorus content of poly-PI (PIP and PIP_2 together) in brain synaptosomes indicated a large (40%) decrease in the level of poly-PI after 1 and 5 min of decapitation ischemic insult to rats (Huang and Sun, 1986). Surprisingly, there was a small increase in the PI level, but levels of other phospholipids were not altered significantly. Subsequent studies by others also indicated the rapid de-

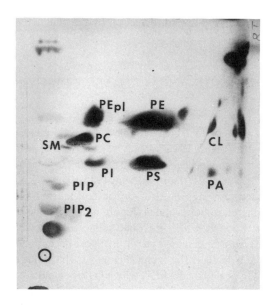

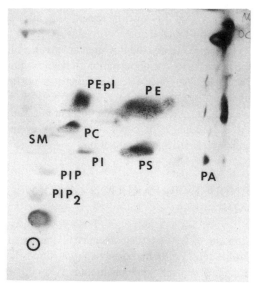

FIGURE 4. HPTLC separation of phospholipids in brain homogenate (upper left) and myelin (lower left) by the improved two-dimensional system described by Sun and Lin (1989). Since phospholipids were prelabeld with [^{32}P]ATP, the righthand panels represent an autoradiogram of the same sample in the left. See the text & the legend in Figure 2 for abbreviations. (Reprinted from Sun and Lin [1989] with permission.)

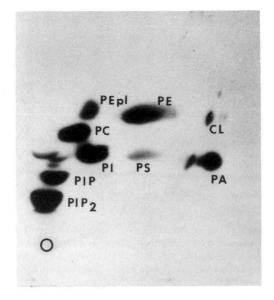

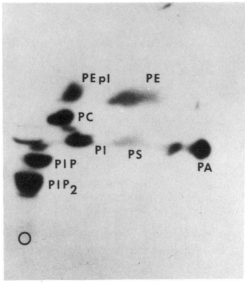

FIGURE 4. (Continued)

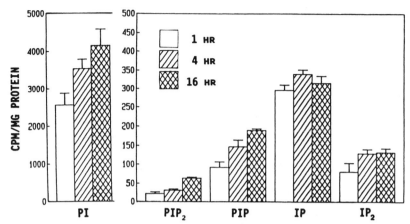

FIGURE 5. Time course of labeling brain phosphoinositides (PI, PIP, and PIP$_2$) and inositol phosphates after intracerebral injection of [^{3}H]inositol. Phosphoinositides were separated by HPTLC, and inositol phosphates were separated by the Dowex ion exchange column (Berridge *et al.*, 1983). Abbreviations: IP, inositol monophosphate; IP$_2$, inositol bisphosphate. (Reprinted from Sun *et al.* [1988*b*] with permission.)

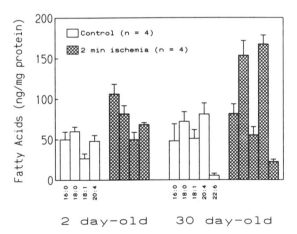

FIGURE 6. Ischemia-induced increase in DG in the developing rat brain: comparison of changes between days 2 and 30. For each age group, rat pups were subjected to a 2-min post-decapitation ischemic treatment and the brain DG content was analyzed by gas liquid chromatographic analysis of the fatty acids. Results are mean ± S.D. from four to six rats in each group. (Data taken from Tang and Sun [1985] with permission.)

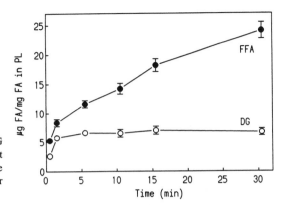

FIGURE 7. Levels of FFA and DG in mouse cerebral cortex at different times after decapitation. Results are mean ± S.D. from three animals for each time point.

crease in poly-PI as a result of cerebral ischemic insults (Ikeda *et al.*, 1986; Abe *et al.*, 1987). Nevertheless, the decrease in poly-PI levels as well as the increase in DG and FFA levels in the ischemic brain are events that can be readily reversed on recirculation (Yoshida *et al.*, 1986).

A substantial improvement for probing the brain poly-PI metabolism is the ability to label these compounds (Sun *et al.*, 1985). The labeling procedure offers greater sensitivity for detection of PIP and PIP_2 and requires less tissue for the assay procedure. Similar to the mass measurement, post-decapitation ischemic treatment (2 and 5 min) was shown to result in a large decrease in labeled poly-PI (Sun and Huang, 1987). Similarly, there was a small increase in the level of labeled PI but no change in other major phospholipids. With the labeling procedure, we could observe a more rapid decline in the level of labeled PIP_2 as compared to that of PIP during the initial period after decapitation (Sun *et al.*, 1988*b*). By 5 min, however, both labeled PIP_2 and PIP essentially reached the same low levels. The large decrease in the level of labeled PIP was unexpected because ATP was severely depleted after 1 min of ischemic treatment and this deprivation would have curtailed the conversion of PIP to PIP_2. On the other hand, the concomitant increase in the level of labeled PI seems to support the notion that some PIP (and possibly PIP_2) may have been retroconverted to PI via the action of phosphomono-esterase.

Using an improved HPTLC procedure, which is especially useful for separating phospholipids that are prelabeld with [32]P (Sun and Lin, 1989), an attempt was made to elucidate the subcellular site(s) of poly-PI breakdown in rat brain after decapitation ischemic insult. In order to isolate subcellular membranes, it was not possible to freeze the brain in liquid nitrogen; therefore, 30 sec was allowed for brain dissection and homogenization in a sucrose medium containing EDTA. When [32]Pi was injected into the rat brain 4 hr prior to decapitation, the ischemia-induced breakdown of poly-PI could be found in the synaptosomal and somal plasma membrane fractions, whereas labeled poly-PI in myelin, free mitochondria, and microsomes were not appreciably affected (Figure 8) (Sun *et al.*, 1990). On further fractionation of the synaptosome fraction, there was a decrease in labeled poly-PI in both synaptic plasma membranes (SPM) and synaptic vesicles (SV) (Figure 8). Since the SV fraction is the primary site for neurotransmitter storage within the nerve endings, it is possible that the poly-PI pool present in this membrane fraction is involved in mediating the vesicular neurotransmitter release or uptake. This notion is supported by the earlier studies of

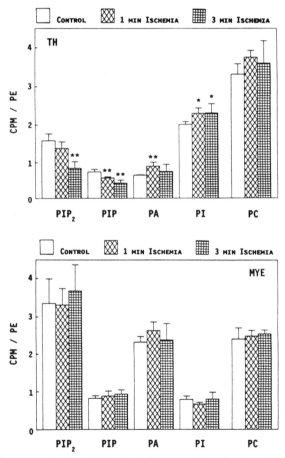

FIGURE 8. Changes in phospholipid labeling in brain subcellular fractions with respect to time of post-decapitation ischemic insult. Subcellular isolation and lipid separation are same as described for Figure 2. Results are mean ± S.D. for four rats for each control and ischemic treatment group.

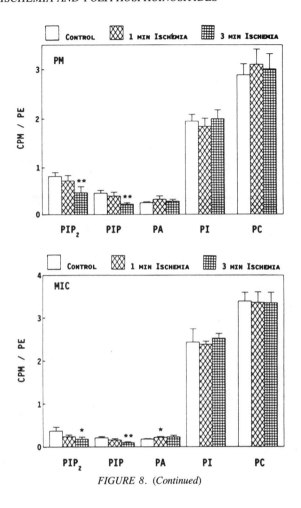

FIGURE 8. (Continued)

Hawthorne and Pickard (1979) who reported that the PI and PA in SV were metabolically active and that these phospholipids may participate in the neurotransmitter release process. Obviously, studies with more purified SV are needed to further clarify the role of poly-PI in these vesicles.

6. CAN POLY-PI DEGRADATION IN ISCHEMIA BE THE PRIMARY SOURCE OF FFA RELEASE?

Results from our laboratory (Huang and Sun, 1986, 1987; Sun and Huang, 1987; Sun et al., 1988b), as well as those of several others (Eichberg and Hauser,

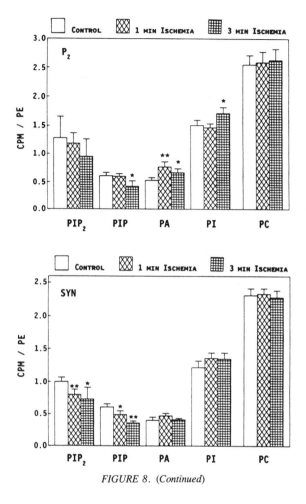

FIGURE 8. (Continued)

1967; Ikeda *et al.*, 1986; Abe *et al.*, 1987), have unequivocally demonstrated the rapid decrease in the level of poly-PI in the brain during the early onset of an ischemic insult. Although poly-PI degradation correlates well with the DG increase, it has not been clearly prove whether any of the DG could become a source of the FFA pool, through sequential hydrolysis by DG and MG lipases. The ischemia-induced release of FFA in the brain has been well demonstrated by Bazan (1970, 1971*b*). Furthermore, arachidonic and stearic acids were preferentially released during the early period of the insult (Bazan, 1976; Tang and Sun, 1982;

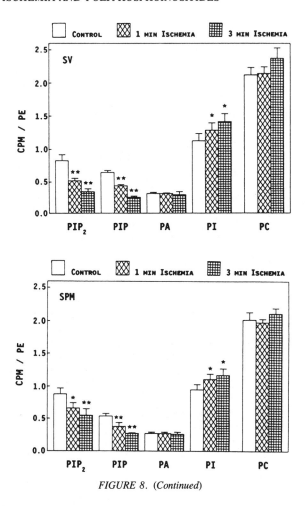

FIGURE 8. (*Continued*)

Ikeda *et al.*, 1986). Although the existence of a direct relationship between poly-PI, DG, and FFA has not been firmly established, the close resemblance between the fatty acids in the FFA pool and those in DG and poly-PI can be used as an evidence to support the relationship between the FFA release and poly-PI break-down during the early phase of ischemic insult. On the other hand, the continuous increase in FFA level in brain after decapitation even at a time when poly-PI are depleted suggests that a large portion of the FFA released during the later time period are derived from some other mechanisms.

7. POLY-PI METABOLISM IN A FOCAL ISCHEMIA MODEL INDUCED BY LIGATION OF THE MIDDLE CEREBRAL ARTERY IN THE RAT

By using the ^{32}P-labeling procedure, poly-PI metabolism in cerebral cortex was tested with a rat focal ischemic model in which the right middle cerebral artery was ligated together with successive occlusion of both common carotid arteries (Chen *et al.*, 1986; Lin *et al.*, 1991). To examine the effect of ligation on the poly-PI in brain cortex, [32]Pi was first injected intracerebrally (stereotactically) into both the left and right side of the rat brain and the label was equilibrated for 2 hr prior to ligation of the right cerebral artery. Sham-operated controls were similarly injected with the labeled precursor, except that the arteries were not ligated. After a brief period of ligation, there was a dramatic decrease (ca. 50%) in the levels of labeled PIP and PIP$_2$ in the right (ischemic) MCA cortex but not in the left MCA cortex and in the sham controls (Figure 9). These results clearly indicate that poly-PI breakdown is a process inherent in the ischemic insult.

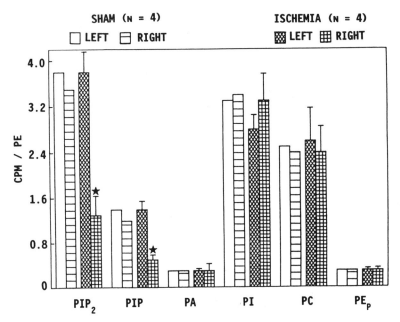

FIGURE 9. Effects of focal ischemia induced by ligation of the right middle cerebral artery of the rat brain on phospholipid labeling. Brain phospholipids were prelabeled with [32]P$_i$ for 2.5 hr prior to ligation for 30 min. Sham controls were similarly operated, but without ligation.

8. ISCHEMIA INDUCES CHANGES IN INOSITOL PHOSPHATES IN THE BRAIN

Agonist stimulation of PIP_2 hydrolysis by phospholipase C is known to give rise to DG and $Ins(1,4,5)P_3$ (Berridge, 1984). In turn, $Ins(1,4,5)P_3$ is rapidly metabolized and converted to other inositol phosphates. With rat brain prelabeled with [^{3}H]inositol, $Ins(1,4,5)P_3$ metabolism can be related to time of the ischemic insult. Experiments with [^{3}H]inositol can be carried out in conjunction with lithium treatment, which causes accumulation of IP_1 by inhibiting the phosphatases for converting IP_1 to inositol (Hallcher and Sherman, 1980; Sherman *et al.*, 1981). In a study in which [^{3}H]inositol was equilibrated in brain for 16 hr prior to injection of lithium (8 meq/kg of body weight for 4 hr), a 5 min decapitation insult decreased the ^{3}H-labeled poly-PI in both lithium-treated and control groups (Sun and Huang, 1987). Nevertheless, an increase in the levels of labeled inositol phosphates was not obvious (Strosznajder *et al.*, 1987). Part of this problem was attributed to the relatively long time for cooling the adult rat brain, even when it was immersed into liquid nitrogen immediately after decapitation. When younger rats (4 to 5 weeks of age) were used, we were able to observe a small and transient appearance of labeled IP_3 at 0.5 min after decapitation (Figure 10) (Sun *et al.*, 1988*b*). The appearance of IP_3 was followed by a marked increase in the level of

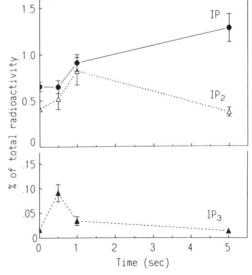

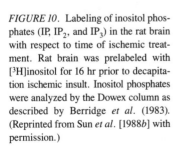

FIGURE 10. Labeling of inositol phosphates (IP, IP_2, and IP_3) in the rat brain with respect to time of ischemic treatment. Rat brain was prelabeled with [^{3}H]inositol for 16 hr prior to decapitation ischemic insult. Inositol phosphates were analyzed by the Dowex column as described by Berridge *et al.* (1983). (Reprinted from Sun *et al.* [1988*b*] with permission.)

labeled IP$_2$, reaching a peak at 1 min before decreasing to the basal level at 5 min. The level of labeled IP$_1$ was not altered during the first 0.5 min, but subsequently showed a biphasic increase reaching a plateau at 5 min (Figure 10). Recently, the time-dependent changes in inositol phosphates after decapitation insult were examined using the ion chromatography (Lin *et al.*, 1990). Results indicated similar transient appearance of the Ins(1,4)P$_2$ which was turned over to Ins(4)P but not Ins(1)P.

It is concluded from these studies that during ischemic insult, the IP$_3$ released from hydrolysis of PIP$_2$ is rapidly converted to IP$_2$ which in turn is further catabolized to IP$_1$ and free inositol. However, more studies are necessary to elucidate the subcellular sites of this event and to understand whether prolonged ischemia insult may cause irreversible changes in these pathways that are critical for maintaining the calcium homeostasis within the neurons.

9. SUMMARY

A review of studies carried out in our laboratory as well as by others has provided a clear indication that poly-PI in brain are degraded during the early period of an ischemic insult. This phenomenon can be demonstrated in all ischemia models tested. Because of ATP deprivation, the brain tissue cannot replenish the poly-PI lost during the ischemic insult. However, a reversal of the changes can be observed shortly after recirculation. These results also stress the importance of ATP for several biochemical steps underlying the signal transduction pathways involving poly-PI turnover. Poly-PI breakdown can account for the increase in DG, and contribute to the FFA release during the early phase of the ischemic insult. Several studies with brain subcellular membrane fractions have given indications that poly-PI breakdown occurs mainly in the synaptic membranes and somal plasma membranes, but not in myelin and microsomes. This is in line with the notion that cerebral ischemia is associated with stimulation of poly-PI breakdown induced by neurotransmitter agonists. In general, the decrease in the level of poly-PI is marked by a transient increase in the levels of inositol phosphates; and the extent of poly-PI decrease and the increase in IP$_1$ can be assessed after lithium administration. Further studies are needed to elucidate the intricate mechanism regulating the metabolism of IP$_3$ because this second messenger is important for regulating the intracellular calcium homeostasis within the neurons.

An imposing question which remains to be answered is the mechanism triggering the breakdown of poly-PI during ischemia. It is natural to think along the lines of neurotransmitter agonists because a large number of neurotransmitters are released during the onset of such an insult. Although it would be difficult to identify the type of neurotransmitters that are directly involved in the ischemic insult, some clue regarding this point may be obtained by examining the poly-PI response in brain regions that are associated with specific neurotransmitter systems.

ACKNOWLEDGMENTS

This research project is supported in part by U.S. Department of Health and Human Services research grants NS 16715 and NS 20836 from NINCDS. The assistance of B. Jones in the preparation of the manuscript is greatly appreciated.

REFERENCES

Abdel-Latif, A. A., 1986, Calcium-mobilizing receptors, polyphosphoinositides, and the generation of second messengers, *Pharmacol. Rev.* **38:**227–272.

Abe, K., and Kogure, K., 1986, Accurate evaluation of 1,2-diacylglycerol in gerbil forebrain using HPLC and in situ freezing technique, *J. Neurochem.* **47:**577–582.

Abe, K., Kogure, K., Yamamoto, H., Imazawa, M., and Miyamoto, K., 1987, Mechanism of arachidonic acid liberation during ischemia in gerbil cerebral cortex, *J. Neurochem.* **48:** 503–509.

Aveldano, M. I., and Bazan, N. G., 1975, Rapid production of diacylglycerols enriched in arachidonate and stearate during early brain ischemia, *J. Neurochem.* **25:**919–920.

Banschbach, M. W., and Geison, R. L., 1974, Post-mortem increase in rat brain cerebral hemisphere diglyceride pool size, *J. Neurochem.* **23:**875–877.

Bazan, N. G., 1970, Effects of ischemia and electroconvulsive shock on free fatty acid pool in the brain, *Biochim. Biophys. Acta* **218:**1–10.

Bazan, N. G., 1971*a*, Modification in the free fatty acids of developing brain, *Acta Physiol. Latinoam.* **21:**15–20.

Bazan, N. G., 1971*b*, Changes in free fatty acids of brain by drug-induced convulsions, electroshock and anesthesia, *J. Neurochem.* **18:**1379–1385.

Bazan, N. G., 1976, Free arachidonic acids and other lipids in the nervous system during early ischemia and after electroshock, *Adv. Exp. Med. Biol.* **72:**317–335.

Berridge, M. J., 1983, Rapid accumulation of inositol triphosphate reveals that agonists hydrolyse polyphosphoinositides instead of phosphatidylinositol, *Biochem. J.* **212:**849–858.

Berridge, M. J., 1984, Inositol triphosphate and diacylglycerol as second messengers, *Biochem. J.* **220:**345–360.

Berridge, M. J., Dawson, R. M. C., Downes, C. P., Henlop, J. P., and Irvine, R. F., 1983, Changes in the levels of inositol phosphates after agonist-dependent hydrolysis of membrane phospho-inositides, *Biochem. J.* **212:**473–483.

Brown, E., Kendall, D. A., and Nahorski, S. R., 1984, Inositol phospholipid hydrolysis in rat cerebral cortical slices: 1. Receptor characterization, *J. Neurochem.* **42:**1379–1387.

Chen, S. T., Hsu, C. Y., Hogan, E. L., Maricq, H., and Balentine, J. D., 1986, A model of focal ischemic stroke in the rat: Reproducible extensive cortical infarction, *Stroke* **17:**738–743.

Chiu, A. S., Li, P. P., and Warsh, J. J., 1988, G-protein involvement in central-nervous-system muscarinic-receptor-coupled polyphosphoinositide hydrolysis, *Biochem. J.* **256:**995–999.

Downes, C. P., 1986, Agonist-stimulated phosphatidylinositol 4,5-bisphosphate metabolism in the nervous system, *Neurochem. Int.* **9**:211–230.

Eichberg, J., and Hauser, G., 1967, Concentration and disappearance post-mortem of polyphosphoinositides in developing rat brain, *Biochim. Biophys. Acta* **144**:415–422.

Eichberg, J., and Hauser, G., 1973, The subcellular distribution of polyphosphoinositides in myelinated and unmyelinated rat brian, *Biochim. Biophys. Acta* **326**:210–223.

Farooqui, A. A., Taylor, W. A., and Horrocks, L. A., 1986, Membrane bound diacylglycerol lipases in bovine brain: Purification and characterization, *in* "Fidia Research Series, vol. 4. Phospholipid Research and the Nervous System: Biochemical and Molecular Pharmacology" (L. A. Horrocks, L. Freysz, and G. Toffano, eds.), pp. 181–190, Liviana Press, Padova, Italy.

Fisher, S. K., and Agranoff, B. W., 1987, Receptor activation and inositol lipid hydrolysis in neural tissue, *J. Neurochem.* **48**:999–1017.

Gonzales, R. A., and Crews, F. T., 1984, Characterization of the cholinergic stimulation of phosphoinositide hydrolysis of rat brain slices, *J. Neurosci.* **4**:3120–3127.

Gonzales, R. A., and Crews, F. T., 1985, Cholinergic- and adrenergic-stimulated inositide hydrolysis in brain: Interaction, regional distribution, and coupling mechanisms, *J. Neurochem.* **45**:1076–1084.

Gonzalez-Sastre, P., Eichberg, J., and Hauser, G., 1971, Metabolic pools of polyphosphoinositides in rat brain, *Biochim. Biophys. Acta* **248**:96–104.

Hallcher, L. M., and Sherman, W. R., 1980, The effects of lithium ion and other agents on the activity of myo-inositol 1-phosphatase from bovine brain, *J. Biol. Chem.* **255**:10896–10901.

Hawthorne, J. N., and Pickard, M. R., 1979, Phospholipids in synaptic function, *J. Neurochem.* **32**:5–14.

Huang, S. F.-L., and Sun, G. Y., 1986, Cerebral ischemia induced quantitative changes in rat brain membrane lipids involved in phosphoinositide metabolism, *Neurochem. Int.* **9**:185–190.

Huang, S. F.-L., and Sun, G. Y., 1987, Acidic phospholipids, diacylglycerols, and free fatty acids in gerbil brain: A comparison of ischemic changes resulting from carotid ligation and decapitation, *J. Neurosci. Res.* **17**:162–167.

Ikeda, M., Yoshida, S., Busto, R., Santiso, M., and Ginsberg, M. D., 1986, Polyphosphoinositides as a probable source of brain free fatty acids accumulated at the onset of ischemia, *J. Neurochem.* **47**:123–132.

Inhorn, R. C., Bansal, V. S., and Majerus, P. W., 1987, Pathway for inositol 1,3,4-triphosphate and 1,4-bisphosphate metabolism, *Proc. Natl. Acad. Sci. USA* **84**:2170–2174.

Kelleher, J. A., and Sun, G. Y., 1989, Effects of free fatty acids and acyl-CoA on diacylglycerol kinase in rat brain, *J. Neuroscience Res.* **23**:87–94.

Keough, K. M. W., MacDonald, G., and Thompson, W., 1972, A possible relation between phosphoinositides and the diacylglyceride pool in the rat, *Biochim. Biophys. Acta* **270**:337–347.

Kobayashi, H., Liest, W. D., and Passonneau, J. V., 1977, Concentrations of energy metabolites and cyclic nucleotides during and after bilateral ischemia in the gerbil cerebral cortex, *J. Neurochem.* **29**:53–59.

Levy, D. E., and Duffy, T. E., 1977, Cerebral energy metabolism during transient ischemia and recovery in gerbil, *J. Neurochem.* **28**:63–70.

Li, P. P., Chiu, A. S., and Warsh, J. J., 1989, Activation of phosphoinositide hydrolysis in rat cortical slices by guanine nucleotides and sodium fluoride, *Neurochem. Int.* **14**:43–48.

Lin, T. N., Sun, G. Y., Premkumar, N., MacQuarrie, R. A., and Carter, S. R., 1990, Decapitation-induced changes in inositol phosphates in rat brain, *Biochem. Biophys. Res. Commun.* **167**:1294–1301.

Lin, T. N., Liu, T. H., Xu, Y., Hsu, C. Y., and Sun, G. Y., 1991, Effect of focal ischemia on polyphosphoinositide breakdown in rat cortex, *Stroke* **22**:495–498.

Litosch, I., 1987, Guanine nucleotide and NaF stimulation of phospholipase C activity in rat cerebral-cortical membranes. Studies on substrate specificity, *Biochem. J.* **244**:35–40.

Lowry, D. H., Passonneau, J. V., Hasselberger, F. Y., and Schulz, D. W., 1964, Effect of ischemia on known substrates and co-factors of the glycolytic pathway in brain, *J. Biol. Chem.* **239:** 18–30.

Manning, R., and Sun, G. Y., 1983, Detergent effects on the phosphatidylinositol-specific phospholipase C in rat brain synaptosomes, *J. Neurochem.* **41:**1735–1743.

Nemoto, E. M., 1985, Brain ischemia, *in* "Handbook of Neurochemistry," vol. 9 (A. Lajtha, ed.), pp. 533–588, Plenum Press, New York.

Nishizuka, Y., 1984, The role of protein kinase C in cell surface signal transduction and tumor promotion, *Nature* **308:**693–698.

Nishizuka, Y., 1986, Studies and perspectives of protein kinase C, *Science* **233:**305–312.

Nowak, T. S., Jr., Fried, R. L., Lust, W. D., and Passonneau, J. V., 1985, Changes in brain energy metabolism and protein synthesis following transient bilateral ischemia in the gerbil, *J. Neurochem.* **44:**487–494.

Sherman, W. R., Leavitt, A. L., Honchar, M. P., Hallcher, L. M., and Phillips, B. E., 1981, Evidence that lithium alters phosphoinositide metabolism. Chronic administration elevates primary D-myo-inositol-phosphate in cerebral cortex of the rat, *J. Neurochem.* **36:**1947–1951.

Smith, R. E., Howell, S., Yourtee, D., Premkumar, N., Sun, G. Y., and MacQuarrie, R. A., 1988, Ion chromatographic determination of sugar phosphates in physiological samples, *J. Chromatogr.* **439:**83–92.

Soukup, J. F., Friedel, R. O., and Shanberg, S. M., 1978, Microwave irradiation fixation for studies of polyphosphoinositide metabolism in brain, *J. Neurochem.* **30:**635–637.

Strosznajder, J., Wikiel, H., Kelleher, J. A., Leu, V. S., and Sun, G. Y., 1986, Diacylglycerol kinase and lipase activities in rat brain subcellular fractions, *Neurochem. Int.* **8:**213–221.

Strosznajder, J., Wikiel, H., and Sun, G. Y., 1987, Effects of cerebral ischemia on [³H]inositol lipids and [³H]inositol phosphates of gerbil brain and subcellular fractions, *J. Neurochem.* **48:**943–948.

Stubbs, E. B., Jr., Kelleher, J. A., and Sun, G. Y., 1988, Phosphatidylinositol, phosphatidylinositol 4-phosphate and diacylglycerol kinase activities in rat brain subcellular fractions, *Biochim. Biophys. Acta* **958:**247–254.

Sun, G. Y., 1988, Phospholipid metabolism in response to cerebral ischemia, *in* "Fidia Research Series, vol. 17. Phospholipids in the Nervous System" (N. Bazan, L. A. Horrocks, and G. Toffano, eds.), pp. 133–149, Liviana Press, Padova, Italy.

Sun, G. Y., and Huang, S. F.-L., 1987, Labeling of phosphoinositides in rat brain membranes: An assessment of changes due to post-decapitative ischemic treatment, *Neurochem. Int.* **10:**361–369.

Sun, G. Y., and Lin, T.-N., 1989, Time course for labeling of brain membrane phosphoinositides and other phospholipids after intracerebral injection of [³²P]-ATP: Evaluation by an improved HPTLC method, *Life Sci.* **44:**689–696.

Sun, G. Y., Yoa, F.-G., and Lin, T.-N., 1990, Response of phosphoinositides in brain subcellular membrane fractions to decapitation ischemia, *Neurochem. Int.* **17:**529–535.

Sun, G. Y., Tang, W., Huang, F. L., and Foudin, L., 1985, Is phosphatidylinositol involved in the release of free fatty acids in cerebral ischemia? *in* "Inositol and Phosphoinositides: Metabolism and Regulation" (J. E. Bleasdale, J. Eichberg, and G. Hauser, eds.), pp. 511–527, Humana Press, Clifton, N. J.

Sun, G. Y., Huang, H.-M., Kelleher, J. A., Stubbs, E. B., Jr., and Sun, A. Y., 1988*a*, Marker enzymes, phospholipids and acyl group composition of a somal plasma membrane fraction isolated from rat cerebral cortex: A comparison with microsomes and synaptic plasma membranes, *Neurochem. Int.* **12:**69–77.

Sun, G. Y., Huang, H.-M., and Chandrasekhar, R., 1988*b*, Turnover of inositol phosphates in brain during ischemia-induced breakdown of polyphosphoinositides, *Neurochem. Int.* **13:**63–68.

Sun, G. Y., Lin, T. N., Premkuma, N., Carter, S. R., and MacQuarrie, R. A., 1990, Separation and quantitation of isomers of inositol phosphates by ion chromatography, *in* "Methods of Inositide Research" (R. Irvine, ed.), pp. 135–144, Raven Press, London.

Tang, W., and Sun, G. Y., 1982, Factors affecting the free fatty acids in rat brain cortex, *Neurochem. Int.* **4**:269–273.

Tang, W., and Sun, G. Y., 1985, Effects of ischemia on free fatty acids and diacylglycerols in developing rat brain, *Int. J. Dev. Neurosci.* **3**:51–56.

Williamson, J. R., Cooper, R. H., Joseph, S. K., and Thomas, A. P., 1985, Inositol triphosphate and diacylglycerol as intracellular second messengers in liver, *Am. J. Physiol.* **248**:C203–C216.

Yoshida, S., Ikeda, M., Busto, R., Santiso, M., Martinez, E., and Ginsberg, M., 1986, Cerebral phosphoinositide, triacylglycerol and energy metabolism in reversible ischemia: Origin and fate of free fatty acids, *J. Neurochem.* **47**:744–757.

CHAPTER 12

PROTECTION AGAINST ISCHEMIC BRAIN DAMAGE BY EXCITATORY AMINO ACID ANTAGONISTS

BRIAN MELDRUM

1. INTRODUCTION

A major goal of research on cerebral ischemia is to identify pharmacological means of preventing ischemic brain damage. Such attempts have commonly been based on altering cerebrovascular dynamics. Drugs based on this approach include those acting on platelets or on the clot itself (e.g., anti-platelet-activating factors, fibrinolysin, plasmin, streptokinase, urokinase, and tissue plasminogen activators) and those acting on the vessel wall (e.g., calcium channel-blocking drugs). The limited success of such approaches (Grotta, 1987) has led to alternative strategies that emphasize biochemical events in neuronal membranes and cyto-

BRIAN MELDRUM • *Department of Neurology, Institute of Psychiatry, London, United Kingdom.*

Neurochemical Correlates of Cerebral Ischemia, Volume 7 of *Advances in Neurochemistry*, edited by Nicolas G. Bazan, Pierre Braquet, and Myron D. Ginsberg. Plenum Press, New York, 1992.

plasm (so-called "parenchymal approaches"). Two of these appear to offer considerable promise. One relates to the supposed role of free radicals in determining cell death (Demopoulos *et al.*, 1980; Halliwell and Gutteridge, 1985; Hall and Braughler, 1989); the other concerns the excitotoxic effect of glutamate and aspartate. This chapter reviews evidence relating to the contribution of the excitotoxic action of dicarboxylic amino acids to brain damage following cerebral ischemia and the possible clinical use of pharmacological agents modifying this action.

1.1. The Concept of Excitotoxicity

The concept of excitotoxicity was introduced to describe the mechanism by which high oral doses of glutamate and some chemical analogues caused lesions in periventricular structures in the mouse brain (Olney *et al.*, 1971). It was observed that there was a correlation between the neurotoxicity of glutamate analogues and their potency as excitants as assessed electrophysiologically in the spinal cord. The concept of excitotoxicity served to define a class of acidic amino acids which possess neurotoxic properties when directly injected into the brain. This class includes compounds acting on each of the subtypes of postsynaptic glutamate receptor now recognized (e.g., kainate and domoate acting on the kainate receptor, N-methyl-D-aspartate (NMDA) and quinolinate acting on the NMDA receptor, quisqualate and d-amino-3-hydroxy-5-methyl-4-isoxazole propionate (AMPA) acting on the ionotropic receptor, and quisqualate and ibotenate acting on the quisqualate metabotropic receptor) (Olney *et al.*, 1974; Garthwaite and Meldrum, 1990).

In cytological terms the characteristic feature of excitotoxic damage is its postsynaptic nature, i.e., that axons of passage and presynaptic terminals are not damaged whereas postsynaptic structures (dendrites and cell bodies) are affected. Acutely this takes the form of focal dendritic swellings and cytoplasmic condensation with multiple vacuolation in the perikarya; in the longer term it involves disappearance of neurones with glial proliferation.

1.2. In Vitro Studies of Excitotoxicity

The concept of excitotoxicity has evolved considerably since it was first introduced. In particular, in vitro studies with cultured neurons or slice preparations have led to specific hypotheses concerning the mechanisms of excitotoxicity. There appear to be at least three distinctive forms of excitotoxic cell death.

(1) High concentrations of excitotoxins (glutamate, NMDA, etc.) act on neurons in culture to induce depolarization and a rapid entry of Na^+ and Cl^-, which apparently act osmotically to draw in H_2O and lead to swelling and death

of the neuron (Rothman, 1985). This type of cell death is seen shortly after brief (5- to 30-min) exposures to glutamate, NMDA, kainate, or quisqualate. It is prevented if Na^+ or Cl^- is substituted by nonpermeable ions; it is not prevented if Ca^{2+} is not present in the superfusing fluid. It is not clear whether this in vitro type of excitotoxicity is ever encountered in vivo.

(2) Low concentrations of excitotoxins (glutamate, NMDA, kainate) lead to slower cell death, which is dependent on Ca^{2+} (Choi, 1985, 1987). This may involve the cytotoxicity of raised intracellular Ca^{2+} concentrations, a mechanism that has been thought to play a role in the degeneration of skeletal, cardiac, and vascular smooth muscle (Wrogemann and Pena, 1976; Emery and Burt, 1980; Garthwaite and Meldrum, 1990). Raised intracellular Ca^{2+} concentrations have multiple consequences including activation of proteinases and phospholipases A and C (Garthwaite and Meldrum, 1990). The latter effect leads to rapid accumulation of arachidonic acid, which acts as a precursor for prostaglandins and leukotrienes. Enhanced lipid peroxidation and free radical formation may thus follow excitatory amino acid (EAA) action.

(3) Low concentrations of quisqualate lead to cell death (in hippocampal pyramidal neurons) that is not dependent on Ca^{2+} or Cl^- and appears to involve activation of both quisqualate metabotropic and ionotropic receptors (Garthwaite and Garthwaite, 1989*a,b*). Release of intracellular calcium from storage sites may play a role in the complex sequence of events leading to cell death under these circumstances.

The toxicity of EAA to cultured neurons can be blocked by appropriate antagonists (Choi *et al.*, 1988). NMDA antagonists are effective against glutamate, indicating that action on the NMDA receptor is particularly significant (Choi *et al.*, 1988). NMDA antagonists are also protective in models of hypoxia-ischemia (exposure to N_2 atmosphere) (Goldberg *et al.*, 1987*a,b*).

2. ISCHEMIC DAMAGE AND EXCITOTOXICITY

The reasons for considering that excitotoxic mechanisms contribute to the abnormalities encountered after cerebral ischemia are discussed below.

2.1. Acute Cytopathology

Experimental material perfusion-fixed shortly after transient cerebral ischemia shows cytopathology similar to that observed in excitotoxicity. Thus, in the rat hippocampus 30 to 90 min after 30 min of forebrain ischemia there is focal dendritic swelling in the apical and basal pyramidal cell zones and pyramidal cell bodies show vacuolation and condensation (Simon *et al.*, 1984*a*; Johansen *et al.*,

1986). Hypoxia-ischemia also produces glutamatelike cytopathology in the neonatal rat brain (Ikonomidou *et al.*, 1989*a,b*).

2.2. Extracellular EAAs

There is a marked rise in extracellular glutamate and aspartate concentrations during ischemia. This has been shown with in vivo microdialysis in animal models of global and focal ischemia. In the rat hippocampus and striatum global ischemia causes the glutamate concentration to rise seven- to eightfold or more and the aspartate concentration fourfold (Benveniste *et al.*, 1984*a*; Hagberg *et al.*, 1985; Globus *et al.*, 1988). Middle cerebral artery occlusion causes more substantial increases in extracellular glutamate concentration (20- to 30-fold) in the striatum (Hillered *et al.*, 1989) and the cortex (Graham *et al.*, 1990). These increases result from a combination of enhanced synaptic release, enhanced cytosolic release, and impaired reuptake (Drejer *et al.*, 1985).

2.3. Deafferentation and Ischemic Damage

An important role in the physiopathogenesis of ischemic damage for excitatory pathways within the hippocampus is indicated by the effect of certain surgical or chemical lesions. The delayed loss of CA1 cells following transient ischemia can be reduced either by lesions to the perforant path or by destruction of the mossyfiber path, the Schaffer collaterals, or the hippocampal commissure (Johansen *et al.*, 1986*b*; Jorgensen *et al.*, 1987; Onodera *et al.*, 1986). Experiments involving combinations of in vivo microdialysis, chemical lesioning of CA3 neurons, and microinjections of glutamate into CA1, show a good correlation between intactness of glutamatergic input, extracellular glutamate concentrations, and delayed ischemic damage to CA1 neurons (Benveniste *et al.*, 1989). It has recently been suggested, however, that nonglutamatergic afferents may also be important in determining the outcome of reversible ischemia in the hippocampus, since fimbria-fornix lesions appear to have a more potent protective effect than perforant path lesions (Buchan and Pulsinelli, 1990*b*).

2.4. EAA Antagonists and Cerebral Protection

Drugs that act as antagonists to the postsynaptic excitatory effect of glutamate can provide protection against damage following global or focal ischemia. The evidence for this is reviewed below and provides strong support for the view that excitation at both NMDA and non-NMDA receptors contributes to the process leading to cell loss.

3. PHARMACOLOGY OF EAA TRANSMISSION

The main subtypes of postsynaptic receptors for glutamate and aspartate differ not only in their preferred (exogenous) agonists but also in their functions and their antagonist pharmacology.

3.1. NMDA Receptor

The NMDA receptor is distinct in terms of its functional effects and its complex modulation. The ionophore that it opens is permeable to Ca^{2+} as well as to Na^+ and K^+ and is subject to a voltage-dependent block by magnesium (at concentrations of Mg^{2+} normally found in cerebrospinal fluid [CSF]). Glycine acts at an allosteric-type site to potentiate the effect of NMDA or glutamate. Since the presence of glycine appears to be obligatory for the activation of the receptor, it may be more appropriate to regard it as a co-agonist.

3.2. NMDA Antagonists

A number of analogues of glutamate that are selective, competitive inhibitors at the NMDA-glutamate receptor have been identified (Watkins and Evans, 1981; Davies et al., 1986; Lehmann et al., 1988; Meldrum et al., 1989). These compounds are all analogues of D-glutamate with a phosphono group in the omega position. The molecular structures of the six most potent and widely used compounds are shown in Figure 1.

Phencyclidine (PCP) and other dissociative anesthetics including ketamine, act as noncompetitive NMDA antagonists, probably by acting at a site within the ionophore. The anticonvulsant MK-801 (Clineschmidt et al., 1982) and the opioid dextrorphan also act at this site, as shown by displacement of ³H-labeled ligands (Wong et al., 1986, 1988). The similarity in the molecular structures of these compounds is shown in Figure 2.

Compounds can also act as NMDA antagonists by competing at the glycine allosteric site. Such compounds include kynurenic acid and 5,7- and 7-chlorokynurenic acids, (+)-HA966, and the quinoxalinediones, 6,7-dinitroquinoxaline-2,3-dione (DNQX) and 6-cyano-7-nitroquinoxaline-2,3-dione (CNQX) (Figure 3).

There may be other sites at which NMDA receptor antagonism can be produced. Zn^{2+} acts as an NMDA antagonist. This appears to depend partially on action at a site at which tricyclic antidepressants also act (Reynolds and Miller, 1988). There is also evidence for a site at which polyamines such as spermidine act (Ransom and Stec, 1988). Spermidine enhances the binding of MK-801 to brain membrane preparations, and this effect is additive to that of glycine or glutamate.

Ifenprodil and SL 82.0715, whose molecular structures slightly resemble

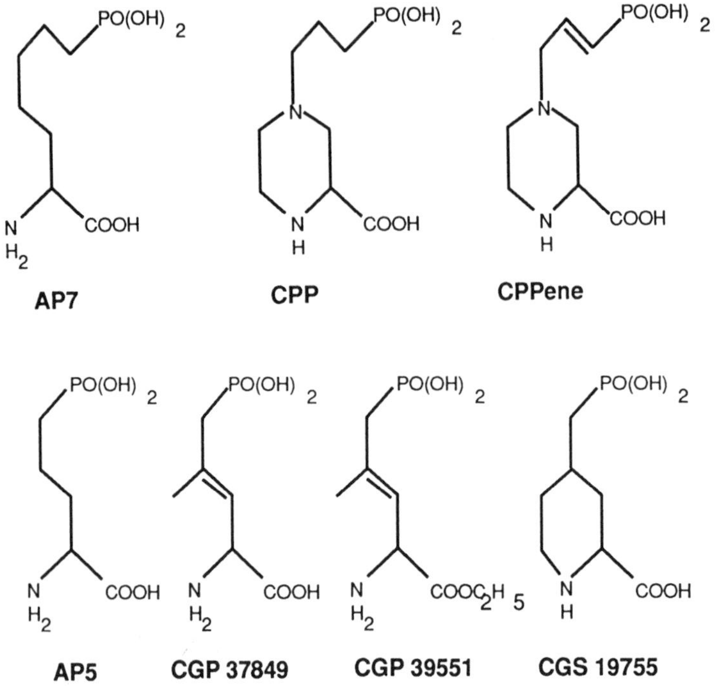

FIGURE 1. Molecular formulae of six competitive antagonists that act selectively on the NMDA receptor: AP5 (2-amino-5-phosphonovaleric acid); AP7 (2-amino-7-phosphonoheptanoic acid); CPP; CPP-ene; CGS 19755; and CGP 37849.

those of the PCP- and MK-801 type of NMDA antagonists, also act as noncompetitive antagonists, but only weakly compete for binding at the PCP/MK-801 site (Carter *et al.*, 1988). It is suggested that they may act at the polyamine site.

3.3. Kainate and AMPA Receptors

Less is known about the properties of the kainate and AMPA receptors. The high-affinity kainate receptor has a very distinctive distribution in the brain, being found in highest density in the mossy-fiber system in the hippocampus and also in the inner laminae of the neocortex and in the striatum (Patel *et al.*, 1988). It is not certain, however, that this is the receptor responsible for postsynaptic excitatory responses induced by kainate. Nevertheless, the high-affinity receptor is involved in the excitotoxic action of kainate, which is most marked in the CA3 neurons receiving the mossy-fiber input.

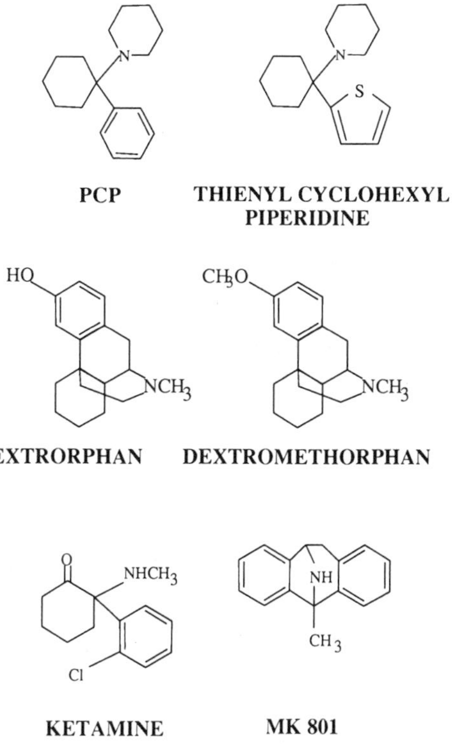

PCP   **THIENYL CYCLOHEXYL**
PIPERIDINE

DEXTRORPHAN   **DEXTROMETHORPHAN**

FIGURE 2. Molecular formulae of non-competitive NMDA antagonists that compete for a membrane-binding site with PCP and MK-801.

KETAMINE   **MK 801**

AMPA receptors represent the principal glutamate receptors mediating synaptic transmission.

Selective antagonists effective in vivo have not been available for the kainate and the AMPA receptor until very recently. Some glutamate analogues (e.g., kynurenic acid) are nonselective antagonists at all three major receptor subtypes. The quinoxalinediones CNQX and DNQX are potent competitive antagonists at both kainate and AMPA receptors (in vitro), with a weaker noncompetitive action at the NMDA receptor (Honoré *et al.*, 1988). A novel quinoxalinedione 2,3-dihydroxy-6-nitro-7-sulfamoylbenzo[*f*]quinoxaline (NBQX) (Figure 3) is a potent AMPA antagonist with central activity following systemic administration (Sheardown *et al.*, 1990).

3.4. Quisqualate/Ibotenate Metabotropic Receptor

Quisqualate also activates a so-called metabotropic receptor system that is linked to a G protein and leads to phosphoinositide hydrolysis (Sugiyama *et al.*,

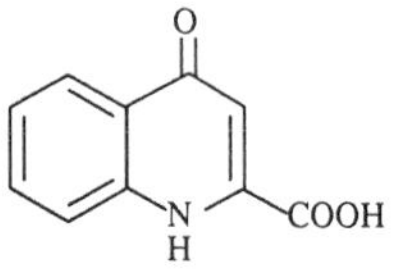

KYNURENIC ACID

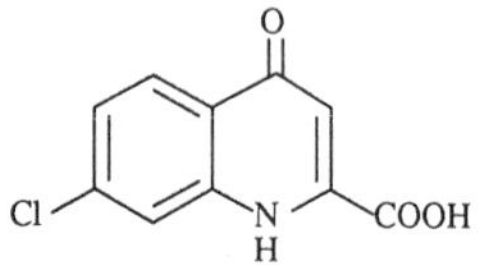

7-Cl-KYNURENIC ACID

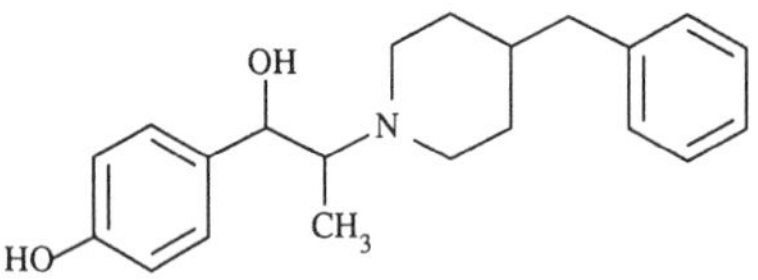

IFENPRODIL

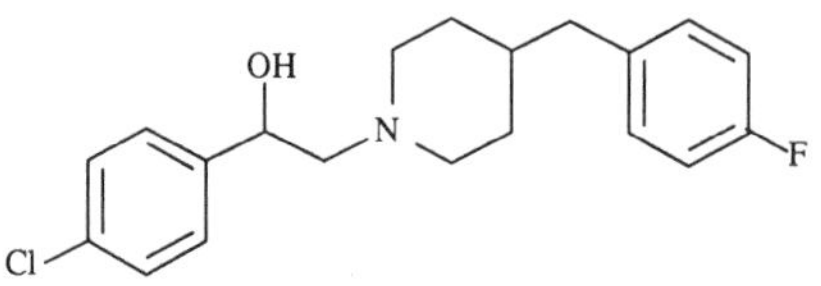

SL 82.0715

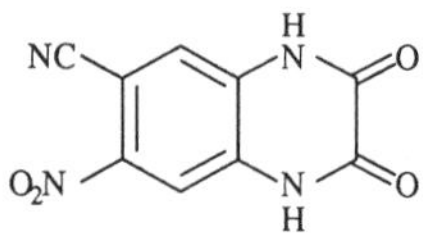

CNQX

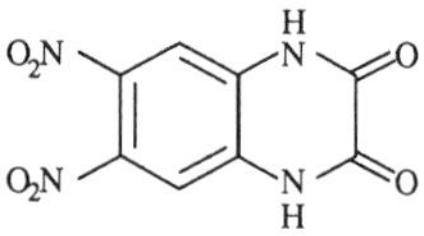

DNQX

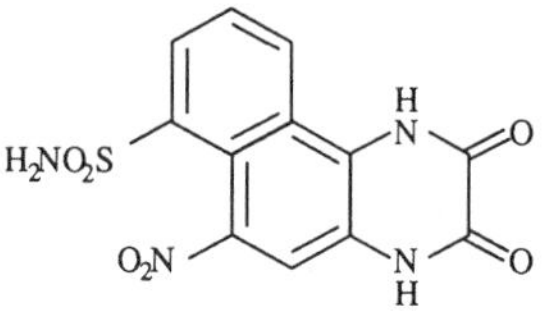

NBQX

FIGURE 3. Molecular formulae of various EAA antagonists. Ifenprodil and SL 82.0715 act as NMDA antagonists by mechanisms not yet fully elucidated, perhaps involving a polyamine site. Kynurenic acid is a competitive antagonist at kainate and quisqualate receptors and also acts as an NMDA receptor antagonist at the glycide site. 7-Chlorokynurenic acid acts at the NMDA glycine site more potently and selectively than does kynurenic acid. DNQX and CNQX are kainate and quisqualate antagonists with a weaker antagonist action at the glycine NMDA site. NBQX is a potent selective inhibitor at the AMPA-quisqualate site, with systemic activity.

1987; Recasens *et al.*, 1988). Glutamate and ibotenate (but not NMDA) also act on this metabotropic receptor. The quinoxalinediones CNQX and DNQX act as antagonists at the kainate and AMPA ionotropic receptors but not at the AMPA metabotropic receptor.

4. CEREBROPROTECTION

Pharmacological intervention to reduce the excitotoxic effects of glutamate during and after ischemia can take many forms. It is possible to modify the synthesis or synaptic release of glutamate by a variety of agents. Adenosine and various adenosine analogues act presynaptically to decrease synaptic release of glutamate. This effect probably contributes to the cerebroprotective effects of intracerebral injection of adenosine analogues (Evans *et al.*, 1987; von Lubitz *et al.*, 1988). However, since the initial report of the cytoprotective effect of 2-amino-7-phosphonoheptanoic acid (Simon *et al.*, 1984*b*), interest has centered mainly on the protective effects of competitive and noncompetititive NMDA antagonists. Such effects have now been shown in a wide range of animal models of cerebral hypoxia-ischemia (Meldrum, 1990). these include studies in infant rats (with unilateral carotid occlusion plus reduction of the O_2 content in the inspired air) to transient global ischemia in adult rats and focal ischemia (middle cerebral artery [MCA] occlusion) in mice, rats, and cats. To date, studies of global ischemia or focal ischemia in mongrel dogs and in monkeys have provided less evidence for protection. Animal models of spinal trauma or cerebral trauma have provided clear evidence of protection by competitive and noncompetitive NMDA antagonists.

4.1. Transient Global Ischemia

Animal models of transient global ischemia involve either cardiac arrest (induced by potassium injection) or transient occlusion of both common carotid arteries with reduction in systemic blood pressure to diminish the flow to the forebrain via the vertebrobasilar system (two-vessel occlusion) or transient occlusion of the carotid arteries with prior permanent occlusion of the vertebral arteries (four-vessel occlusion). Most of the positive results have been obtained with two-vessel occlusion in the gerbil and the rat. Protective effects include suppression of the usual postischemic enhanced motor activity 24 hr after ischemia and prevention of delayed cell loss in the CA1 region of the hippocampus (assessed 4 to 7 days after ischemia). The phenomenon of delayed pyramidal cell loss was first described in the gerbil (Kirino, 1982; Kirino and Sano, 1984) and rat (Pulsinelli *et al.*, 1982) but has been subsequently observed in humans (Petito *et al.*, 1987). Studies in the gerbil are subject to two major criticisms: first, gerbils are particularly prone to postischemic epileptic activity, which may contribute to hippocampal abnormalities (and be suppressed by the anticonvulsant effect of NMDA antagonists), and second, hypothermia during and after ischemia may be induced by NMDA antagonists and may contribute to cerebroprotection (Buchan and Pulsinelli, 1990*a*).

Data concerning pyramidal cell loss in rats and gerbils are summarized in Table 1. 2-amino-7-phosphonoheptanoic acid (2-APH), 3-(2-carboxypiperazine-4-yl)-propyl-1-phosphonic acid (CPP), and cis-4-phosphonomethyl-2-piperidine carboxylic acid (CGS 19755) show comparable potencies in rats and gerbils, and their relative cerebroprotective potencies match their relative anticonvulsant potencies, although significantly higher doses are required for cerebroprotection than for anticonvulsant action. Noncompetitive antagonists such as MK-801 and dextrorphan are also effective. The non-NMDA antagonist NBQX protects CA_1 pyramidal cells in gerbils and rats even when administration is delayed for 1 hour post-ischemia.

With NMDA antagonists in the rat, however, protection is observed with 15- or 20-min delays but not subsequently following 2-vessel occlusions (Swan and Meldrum, 1990; Rod and Auer, 1989). Protection is not seen with NMDA antagonists in the four-vessel occlusion model in the rat (Block and Pulsinelli, 1988).

TABLE 1. Prevention of Pyramidal Cell Loss in the Rat and Gerbil Hippocampus Following Transient Forebrain Ischemia

Antagonist	Dose (mg/kg)	Species	Ischemia duration (min)	Time pre- or postischemia (hr)	Reference
APH	100 × 4	Gerbil	20	0, 2, 4, 6	Boast et al. (1987)
APH	675 × 3	Rat	10	0, 4, 10	Swan et al. (1988)
APH	300 × 2	Rat	10	0.25, 5	Swan and Meldrum (1990)
CGS 19755	10 × 4	Gerbil	20	−0.25, 2, 4, 6	Boast et al. (1988)
CGS 19755	30 × 4	Gerbil	20	1, 3, 5, 7	Boast et al. (1988)
CGS 19755	10 × 2	Rat	10	0.25	Swan and Meldrum (1990)
CPP	30 × 4	Gerbil	20	−0.25, 2, 4, 6	Boast et al. (1988)
CPP	10 × 2	Rat	10	0.25, 5	Swan and Meldrum (1990)
Dextrorphan	54 × 2	Rat	10	0.25, 5	Swan and Meldrum (1990)
MK-801	0.3–1.0	Gerbil	5	−1	Gill et al. (1987)
MK-801	3 or 10	Gerbil	5	2 or 24	Gill et al. (1988)
MK-801	1	Rat		0.33	Rod and Auer (1989)
PCP	2	Rat	10		Sauer et al. (1988)
NBQX	30 × 3	Gerbil	10	0 or 1	Sheardown et al. (1990)
NBQX	30 × 3	Rat	15	0 or 1	Diemer et al. (1990)

In the models of complete global ischemia in the cat, dog, and monkey, dizocilpine (MK-801) has failed to show a cerebroprotective effect (Fleischer *et al.*, 1989; Michenfelder *et al.*, 1989; Lanier *et al.*, 1990). It appears likely that the NMDA antagonists have little or no protective actions against delayed cell loss following complete global ischemia.

4.2. Neonatal Cerebral Ischemia

Studies of cerebroprotection have utilized the modified Levine model (Rice *et al.*, 1981), in which 7-day-old rats have one carotid artery tied in the neck and are then exposed to a reduced partial pressure of oxygen (e.g., 8% O_2, 92% N_2) for 2 to 3 hr. The outcome can be assessed by comparing hemisphere weights after 5 to 14 days. With 3 hr of hypoxia in such a test system, McDonald *et al.* (1987) found protection when administering MK-801 (1 mg/kg) either before or at 1.25 hr after hypoxia onset. Delaying the administration of MK-801 to 2.5 hr after hypoxia onset offered no protection. With a 2-hr hypoxic period, Andiné *et al.* (1988) found protection when kynurenic acid (300 mg/kg) was administered directly after the hypoxic period. The protective effect of MK-801 is enhanced by hypothermia (Ikonomidou *et al.*, 1989*b*).

4.3. Focal Ischemia

Experimental studies have principally involved middle cerebral artery occlusion in the mouse, rat, cat, dog, and monkey. The severity and variability of the infarcted volume show not only considerable species variation but also systematic differences according, for example, to the strain of rat used (Duverger and McKenzie, 1988). Techniques of occlusion and methods of evaluation have varied widely. In particular, short survival periods have sometimes been used with histological or biochemical evaluation. Two particular nonhistological evaluations have been successfully employed. These are intravital staining with 2,3,5-triphenyltetrazolium chloride (TTC) (which is converted by intact mitochondria to a deep red fat-soluble formazan compound) (Bederson *et al.*, 1986; Germano *et al.*, 1987) and measurement of the peripheral or omega benzodiazepine-binding sites (Benavides *et al.*, 1987), which occur on reactive astrocytes; when assessed after a 7-day survival period, measurement of these sites provides a quantitative measure that correlates with the extent of cortical pathology.

Results obtained with a number of different EAA antagonists are summarized in Table 2. In most cases the antagonist was administered prior to or 30 min after onset of MCA occlusion. The effect of delayed administration has not been systematically studied. Not included in the table are several positive studies in which unconventional protocols were followed. Dextrorphan and dextromethorphan have been shown to dramatically decrease neocortical ischemic damage in

TABLE 2. EAA Antagonists Providing Cortical Sparing in Permanent MCA Occlusion

Drug	Dose (mg/kg)	Species	Survival time	Protection (%)	Reference
Kynurenate	300 × 3	Rat	24 hr	43	Germano et al. (1987)
MK-801	5	Cat	6 hr	50	Ozyurt et al. (1988)
MK-801	0.5	Rat	3 hr	52	Park et al. (1988)
Ifenprodil	3	Cat	4 days	42	Gotti et al. (1988)
SL 82.0715	1, 10	Rat	2 days	34, 48	Gotti et al. (1988)
TCP	1	Rat	2 days	27	Gotti et al. (1988)
D-CPPene	15	Cat	6 hr	65	Bullock et al. (1990)

rabbits subjected to a 1-hr occlusion of the left internal carotid and anterior cerebral arteries (Steinberg et al., 1988, 1989).

A striking and uniform feature of these studies is the widespread protection afforded to the neocortex, sparing of 40 to 50% by area or volume being commonly reported. In contrast, there is little sparing of the striatum. The difference is presumably because the lenticulostriate arteries are end-terminal arteries, whereas the cortex is supplied via collateral systems. The failure of collateral flow to sustain cortical viability following MCA occlusion involves an action of endogenous agents on NMDA receptors. This is probably not a direct effect on vessels. It is not necessarily a direct excitotoxic effect, and changes in extracellular ion concentration and swelling of astrocytic processes could be involved.

4.4. Cerebral and Spinal Trauma

In a rodent model of spinal cord trauma the administration of MK-801 (1 mg/ kg) 15 min after injury improved the neurological outcome (Faden and Simon, 1988). A protective effect has also been demonstrated when CPP and MK-801 are administered following head injury in rats (Faden et al., 1989).

4.5. Cerebroprotection by Indirect Means

It is evident that the complex sequence of events linking cerebral ischemia to neuronal death frequently includes activation of EAA receptors. The assumption that cerebroprotection following administration of EAA antagonists is due to a direct action at EAA receptors on threatened neurons may not, however, be justified. EAA antagonists have a wide range of systemic effects, some of which derive from actions on glutamate receptors in brain stem centers controlling respiration and blood pressure. Noncompetitive NMDA antagonists tend to raise the body temperature in conscious rodents (Chapman and Meldrum, 1989). In anesthetized or postischemic animals in a cold environment, the body temperature can fall. Even small decreases in brain temperature ($> 2°C$) can produce cerebroprotection (Busto *et al.*, 1987). The EAA antagonists may have antidiuretic or other osmotic effects that are cerebroprotective. Endocrine effects may be significant; plasma catecholamines and corticosterone levels influence hippocampal survival (Koide *et al.*, 1986; Sapolsky and Pulsinelli, 1985). Plasma glucose levels during and after ischemia modify the pathological outcome (Voll and Auer, 1988), and EAA antagonists may influence blood glucose levels. There is also the possibility of indirect intracerebral effects. These include (1) effects of EAAs and their antagonists on ascending dopaminergic and noradrenergic systems (which modify striatal and hippocampal vulnerability to ischemic damage) (Globus *et al.*, 1987) and (2) effects on systems that modulate excitability within the limbic system such as the basal ganglia outputs via the substantia nigra pars reticulata and globus pallidus (Meldrum *et al.*, 1988).

Additionally, there are complex interactions between excitotoxic phenomena and other metabolic processes. Impaired energy metabolism reduces reuptake of extracellular EAAs. The toxicity of glutamate is enhanced when energy levels are impaired (Novelli *et al.*, 1988). Free radical formation may enhance EAA release (Pellegrini-Giampietro *et al.*, 1988).

5. THERAPEUTIC POSSIBILITIES

It would appear from the animal data that there is a good prospect of a significant therapeutic effect for focal ischemia, perinatal asphyxia, and cerebral trauma. Clinical trial data for NMDA or AMPA antagonists are, however, not yet available. There are various reasons for this. First, in the past promising experimental data have not been reliably reflected in clinical trials. Second, the greatest clinical need is for an effective therapy that can be given in the hours following a stroke. Here the difficulty is defining the therapeutic window. It is unlikely that this can be defined by studies in rodents. The window may be relatively short, which would present major practical problems, since there are commonly long delays before stroke patients arrive in hospital. In this respect, head injury patients may be a better prospect since emergency care is commonly provided early and the therapeutic window may be longer, because the cerebral ischemia is commonly a delayed secondary event. Cardiac arrest commonly occurs in hospital, and resuscitation is immediate. Therefore, treatment could be initiated within a few minutes. Similarly, the neurological impairments following cardiac bypass operations or cerebral aneurysm could be treated prophylactically with NMDA antagonists.

The side effects of competitive NMDA antagonists include ataxia, muscle weakness, and sedation. Cognitive effects including perhaps impaired spatial learning may also be produced. The PCP-like noncompetitive NMDA antagonists are likely to produce more profound cognitive disturbances, possibly including psychotomimetic effects. How significant a problem this would be in the intensive care setting remains to be determined. However, the basic side effects of ataxia, muscle relaxation, and reflex depression would be a significant problem if the antagonists were used in the newborn child.

6. SUMMARY

The early cytopathology in the hippocampus following transient forebrain ischemia in the rodent closely resembles excitotoxic changes induced by agonists acting on NMDA, kainate, or AMPA receptors. Delayed cell loss in the hippocampus following forebrain ischemia can be prevented by lesions of the excitatory (glutamatergic) pathways within the hippocampal formation.

Pharmacological antagonism of glutamatergic activation can be produced by agents affecting neurotransmitter release or by agents acting postsynaptically. The latter may be nonselective in terms of receptor subtype or selective, as with the highly potent competitive NMDA antagonists [CPP, 3-(2-carboxypiperazine-4-yl)-propenyl-1-phosphonic acid (D-CPPene), CGS 19755, DL-(E)-2-amino-4-methyl-5-phosphon-3-pentenoic acid (CGP 37849)] and noncompetitive NMDA antagonists (such as MK-801 and other agents acting on the PCP receptor).

Administration of NMDA antagonists prior to or directly after the ischemic episode protects against delayed neuronal loss following transient forebrain ischemia in the gerbil and rat. The same agents also provide dramatic and highly consistent protection against cortical damage in MCA occlusion in rats, mice, and cats. In vitro experiments with cultured neurons show that concentrations of the antagonists similar to the peak concentrations achieved in vivo also protect against neuronal death induced by hypoxia, supporting the concept that the antagonists are protecting in vivo by a direct action on receptors of vulnerable neurons. Nevertheless, indirect actions, such as suppression of epileptic activity may contribute to the protective effect.

REFERENCES

Andiné, P., Lehmann, A., Ellren, K., Wennberg, E., Kjellmer, I., Nielsen, T., and Hagberg, H., 1988, The excitatory amino acid antagonist kynurenic acid administered after hypoxia-ischemia in neonatal rats offers neuroprotection, *Neurosci. Lett.* **90:**208–212.

Bederson, J. B., Pitts, L. H., and Germano, S. M., 1986, Evaluation of 2,3,5-triphenyltetrazolium chloride as a stain for detection and quantification of experimental cerebral infarction in rats, *Stroke* **17**:1304–1308.

Benavides, J., Fage, D., Carter, C., and Scatton, B., 1987, Peripheral type benzodiazepine binding sites are a sensitive indirect index of neuronal damage, *Brain Res.* **421**:167–172.

Benavides, J., Cornu, T., Dubois, A., Gotti, D., MacKenzie, E. T., and Scatton, B., 1989, Omega3 binding sites as a tool for the detection and quantification of brain lesions: Application to the evaluation of neuroprotective agents, *in* "Pharmacology of Cerebral Ischemia, 1988" (J. Krieglstein, ed.), pp. 187–196, CRC Press, Boca Raton, Fla.

Benveniste, H., Drejer, J., Schousboe, A., and Diemer, N. H., 1984*a*, Elevation of the extracellular concentrations of glutamate and aspartate in rat hippocampus during transient cerebral ischemia monitored by intracerebral microdialysis, *J. Neurochem.* **43**:1369–1374.

Benveniste, M., Drejer, J., Schousboe, A., and Diemer, N. H., 1984*b*, Elevation of the extracellular concentrations of glutamate and aspartate in rat hippocampus during transient cerebral ischemia monitored by intracerebral microdialysis, *J. Neurochem.* **43**:369–374.

Benveniste, H., Jórgensen, B., Sandberg, M., Christensen, T., Hagberg, H., and Diemer, N. H., 1989, Ischaemic damage in hippocampal CA1 is dependent on glutamate release and intact innervation from CA3, *J. Cereb. Blood Flow Metab.* **9**:629–639.

Block, G. A., and Pulsinelli, W. A., 1988, Excitatory amino acid and purinergic transmitter involvement in ischemia-induced selective neuronal death, *in* "Mechanisms of cerebral hypoxia and stroke" (G. Somjen, ed.), pp. 359–365, Plenum Press, New York.

Boast, C. A., Gerhardt, S. C., and Janak P., 1987, Systemic AP7 reduces ischaemic brain damage in gerbils, *In* "Excitatory Amino Acid Transmission" (T. P. Hicks, D. Lodge, and H. McLennan, eds.), pp. 249–252, Alan R. Liss, New York.

Boast, C. A., Gerhardt, S. C., Pastor, G., Lehmann, J., Etienne, P. E., and Liebman, J. M., 1988, The *N*-methyl-D-aspartate antagonists CGS 19755 and CPP reduce ischemic brain damage in gerbils, *Brain Res.* **442**:345–348.

Buchan, A., and Pulsinelli, W. A., 1990*a*, Hypothermia but not the N-methyl-D-aspartate antagonist, MK-801, attenuates neuronal damage in gerbils subjected to transient global ischemia, *J. Neurosci.* **10**:311–316.

Buchan, A. M., and Pulsinelli, W. A., 1990*b*, Septo-hippocampal deafferentation protects CA1 neurons against ischemic injury, *Brain Res.* **512**:7–14.

Bullock, R., Graham, D. I., Chen, M.-H., Lowe, D., and McCulloch, J., 1990, Focal cerebral ischemia in the cat: Pretreatment with a competitive NMDA receptor antagonist, D-CPPene, *J. Cereb. Blood Flow Metab.* **10**:665–674.

Busto, R., Dietrich, W. D., Globus, M. Y. T., Valdes, I., Scheinberg, P., and Ginsberg, M. D., 1987, Small differences in intraischemic brain temperature critically determine the extent of ischemic neuronal injury, *J. Cereb. Blood Flow Metab.* **7**:729–738.

Carter, C., Benavides, J., Legendre, P., Vincent, J. D., Noel, F.,Thuret, F., Lloyd, K. G., Arbilla, S., Zivkovic, B., MacKenzie, E. T., Scatton, B., and Langer, S. Z., 1988, Ifenprodil and SL 82.0715 as cerebral anti-ischemic agents. II. Evidence of N-methyl-D-aspartate receptor antagonist properties, *J. Pharmacol. Exp. Ther.* **247**:1222–1232.

Chapman, A. G., and Meldrum, B. S., 1989, Non-competitive N-methyl-D-aspartate antagonists protect against sound-induced seizures in DBA/2 mice, *Eur. J. Pharmacol.* **166**:201–211.

Choi, D. W., 1985, Glutamate neurotoxicity in cortical cell culture is calcium dependent, *Neurosci. Lett.* **58**:293–297.

Choi, D. W., 1987, Ionic dependence of glutamate neurotoxicity, *J. Neurosci.* **7**:369–379.

Choi, D. W., Peters, S., and Viseskul, V., 1987, Dextrorphan and levorphanol selectively block *N*-methyl-D-aspartate receptor-mediated neurotoxicity on cortical neurons, *J. Pharmacol. Exp. Ther.* **242**:713–720.

Choi, D. W., Koh, J.-Y., and Peters, S., 1988, Pharmacology of glutamate neurotoxicity in cortical cell culture: Attenuation by NMDA antagonists, *J. Neurosci.* **8:**185–196.

Clineschmidt, B. V., Martin, G. E., and Bunting, P. R., 1982, Anticonvulsant activity of MK 801, a substance with potent anticonvulsant central sympathomimetic and apparent anxiolytic properties, *Drug Dev. Res.* **2:**123–134.

Davies, J., Evans, R. H., Herrling, P. L., Jones, A. W., Olverman, H. J., Pook, P., and Watkins, J. C., 1986, CPP, a new potent and selective NMDA antagonist. Depression of central neuron responses, affinity of [^{3}H]D-AP5 binding sites on brain membranes and anticonvulsant activity, *Brain Res.* **382:**169–173.

Demopoulos, H. B., Flamm, E. S., Pietronigro, D. D., and Seligman, M. L., 1980, The free radical pathology and the microcirculation in the major central nervous system disorders, *Acta Physiol. Scand.* **492:**91–119.

Diemer, N. H., Johansen, F. F., and Jorgensen, M. B., 1990, N-methyl-D-aspartate and non-N-methyl-D-aspartate antagonists in global cerebral ischemia, *Stroke* **21**(Suppl. III):39–42.

Drejer, J., Benveniste, H., Diemer, N. H., and Schousboe, A., 1985, Cellular origin of ischemia-induced glutamate release from brain tissue in vivo and in vitro, *J. Neurochem.* **45:**145–151.

Duverger, D., and McKenzie, E. T., 1988, The quantification of cerebral infarction following focal ischemia in the rat: Influence of strain, arterial pressure, blood glucose concentration, and age, *J. Cereb. Blood Flow Metab.* **8:**449–461.

Emery, A. E. H., and Burt, D., 1980, Intracellular calcium and pathogenesis and antenatal diagnosis of Duchenne muscular dystrophy, *Br. Med. J.* **280:**355–357.

Evans, M. C., Swan, J. H., and Meldrum, B. S., 1987, An adenosine analogue, 2-chloroadenosine, protects against long term development of ischaemic cell loss in the rat hippocampus, *Neurosci. Lett.* **83:**287–292.

Faden, A. I., and Simon, R. P., 1988, A potential role for excitotoxins in the pathophysiology of spinal cord injury, *Ann. Neurol.* **23:**623–626.

Faden, A. I., Demediuk, P., Panter, S. S., and Vink, R., 1989, The role of excitatory amino acids and NMDA receptors in traumatic brain injury, *Science* **244:**798–800.

Fleischer, J. E., Tateishi, A., Drummond, J. C., Scheller, M. S., Grafe, M. R., Zornow, M. H., Shearman, G. T., and Shapiro, H. M., 1989, MK-801, an excitatory amino acid antagonist, does not improve neurologic outcome following cardiac arrest in cats, *J. Cereb. Blood Flow Metab.* **9:**795–804.

Garthwaite, G., and Garthwaite, J., 1989*a*, Differential dependence on Ca^{2+} of N-methyl-D-aspartate and quisqualate neurotoxicity in young rat hippocampal slices, *Neurosci. Lett.* **97:**316–322.

Garthwaite, G., and Garthwaite, J., 1989*b*, Quisqualate neurotoxicity: A delayed, CNQX-sensitive process triggered by a CNQX-insensitive mechanism in young rat hippocampal slices, *Neurosci. Lett.* **99:**113–118.

Garthwaite, J., and Meldrum, B. S., 1990, Excitatory amino acid neurotoxicity and neurodegenerative disease, *Trends Pharmacol. Sci.* **11:**379–387.

Germano, I. M., Pitts, L. H., Meldrum, B. S., Bartkowski, H. M., and Simon, R. P., 1987, Kynurenate inhibition of cell excitation decreases stroke size and deficits, *Ann. Neurol.* **22:**730–734.

Gill, R., Foster, A. C., and Woodruff, G. N., 1987, Systemic administration of MK-801 protects against ischemia-induced hippocampal neurodegeneration in the gerbil, *J. Neurosci.* **7:**3343–3349.

Gill, R., Foster, A. C., and G. N., Woodruff, 1988, MK-801 is neuroprotective in gerbils when administered during the post-ischemic period, *Neuroscience* **25:**847–856.

Globus, M. Y. T., Ginsberg, M. D., Dietrich, W. D., Busto, R., and Scheinberg, P., 1987, Substantia nigra lesion protects against ischemic damage in the striatum, *Neurosci. Lett.* **80:**251–256.

Globus, M. Y. T., Busto, R., Dietrich, W. D., Martinez, E., Valdes, I., and Ginsberg, M. D., 1988, Effect of ischemia on the in vivo release of striatal dopamine glutamate, and γ-aminobutyric acid studied by intracerebral microdialysis, *J. Neurochem.* **51:**1455–1464.

Goldberg, M. P., Pham, P.-C., and Choi, D. W., 1987a, Dextrorphan and dextromethorphan attenuate hypoxic injury in neuronal culture, *Neurosci. Lett.* **80**:11–15.

Goldberg, M. P., Weiss, J. H., Pham, P. C., and Choi, D. W., 1987b, N-methyl-D-aspartate receptors mediate hypoxic neuronal injury in cortical culture, *J. Pharmacol. Exp. Ther.* **243**:784–791.

Gotti, B., Duverger, D., Bertin, J., Carter, C., Dupont, R., Frost, J., Gaudilliere, B., MacKenzie, E. T., Rousseau, J., Scatton, B., and Wick, A., 1988, Ifenprodil and SL 82.0715 as cerebral anti-ischemic agents. I. Evidence for efficacy in models of focal cerebral ischemia, *J. Pharmacol. Exp. Ther.* **247**:1211–1221.

Graham, S. H., Shiraishi, K., Panter, S. S., Simon, R. P., and Faden, A. I., 1990, Changes in extracellular amino acid neurotransmitters produced by focal cerebral ischemia, *Neurosci. Lett.* **110**:124–130.

Grotta, J. C., 1987, Current medial and surgical therapy for cerebrovascular disease, *N. Engl. J. Med.* **317**:1505–1516.

Hagberg, H., Lehmann, A., Sandberg, M., Nyström, B., Jacobson, I., and Hamberger, A., 1985, Ischemia-induced shift of inhibitory and excitatory amino acids from intra- to extracellular compartments, *J. Cereb. Blood Flow Metab.* **5**:413–419.

Hall, E. D., and Braughler, J. M., 1989, Central nervous system trauma and stroke. II. Physiological and pharmacological evidence for involvement of oxygen radicals and lipid peroxidation, *Free Radical Biol. Med.* **6**:303–313.

Halliwell, B., and Gutteridge, J. M. C., 1985, The importance of free radicals and catalytic metal ions in human diseases, *Mol. Aspects Med.* **8**:89–193.

Hillered, L., Hallström, A., Segersvård, S., Persson, L., and Ungerstedt, U., 1989, Dynamics of extracellular metabolites in the striatum after middle cerebral artery occlusion in the rat monitored by intracerebral microdialysis, *J. Cereb. Blood Flow Metab.* **9**:607–616.

Honoré, T., Davies, S. N., Drejer, J., Fletcher, E. J., Jacobsen, P., Lodge, D., and Nielsen, F. E., 1988, Quinoxalinediones: Potent competitive non-NMDA glutamate receptor antagonists, *Science* **241**:701–703.

Ikonomidou, C., Mosinger, J. L., and Olney, J. W., 1989a, Hypothermia enhances protective effect of MK-801 against hypoxic-ischemic brain damage in infant rats, *Brain Res.* **487**:184–187.

Ikonomidou, C., Price, M. T., Mosinger, J. L., Frierdich, G., Labruyere, J., Shahid Salles, K., and Olney, J. W., 1989b, Hypobaric-ischemic conditions produce glutamate-like cytopathology in infant rat brain, *J. Neurosci.* **9**:1693–1700.

Johansen, F. F., Jorgensen, M. B., and Diemer, N. H., 1986a, Ischaemic CA1 pyramidal cell loss is prevented by preischaemic colchicine destruction of dentate gyrus granule cells, *Brain Res.* **377**:344–347.

Johansen, F. F., Jorgensen, M. B., Ekstrom von Lubitz, K. J., and Diemer, N. H., 1986b, Selective dendrite damage in hippocampal CA1 stratum radiatum with unchanged axon ultrastructure and glutamate uptake after transient cerebral ischaemia in the rat, *Brain Res.* **291**:373–377.

Jorgensen, M. B., Johansen, F. F., and Diemer, N. H., 1987, Removal of the entorhinal cortex protects hippocampal CA-1 neurons from ischemic damage, *Acta Neuropathol.* **73**:189–194.

Kirino, T., 1982, Delayed neuronal death in the gerbil hippocampus following ischaemia, *Brain Res.* **239**:57–69.

Kirino, T., and Sano, K., 1984, Selective vulnerability in the gerbil hippocampus following transient ischaemia, *Acta Neuropathol.* **62**:201–208.

Koide, T., Wieloch, T. W., and Siesjö, B., 1986, Circulating catecholamines modulate ischemic brain damage, *J. Cereb. Blood Flow Metab.* **6**:559–565.

Lanier, W. L., Perkins, W. J., Karlsson, B. R., Milde, J. H., Scheithauer, B. W., Shearman, G. T., and Michenfelder, J. D., 1990, The effects of dizocilpine maleate (MK-801), an antagonist of the N-methyl-D-aspartate receptor, on neurologic recovery and histopathology following complete cerebral ischemia in primates, *J. Cereb. Blood Flow Metab.* **10**:252–261.

Lehmann, J., Chapman, A. G., Meldrum, B. S., Hutchison, A., Tsai, C., and Wood, P. L., 1988, CGS

19755 is a potent and competitive antagonist at NMDA-type receptors in vitro and in vivo, *Eur. J. Pharmacol.* **15**:89–93.

McDonald, J. W., Silverstein, F. S., and Johnston, M. V., 1987, MK 801 protects the neonatal brain from hypoxic-ischemic damage, *Eur. J. Pharmacol.* **140**:359–361.

Meldrum, B. S., 1990, Protection against ischaemic neuronal damage by drugs acting on excitatory neurotransmission, *Cerebrovasc. Brain Metab. Rev.* **2**:27–57.

Meldrum, B. S., and Swan, J. H., 1989, Competitive and non-competitive NMDA antagonists as cerebroprotective agents, *in* "Pharmacology of Cerebral Ischemia, 1988" (J. Krieglstein, ed.), pp. 157–163, CRC Press, Boca Raton, Fla.

Meldrum, B. S., Chapman, A. G., Patel, S., and Swan, J. H., 1989, Competitive NMDA antagonists as drugs, *in* "The NMDA Receptors" (J. C. Watkins and G. L. Collingridge, eds.), pp. 207–216, IRL Press, Oxford.

Meldrum, B., Millan, M., Patel, S., and DeSarro, G., 1988, Anti-epileptic effects of focal micro-injection of excitatory amino acid antagonists, *J. Neurol. Transm.* **72**:191–200.

Michenfelder, J. D., Lanier, W. L., Scheithauer, B. W., Perkins, W. J., Shearman, G. T., and Milde, J. H., 1989, Evaluation of the glutamate antagonist dizocilpine maleate (MK-801) on neurologic outcome in a canine model of complete cerebral ischemia: Correlation with hippocampal histopathology, *Brain Res.* **481**:228–234.

Novelli, A., Reilly, J. A., Lysko, P. G., and Henneberry, R. C., 1988, Glutamate becomes neurotoxic via the N-methyl-D-aspartate receptor when intracellular energy levels are reduced, *Brain Res.* **451**:205–212.

Olney, J. W., Ho, O. C., and Rhee, V., 1971, Cytotoxic effects of acidic and sulphur containing amino acids on the infant mouse central nervous system, *Exp. Brain Res.* **14**:61–76.

Olney, J. W., Rhee, V., and Ho, O. L., 1974, Kainic acid: A powerful neurotoxic analogue of glutamate, *Brain Res.* **77**:507–512.

Onodera, H., Sata, G., and Kogure, K., 1986, Lesions to Schaffer collaterals prevent ischaemic death of CA1 pyramidal cells, *Neurosci. Lett.* **68**:169–174.

Ozyurt, E., Graham, D. I., Woodruff, G. N., and McCulloch, J., 1988, Protective effect of the glutamate antagonist, MK-801, in focal cerebral ischemia in the cat, *J. Cereb. Blood Flow Metab.* **8**:138–143.

Park, C. K., Nehls, D. G., Graham, D. I., Teasdale, G. M., and McCulloch, J., 1988, The glutamate antagonist MK801 reduces focal ischemic damage in the rat, *Ann. Neurol.* **24**:543–551.

Patel, S., Meldrum, B. S., and Collins, J. F., 1986, Distribution of [³H]kainic acid binding sites in the rat brain: In vivo and in vitro receptor autoradiography, *Neurosci. Lett.* **70**:301–307.

Patel, S., Chapman, A. G., Millan, M. H., and Meldrum, B. S., 1988*a*, Epilepsy and excitatory amino acid antagonists, *in* "Excitatory Amino Acids in Health and Disease" (D. Lodge, ed.), pp. 353–378, John Wiley, Chichester, England.

Patel, S., Millan, M. H., and Meldrum, B. S., 1988*b*, Decrease in excitatory transmission within the lateral habenula and the mediodorsal thalamus protects against limbic seizures in rats, *Exp. Neurol.* **101**:63–75.

Pellegrini-Giampietro, D. E., Cherici, G., Alesiani, M., Carla, V., and Moroni, F., 1988, Excitatory amino acid release and free radical formation may cooperate in the genesis of ischemia-induced neuronal damage, *J. Neurosci.* **10**:1035–1041.

Petito, C. K., Feldmann, E., Pulsinelli, W. A., and Plum, F., 1987, Delayed hippocampal damage in humans following cardiorespiratory arrest, *Neurology* **37**:1281–1286.

Pulsinelli, W. A., Bierley, J. B., and Plum, F., 1982, Temporal profile of neuronal damage in a model of transient forebrain ischaemia, *Ann. Neurol.* **11**:491–499.

Ransom, R. W., and Stec, N. L., 1988, Co-operative modulation of [³H]MK 801 binding to the N-methyl-D-aspartate receptor-ion channel complex by *L*-glutamate, glycine, and polyamines, *J. Neurochem.* **51**:830–836.

Recasens, M., Guiramand, J., Nourigat, A., Sassetti, I., and Devilliers, G., 1988, A new quisqualate receptor subtype (sAA2) responsible for the glutamate-induced inositol phosphate formation in rat brain synaptoneurosomes, *Neurochem. Int.* **13**:463–467.

Reynolds, I. J., and Miller, R. J., 1988, Tricyclic antidepressants block N-methyl-D-aspartate receptors: Similarities to the action of zinc, *Br. J. Pharmacol.* **95**:95–102.

Rice, J. E., Vannucci, R. C., and Brierley, J. B., 1981, The influence of immaturity on hypoxic-ischemic brain damage in the rat, *Ann. Neurol.* **9**:131–141.

Rod, M. R., and Auer, R. N., 1989, Pre- and post-ischemic administration of dizocilpine (MK 801) reduces cerebral necrosis in the rat, *Can. J. Neurol. Sci.* **16**:340–344.

Rothman, S. M., 1985, The neurotoxicity of excitatory amino acids is produced by passive chloride influx, *J. Neurosci.* **5**:1483–1489.

Sapolsky, R., and Pulsinelli, W., 1985, Glucocorticoids potentiate ischemic injury to neurons: Therapeutic implications, *Science* **229**:1397–1400.

Sauer, D., Nuglisch, J., and Rossberg, C., 1988, Phencyclidine reduces postischemic neuronal necrosis in rat hippocampus without changing blood flow, *Neurosci. Lett.* **91**:327–332.

Sheardown, J. J., Nielsen, E. O., Hansen, A. J., Jacobsen, P., and Honoré, T., 1990, 2,3-Dihydroxy-6-nitro-7-suflamoylbenzo(F)quinoxaline: A neuroprotectant for cerebral ischemia, *Science* **247**: 571–574.

Simon, R. P., Griffiths, T., Evans, M. C., Swan, J. H., and Meldrum, B. S., 1984a, Calcium overload in selectively vulnerable neurons of the hippocampus during and after ischaemia: An electron microscopy study in the rat, *J. Cereb. Blood Flow Metab.* **4**:350–361.

Simon, R. P., Swan, J. H., Griffiths, T., and Meldrum, B. S., 1984b, Blockade of N-methyl-D-aspartate receptors may protect against ischaemic damage in the brain, *Science* **226**:850–852.

Steinberg, G. K., George, C. P., DeLaPaz, R., Shibata, D. K., and Gross, T., 1989a, Dextromethorphan protects against cerebral injury following transient focal ischemia in rabbits, *Stroke* **19**:1112–1118.

Steinberg, G. K., Saleh, J., and Kunis, D., 1988b, Delayed treatment with dextromethorphan and dextrorphan reduces cerebral damage after transient focal ischaemia, *Neurosci. Lett.* **89**:193–197.

Sugiyama, H., Ito, I., and Hirono, C., 1987, A new type of glutamate receptor linked to inositol phospholipid metabolism, *Nature* **325**:531–533.

Swan, J. H., and Meldrum, B. S., 1990, Protection by NMDA antagonists against selective cell loss following transient ischaemia, *J. Cereb. Blood Flow Metab.* **10**:343–351.

Swan, J. H., Evans, M. C., and Meldrum, B. S., 1988, Long term development of selective neuronal loss and the mechanism of protection by 2-amino-7-phosphonoheptanoate in a rat model of incomplete forebrain ischaemia, *J. Cereb. Blood Flow Metab.* **8**:64–78.

Voll, C. L., and Auer, R. N., 1988, The effect of postischemic blood glucose levels on ischemic brain damage in the rat, *Ann. Neurol.* **24**:638–646.

von Lubitz, D. K. J. E., Dambrosia, J. M., Kempski, O., and Redmond, D. J., 1988, Cyclohexyl adenosine protects against neuronal death following ischemia in the CA1 region of gerbil hippocampus, *Stroke* **19**:1133–1139.

Watkins, J. C., and Evans, R. H., 1981, Excitatory amino acid transmitters, *Annu. Rev. Pharmacol. Toxicol.* **21**:165–204.

Wong, E. H. F., Kemp, J. A., Priesley, T., Knight, A. R., Woodruff, G. N., and Iversen, L. L., 1986, The anticonvulsant MK-801 is a potent N-methyl-D-aspartate antagonist, *Proc. Natl. Acad. Sci. USA* **83**:7104–7108.

Wong, E. H. F., Knight, A. R., and Woodruff, G. N., 1988, [^{3}H]MK-801 labels a site on the N-methyl-D-aspartate receptor channel complex in rat brain membranes, *J. Neurochem.* **50**: 274–281.

Wrogemann, K., and Pena, S. D. J., 1976, Mitochondrial calcium overload. A general mechanism for cell necrosis in muscle diseases, *Lancet* **i**:672–674.

CHAPTER 13

ACUTE ALTERATIONS IN PHOSPHOINOSITIDE TURNOVER

FAYE S. SILVERSTEIN, CHU KUANG CHEN, STEPHEN K. FISHER, DANIEL STATMAN, and MICHAEL V. JOHNSTON

1. INTRODUCTION

In the developing nervous system, selected excitatory amino acid (EAA) recognition sites are coupled to activation of phospholipase C, the enzyme that catalyzes the hydrolysis of membrane inositol phospholipids (PPI) (Nicoletti *et al.*, 1986*b*; Sladeczek *et al.*, 1985). Phospholipase C-mediated phosphodiesteratic cleavage of phosphatidylinositol 4,5-bisphosphate yields the two potent intracellular second-

FAYE S. SILVERSTEIN, CHU KUANG CHEN, and DANIEL STATMAN • Departments of Pediatrics and Neurology, Neuroscience Program, University of Michigan, Ann Arbor, Michigan.   STEPHEN K. FISHER • Department of Pharmacology, University of Michigan, Ann Arbor, Michigan.   MICHAEL V. JOHNSTON • Departments of Pediatrics and Neurology, Johns Hopkins University and Kennedy Institute, Baltimore, Maryland.

Neurochemical Correlates of Cerebral Ischemia, Volume 7 of Advances in Neurochemistry, edited by Nicolas G. Bazan, Pierre Braquet, and Myron D. Ginsberg. Plenum Press, New York, 1992.

messenger molecules inositol 1,4,5-triphosphate (IP_3) and diacylglycerol (Berridge and Irvine, 1984; Berridge et al., 1982; Fisher and Agranoff, 1987).

The pharmacology of EAA receptor agonists and antagonists is complex. At least three glutamate receptor subtypes have been delineated on the basis of their preferential activation by the selective agonists N-methyl-D-aspartate (NMDA), quisqualic acid (QUIS), and kainic acid (Watkins and Evans, 1981). Another classification scheme for EAA receptors is based on their mechanisms for signal transduction—which include ion channel-linked ("ionotropic") and second-messenger-linked ("metabolotropic") mechanisms (Costa et al., 1988). Sladeczek et al. (1985) observed that glutamic acid stimulated inositol phosphate (IP) release in striatal neurons in culture. Nicoletti et al. (1986b) reported that ibotenic acid, traditionally classified as an NMDA agonist, stimulates PPI turnover in the striatum and hippocampus, as do QUIS and, to a lesser extent, glutamate. Both ibotenic acid and QUIS stimulate PPI hydrolysis in the hippocampus and striatum of neonatal rat brain to a much greater extent than in adult brain (Nicoletti et al., 1986b).

Recent experimental evidence implicates overexcitation of EAA receptors in the pathogenesis of irreversible neuronal damage due to hypoxia-ischemia (Meldrum, 1985; Rothman and Olney, 1986). We have used a well-characterized in vivo model of perinatal hypoxic-ischemic encephalopathy to examine the role of glutamate and related EAA in the pathogenesis of neuronal injury in the perinatal period.

In this model, right carotid artery ligation (RCL) followed by exposure to 8% oxygen for 2.5 hr in 7-day-old rat pups elicits unilateral forebrain injury ipsilateral to ligation (see Johnston and Silverstein [1987] for a review). A considerable amount of information about the pathophysiologic and neurochemical features of the model is available. The evolution of injury is attributable to progressive ischemia with increasing duration of hypoxia.

Our data indicate that in this model of perinatal hypoxic-ischemic encephalopathy, there is considerable acute functional disruption of glutamatergic synapses. For example, in synaptosomes derived from brains in which lesions had been formed, there is an early, reversible suppression of high-affinity glutamate uptake; since glutamate is removed from the synapse predominantly by reuptake, this suppression could lead to accumulation of glutamate in the synaptic cleft. Postsynaptic abnormalities evolve concurrently; autoradiography studies with [3H]glutamate ([3H]Glu) as the ligand demonstrate that in target areas for irreversible injury, acute reductions in binding become apparent in the first 24 hr after ligation (Silverstein et al., 1987). Furthermore, systemic administration of the noncompetitive NMDA antagonist MK-801 limits the extent of tissue injury (McDonald et al., 1987).

There is little information about the effects of hypoxia-ischemia on EAA-coupled stimulation of PPI turnover. On the basis of the observations that [3H]Glu binding was reduced unilaterally in the hippocampus and striatum 24 hr after the initial hypoxic-ischemic insult, we sought to determine whether these changes would be reflected in an altered ability of the selective agonist QUIS to stimulate PPI metabolism in brains containing lesions.

We measured agonist-stimulated [³H]IP release in tissues labeled with *myo*-[2-³H]inositol to examine this question. In vivo, IP₃ is quickly dephosphorylated. In vitro, in the presence of lithium, inositol 1-phosphatase is inhibited and inositol monophosphate (IP₁) accumulates (Berridge *et al.*, 1983). Thus, in tissues labeled with *myo*-[2-³H]-inositol, the measurement of total [³H]inositol phosphates or [³H]IP₁ accumulation in the presence of lithium provides a sensitive index of the extent of membrane PPI hydrolysis.

We assayed basal and QUIS-stimulated PPI turnover in the hippocampus and striatum 24 hr after RCL followed by hypoxic exposure. To evaluate the specificity of any observed alterations in QUIS-stimulated PPI turnover, in selected experiments muscarinic agonist-stimulated PPI turnover was assayed concurrently. We found that hypoxic-ischemic injury resulted in a selective enhancement of QUIS-stimulated PPI turnover in both hippocampal and striatal slices (Chen *et al.*, 1987).

2. METHODS

2.1. Animal Preparation

Seven-day-old Sprague-Dawley rat pups were anesthetized with ether, and the right carotid artery was exposed and ligated (Johnston and Silverstein, 1987). After surgery, pups had a 1-hr recovery period with the dam and were then placed in a plastic chamber, warmed to 37°C, and exposed to 8% oxygen-92% nitrogen for 2.5 hr. Mortality was typically less than 10%. Pups were returned to the dam 1 hr after hypoxic exposure. Pups and littermate controls were killed by decapitation 24 hr later. Experience with this model reveals that there is typically both inter- and intralitter variability in the severity of the resulting lesion. The factors that account for this variability are often difficult to identify; inclusion of control groups is essential for data interpretation in experiments in which this preparation are used. In each experiment, tissue was obtained from 14 to 16 treated pups and 8 unoperated littermate controls.

2.2. Assay of [³H]IP Release

Cross-chopped brain slices (350 × 350 μm) were prepared from hippocampal and striatal tissue. For each region, there were three pooled tissue samples from the side of the ligation (ipsilateral), from the contralateral hemisphere, and from unoperated controls. A continuous-labeling paradigm was used to assay PPI turnover in these experiments because of the simplicity and sensitivity of this approach.

In brief, slices were suspended in a buffer which included 142 mM NaCl, 5.6 mM KCl, 2.2 mM $CaCl_2$, 3.6 mM $NaHCO_3$, 1 mM $MgCl_2$, 5 mM D-glucose, and 30 mM 4-(2-hydroxyethyl)-1-piperazineethanesulfonic acid sodium salt (HEPES-Na^+) (pH 7.4) and were incubated at 37°C for 10 min. After the slices settled, 50-μl aliquots of tissue (0.6 to 1 mg of protein) were transferred to 10-ml test tubes containing 4.0 μCi of *myo*-[2-^{3}H]inositol (15 Ci/mmol; American Radiolabeled Chemicals, St. Louis, Mo) and 10 mM LiCl in a final volume of 500 μl of buffer.

PPI turnover was assayed in the absence (basal state) or in the presence of specified agonists (QUIS or carbachol [CCh]). After a 2-hr incubation period at 37°C, reactions were stopped by the addition of 1.7 ml of chloroform-methanol (1:2 by volume). A total water-soluble IP fraction was separated from *myo*-[2-^{3}H]inositol by ion exchange chromatography and quantitated as previously described (Fisher *et al.*, 1984). For separation of the [^{3}H]inositol metabolites, the water-soluble extracts were applied to ion exchange columns containing Dowex-1 × 8 resin (formate form; Bio-Rad Laboratories, Richmond, Calif.) and individual IP fractions were eluted sequentially as described by Berridge *et al.* (1983). To monitor the incorporation of labeled *myo*-inositol into the phospholipid fraction, a 0.2-ml aliquot from the lower organic phase was removed and allowed to evaporate, and then radioactivity was determined by liquid scintillation spectrometry.

3. RESULTS

In both hippocampus and striatum, optimal stimulation of PPI turnover (8- to 10-fold increase) was seen at 10^{-4} to 10^{-6} M QUIS. Of note, a higher concentration of QUIS (10^{-3} M) produced a paradoxical inhibition of PPI turnover, possibly as a result of direct tissue toxicity. We also determined that there was a linear increase in agonist-stimulated [^{3}H]IP accumulation as the incubation period was increased from 0.5 to 2 hr (Figure 1). In these experiments, the largest fraction (40 to 65%) of the label was recovered in [^{3}H]IP$_1$, and a substantial fraction (37 to 41%) was found in glycero-phosphorylinositol (GPI). In both control and lesion-containing brains, QUIS and CCh stimulated [^{3}H]IP$_1$ accumulation (expressed as a fraction of total IP release in that tissue) to a similar extent. The relatively large proportion of label in GPI may have resulted from the deacylation of phosphatidylinositol that occurs in long-term incubations. Less than 10% of the label was recovered in either [^{3}H]IP$_2$ or [^{3}H]IP$_3$. No significant increases in agonist-stimulated [^{3}H]IP$_2$ and [^{3}H]IP$_3$ accumulation were detected, presumably because of rapid dephosphorylation of these compounds.

In these experiments, we expressed values for [^{3}H]IP release as a percentage

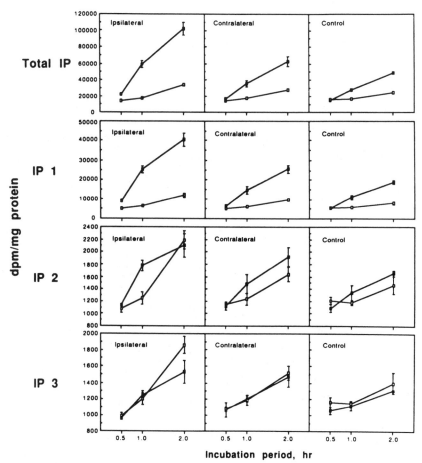

FIGURE 1. Time course for QUIS-stimulated release of IP, IP_1, IP_2, and IP_3 in hippocampal slices from the side of ligation (ipsilateral), the opposite hemisphere (contralateral), and control groups. Tissue slices were incubated with *myo*-[2-^{3}H]inositol in the presence of 10^{-4} M QUIS for three incubation periods: 0.5, 1, and 2 h. Values are expressed as dpm per milligram of protein; each value is the mean ± SEM of three determinations. There is a linear increase in IP_1 accumulation with increasing duration of the incubation period in both control and lesion-containing brain. Open squares represent basal values; filled squares represent values from tissue incubated with 10^{-4} M QUIS. (From Chen *et al.*, 1987.)

of basal values (i.e., in the absence of agonist in that tissue). This approach enabled us to more readily incorporate results from multiple assays. We found that the preceding hypoxic-ischemic insult had no apparent effect on basal [³H]IP release 24 hr later. Of interest, in another experimental model of excitotoxic focal brain injury in the immature brain, produced by direct intrastriatal injection of QUIS, we have observed stimulation of basal [³H]IP release in lesion-containing tissue for up to 48 hr after the initial insult (unpublished observation).

When QUIS-stimulated [³H]IP release was expressed as a percentage of basal release, a selective ability of QUIS to stimulate PPI turnover in tissues obtained from hypoxic-ischemic brains was apparent (Figure 2). In hippocampal slices prepared from the hemisphere ipsilateral to the ligation, a 10-fold increase in the amount of [³H]IP release was observed; in contrast, 5- to 6-fold increases were observed in tissue obtained from the contralateral hippocampus or from control animals. Similarly, in the presence of QUIS, [³H]IP release increased by eightfold in the striatum ipsilateral ligation and only by fivefold in tissue obtained from the contralateral side or from control animals. The results demonstrate that the tissue

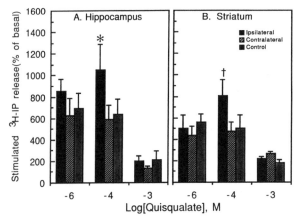

FIGURE 2. (A) QUIS-stimulated release of IP in hippocampal tissue slices. Seven-day-old rat pups underwent RCL and subsequent exposure to 8% oxygen for 2.5 hr ($n = 14$ to 16 pups per experiment; values from nine experiments included). Pups were killed by decapitation 24 hr later. Hippocampal slices were prepared from the hippocampus ipsilateral to ligation, from the contralateral hemisphere, and from untreated littermate controls ($n = 8$ pups per experiment). Tissue slices were incubated with *myo*-[2-³H]inositol in the presence of three concentrations of QUIS: 10^{-6} M ($n = 3$); 10^{-4} ($n = 9$); 10^{-3} M ($n = 2$). Reactions were stopped after 120 min, and the radioactivity in the total IP fraction was determined. [³H]IP release in the presence of QUIS was expressed as a percentage of [³H]IP release in the absence of agonist (basal). (B) Corresponding values for QUIS-stimulated IP release in striatum assayed concurrently. *, $P < 0.005$; †, $P < 0.05$, comparison of tissue derived from hypoxic-ischemic brain with tissue from the contralateral hemisphere by Student's t test. (From Chen *et al.*, 1987.)

remains viable over this 2-hr incubation period and that 10^{-4} M QUIS does not exert significant in vitro neurotoxicity.

The muscarinic cholinergic agonist (CCh) yielded a different pattern of [^{3}H]IP release. CCh stimulated PPI hydrolysis to a similar extent in all tissues (Figure 3).

Examination of [^{3}H]IP$_1$ release revealed similar trends. In hippocampal tissue, [^{3}H]IP$_1$ accumulation, expressed as a percentage of basal release, was 1048% $\pm$ 348% in hypoxic-ischemic tissue, 611% $\pm$ 201% in tissue from the contralateral hemisphere, and 466% $\pm$ 128% in control samples, paralleling total [^{3}H]IP accumulation in each of these tissues. In the striatum, the [^{3}H]IP$_1$ content, expressed as a percentage of basal values, was 952% $\pm$ 345% in hypoxic-ischemic tissue, 545% $\pm$ 145% in the contralateral striatum, and 449% $\pm$ 192% in controls. Similarly, CCh-stimulated [^{3}H]IP$_1$ accumulation paralleled total [^{3}H]IP release and was similar in all tissues assayed.

Of note, under basal conditions hypoxia-ischemia also caused an increased incorporation (approximately 80%) of myo-[2-^{3}H]inositol into membrane phospholipids (271,000 $\pm$ 56,000 ipsilateral to ligation, 147,000 $\pm$ 27,000 contra-

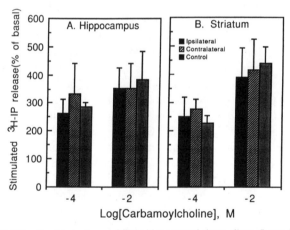

FIGURE 3. (A) CCh-stimulated release of IP in hippocampal tissue slices. Seven-day-old rat pups underwent RCL and subsequent exposure to 8% oxygen for 2.5 hr (n = 14 to 16 pups per experiment, values from eight experiments included). Pups were killed by decapitation 24 hr later. Hippocampal slices were prepared from the hipppocampus ipsilateral to ligation, from the contralateral hemisphere, and from untreated littermate controls (n = 8 pups per experiment). Tissue slices were incubated with myo-[2-^{3}H]inositol in the presence of 10^{-4} M CCh (n = 3) or 10^{-2} M CCh (n = 4). Reactions were stopped after 2 hr, and radioactivity in the total IP fraction was determined. Values are expressed as the percent basal release in the absence of agonist ($\pm$ SEM). (B) Corresponding values for CCh-stimulated IP release in the striatum assayed concurrently. In both brain regions, at each concentration of CCh, no significant differences in CCh-stimulated [^{3}H]IP release were found. (From Chen $et\ al.$, 1987.)

lateral to ligation, and 150,000 ± 27,000 in control [expressed as dpm per milligram of protein for $n = 11$]).

4. DISCUSSION

These results demonstrate that in the perinatal rodent brain an acute hypoxic-ischemic insult augments the subsequent responsiveness of injured hippocampal and striatal tissue to the glutamate agonist QUIS. Incubation with QUIS consistently elicits greater [³H]IP release from injured brain than from control tissue. In contrast, muscarinic stimulation of PPI hydrolysis in the injured tissue is not increased. This suggests that hypoxia-ischemia causes a specific change in the QUIS receptor-PPI second-messenger complex. The enhanced response to QUIS in ischemic tissue is most prominent at 10^{-4} M.

One possible explanation for the increased effectiveness of QUIS would be the availability of an increased number of higher affinity of glutamate receptors in the injured tissue. However, previously, in this experimental model, we found that at the corresponding time interval after ligation [³H]Glu binding is reduced by 24 to 40% in the ipsilateral hippocampus and by 20% in the striatum (Silverstein et al., 1987). Functional loss of Glu recognition sites at 24 hr after unilateral hypoxia-ischemia appears to be a marker for brain regions destined for irreversible neuronal damage. We assayed [³H]Glu binding in these studies by in vitro autoradiography. The recognition sites were visualized after incubation in [³H]Glu in CaCl₂-containing buffer, which optimizes binding to QUIS-preferring sites. The relationship between the glutamate recognition sites visualized by autoradiography, and the receptor subtype linked to PPI turnover is uncertain (Nicoletti et al., 1986a,b). There are no autoradiographic methods presently available which selectively label the Glu recognition sites that are coupled to enhanced PPI turnover, and it is conceivable that there is an isolated increase in the number or affinity of this receptor subtype which we could not measure. In more recent autoradiography studies aimed at identification of Glu receptor subtype changes, we have not found any selectivity (unpublished observations). Therefore, it is more likely that a proportion of the [³H]Glu sites which were lost following hypoxia-ischemia are coupled with PPI hydrolysis.

There is a possible confounding issue in determining whether responses to QUIS and CCh are directly comparable. Glutamatergic and muscarinic cholinergic receptors are widely distributed in the immature brain. Although the two agonists were assayed in the same tissue preparations, we cannot determine whether glutamatergic and muscarinic receptors are located on the same cell bodies. With in vitro autoradiography there is marked overlap in the distribution of [³H]quinuclidinyl benzilate (muscarinic) and [³H]Glu binding in the striatum and hippocampus, but there is no detailed information about the cellular distribution of these receptors. If cells bearing Glu receptors are selectively vulnerable to ischemic injury, the differences in agonist-stimulated PPI turnover we observed may reflect local variations in severity of cellular damage. [^{3}H]IP release stimulated by QUIS (10^{-4} M) and CCh (10^{-2} M) are additive in vitro (Statman and Silverstein, unpublished), suggesting that these agonists influence different phospholipid pools.

It is conceivable that preferential labeling of membrane phospholipids from injured cells accounts for some of the differential effects observed. Increased incorporation of myo-[2-^{3}H]inositol into membrane phospholipids of injured tissue could result in an apparent enhanced response to agonist in hypoxic-ischemic brain. We found a consistent increase in myo-[2-^{3}H]inositol labeling of membrane phospholipids in both the hippocampus and striatum ipsilateral to ligation. This increased myo-[2-^{3}H]inositol incorporation could reflect compensatory resynthesis after hypoxia-ischemia-induced membrane PPI degradation (Yochida et al., 1986). However, this effect does not appear to be of sufficient magnitude to account for the enhanced response to QUIS which we observed.

Another possibility that must be considered is that the enhanced stimulation of [^{3}H]IP release in injured tissue reflects a glial reaction rather than a specific neuronal response. In cultured astrocytes, both Glu and muscarinic agonists stimulate PPI metabolism (Pearce et al., 1986a,b). There would be no reason to expect selective changes in QUIS-coupled PPI metabolism.

A variety of metabolic derangements in the ischemic brain could also directly influence PPI hydrolysis. For example, elevated potassium levels, in the range seen in the extracellular fluid of an ischemic brain, can potentiate PPI hydrolysis in vitro (Eva and Costa, 1986). Intracellular levels of calcium rise in ischemic tissue (Simon et al., 1984) and may directly stimulate inositide phosphodiesterase (Fisher and Agranoff, 1987).

Conversely, enhanced Glu-stimulated PPI hydrolysis elicited by hypoxia-ischemia may, in turn, contribute to potentially detrimental intracellular events. The inositol lipids are a rich source of arachidonic acid, an important substrate for free-radical formation (Bazan, 1970; Ikeda et al., 1986; Westerberg and Wieloch, 1986). Furthermore, the metabolic cost of the futile cycle of receptor-mediated breakdown of PPI and its subsequent resynthesis is high; for each mole of phosphatidylinositol 4,5-biphosphate degraded and resynthesized, four high-energy phosphates are consumed.

We have also examined QUIS-coupled PPI hydrolysis in immature rodent brain after induction of a unilateral excitotoxic striatal lesion (Statman et al., 1988). The extent of [^{3}H]IP release was measured in a similar fashion in striatal tissue derived from animals sacrificed up to 5 days after a right intrastriatal injection of a neurotoxic dosage of QUIS acid (100 nmol). This lesion results in an acute decrease in [^{3}H]Glu binding in the striatum at 1 to 5 days after the injection (Silverstein et al., 1986). However, we again found that excitotoxic injury markedly enhanced QUIS-stimulated PPI hydrolysis; the peak effect was detected at 2 days; 5 days later there still was significantly higher [^{3}H]IP release in lesion-containing than in control striatum (Statman *et al.*, 1988). CCh-stimulated PPI hydrolysis was unaffected by the lesion in assays carried out concurrently 2 or 5 days later.

Alterations in the functional activity of metabolotropic QUIS receptors may play an important role in the neuronal response to excitotoxic injury in the developing brain. It is important to note that a similar enhancement of ibotenate-coupled PPI hydrolysis is elicited by kindling or excitoxin lesions in mature brain (Iadarola *et al.*, 1986). The underlying molecular mechanisms are unknown. EAA and muscarinic receptor coupling to PPI turnover is regulated developmentally; both receptors are coupled more efficiently to PPI hydrolysis at early developmental stages (Heacock *et al.*, 1987; Nicoletti *et al.*, 1986b). Enhanced activity could reflect changes in the neurotransmitter recognition site or in a protein coupling the receptor with phospholipase C. The enhanced EAA receptor coupling we observed in injured brain may reflect an adaptive, possibly compensatory, response of surviving neurons.

ACKNOWLEDGMENTS

This work was supported by PHS grants 1 PO1 NS 19613 (M. V. J.), 1 KO8 NS01171 (F. S. S.), and NS 23831 (S. K. F.); grant R-326 from the United Cerebral Palsy Foundation (M. V. J.), and a basic research grant from the March of Dimes Birth Defects Foundation (M. V. J.).

REFERENCES

Bazan, N., 1970, Effects of ischemia and electroconvulsive shock on free fatty acid pool in the brain, *Biochim. Biophys. Acta* **218**:1–10.

Berridge, M. J., and Irvine, R. F., 1984, Inositol triphosphate, a novel second messenger in cellular signal transduction, *Nature* **312**:315–321.

Berridge, M. J., Downes, P. C., and Hanley, M. R., 1982, Lithium amplifies agonist dependent phosphatidyl inositol response in brain and salivary gland, *Biochem. J.* **206**:587–595.

Berridge, M. J., Dawson, R. M. C., Downes, C. P., Heslop, J. T., and Irvine, R. F., 1983, Changes in the levels of inositol phosphates after agonist-dependent hydrolysis of membrane phospho-inositides, *Biochem. J.* **212**:473–482.

Chen, C.-K., Silverstein, F. S., Fisher, S. K., Statman, D., and Johnston, M. V., 1987, Perinatal hypoxia-ischemia enhances quisqualic acid stimulated phosphoinositide turnover, *J. Neurochem.* **51**:353–359.

Costa, E., Fadda, E., Kozikowski, A. P., Nicoletti, F., and Wroblewski, J. T., 1988, Classification and allosteric modulation of EAA signal transduction in brain slices and primary cultures of cerebellar neurons, *in* "Neurobiology of Amino Acids, Peptides and Trophic Factors" (J. Ferendelli, R. Collins, and E. Johnson, eds.), pp. 35–50, Martinus Nijhoff Publishers, Boston.

Eva, C., and Costa, E., 1986, Potassium ion facilitation of phosphoinositide turnover activation by muscarinic receptor agonists in rat brain, *J. Neurochem.* **46**:1429–1435.

Fisher, S. K., and Agranoff, B. W., 1987, Receptor activation and inositol lipid hydrolysis in neural tissue, *J. Neurochem.* **48**:999–1017.

Fisher, S. K., Figueiredo, J. C., and Bartus, R. T., 1984, Differential stimulation of inositol phospholipid turnover in brain by analogs of oxotremorine, *J. Neurochem.* **43**:1171–1179.

Heacock, A. M., Fisher, S. K., and Agranoff, B. W., 1987, Enhanced coupling of neonatal muscarinic receptors in rat brain to phosphoinositide turnover, *J. Neurochem.* **48**:1904–1911.

Iadarola, M. J., Nicoletti, F., Naranjo, J. R., Putnam, F., and Costa, E., 1986, Kindling enhances the stimulation of inositol phospholipid hydrolysis elicited by ibotenic acid in rat hippocampal slices, *Brain Res.* **374**:174–178.

Ikeda, M., Yoshidea, S., Busto, R., Santiso, M., and Ginsberg, M. D., 1986, Polyphosphoinositides as a probable source of brain free fatty acids accumulated at the onset of ischemia, *J. Neurochem.* **47**:123–132.

Johnston, M. V., and Silverstein, F. S., 1987, Perinatal anoxia, *Neurol. Neurobiol.* **33**:223–252.

McDonald, J. T., Silverstein, F. S., and Johnston, M. V., 1987, MK-801 protects the neonatal brain from hypoxia-ischemic damage, *Eur. J. Pharmacol.* **140**:359–361.

Meldrum, B., 1985, Excitatory amino acids and anoxic-ischemic brain damage, *Trends Neurosci.* **8**: 47–48.

Nicoletti, F., Iadorola, J. J., Wroblewski, J. T., and Costa, E., 1986a, Coupling of inositol phospholipid metabolism with excitatory amino acid recognition sites in rat hippocampus, *J. Neurochem.* **46**: 40–46.

Nicoletti, F., Iadarola, M. J., Wroblewski, J. T., and Costa, E., 1986b, Excitatory amino acid recognition sites coupled with inositol phospholipid metabolism: Developmental changes and interaction with α-1 adrenoreceptors, *Proc. Natl. Acad. Sci. USA* **83**:1931–1935.

Pearce, B., Albrecht, B., Morrow, C., and Murphy, S., 1986a, Astrocyte glutamate receptor activation promotes inositol phospholipid turnover and calcium flux, *Neurosci. Lett.* **72**:335–340.

Pearce, B., Morrow, C., and Murphy, S., 1986b, Receptor mediated inositol phospholipid hydrolysis in astrocytes, *Eur. J. Pharmacol.* **121**:231–243.

Rothman, S., and Olney, J., 1986, Glutamate and the pathophysiology of hypoxic-ischemic brain damage, *Ann. Neurol.* **19**:105–111.

Silverstein, F. S., Hick, P., Chen, R., and Johnston, M. V., 1986, Quisqualic acid produces focal disruption of glutamate receptors in developing brain, *Neurology* **37**:(Suppl. 1):3.

Silverstein, F. S., Torke, L., Barks, J., and Johnston, M. V., 1987, Hypoxia-ischemia produces focal disruption of glutamate receptors in developing brian, *Dev. Brain Res.* **34**:33–39.

Simon, R. P., Griffiths, T., Evans, M. C., Swan, J. H., and Meldrum, B. S., 1984, Calcium overload in selectively vulnerable neurons of the hippocampus during and after ischemia: An electron microscopy study in the rat, *J. Cereb. Blood Flow Metab.* **4**:350–361.

Sladeczek, F., Pin, J. P., Recasens, M., Bockart, J., and Weiss, S., 1985, Glutamate stimulates inositol phosphate formation in striatal neurons, *Nature* **317**:717–719.

Statman, D., Chen, C.-K., Johnston, M. V., and Silverstein, F. S., 1988, Excitotoxic brain injury enhances quisqualic acid stimulated phosphoinositide turnover in developing brain, *Soc. Neurosci. Abstr.* **14**:168.8.

Watkins, J. C., and Evans, R. H., 1981, Excitatory amino acid transmitters, *Annu. Rev. Pharmacol. Toxicol.* **21**:165–205.

Westerberg, E., and Wieloch, T., 1986, Lesions to the corticostriatal pathways ameliorate hypoglycemia-induced arachidonic acid release, *J. Neurochem.* **47**:1507–1511.

Yochida, S., Ikeda, M., Busto, R., Santiso, M., Martinez, E., and Ginsberg, M., 1986, Cerebral phosphoinositide, triacylglycerol, and energy metabolism in reversible ischemia. Origin and fate of free fatty acids, *J. Neurochem.* **47**:744–757.

CHAPTER 14

NEW INSIGHTS INTO THE ROLE OF OXYGEN RADICALS IN CEREBRAL ISCHEMIA

PAK H. CHAN, SYLVIA CHEN,
SHIGEKI IMAIZUMI, LILLIAN CHU,
JUDITH A. KELLEHER,
GEORGE A. GREGORY, and THELMA CHAN

1. INTRODUCTION

During the past few decades, a large body of experimental data has accumulated indicating that the biological reduction of molecular oxygen could yield dangerously reactive free radical intermediates (Fridovich, 1986). In mammalian cells, various subcellular membranous structures and cytosolic compartments are sites of production of oxygen radicals (Freeman and Crapo, 1982). It has been

---

PAK H. CHAN, SYLVIA CHEN, SHIGEKI IMAIZUMI, LILLIAN CHU, JUDITH A. KELLEHER, GEORGE A. GREGORY, and THELMA CHAN • *CNS Injury and Edema Research Center, Department of Neurology, School of Medicine, University of California, San Francisco, California.*

Neurochemical Correlates of Cerebral Ischemia, Volume 7 of *Advances in Neurochemistry*, edited by Nicolas G. Bazan, Pierre Braquet, and Myron D. Ginsberg. Plenum Press, New York, 1992.

demonstrated that about 2 to 5% of the electron flow in isolated brain mitochondria goes to produce superoxide (O_2^-) and hydrogen peroxide (H_2O_2) (Boveris and Chance, 1973). Under normal metabolic conditions, these oxygen radicals formed by mitochondria and other sources are constantly scavenged by endogenous enzymes (superoxide dismutase [SOD], catalase, glutathione peroxidase, etc.) and antioxidants (vitamin E, glutathione, vitamin C, etc.). However, pathological insults, such as ischemia and reperfusion, cause perturbation of this defense mechanisms and the overproduction of oxygen radicals and lipid peroxidation (Chan, 1988; Demopoulos *et al.*, 1982; Flamm *et al.*, 1978; Kogure *et al.*, 1982). Moreover, the release of free polyunsaturated fatty acids (PUFAs) from phospholipids of damaged membranes also contributes to the formation of oxygen radicals (Kuehl and Egan, 1980; Samuelsson, 1983). The pathological role of these oxygen radicals in central nervous system (CNS) ischemia and injury is not completely clear. The purpose of this chapter is to review the current status of the involvement of oxygen free radicals and lipid peroxidation in CNS injury.

2. EXPERIMENTAL APPROACHES TO THE STUDY OF OXYGEN RADICALS IN CEREBRAL ISCHEMIA

There is conflicting evidence regarding the involvement of free radicals in brain ischemia in vivo. Several experimental approaches have been used to identify the effects of free radicals. First, a direct approach is used to measure free radical levels during both the ischemic and reperfusion periods. This technique has proven to be somewhat difficult owing to the transient nature of free radicals and the inaccuracy in the measurement of minute quantities of free radicals in rather heterogeneous brain compartments. Nevertheless, Demopoulos *et al.* (1982) and Yoshida *et al.* (1982) have successfully demonstrated the elevated level of ubiquinone (coenzyme Q) radicals derived from inner mitochondrial membrane in ischemic brain tissue. Another approach is to measure the rate of consumption of endogenous antioxidants such as vitamin E, ascorbic acid, and the reduced form of glutathione (GSH) as an index of the effects of free radicals. It has been demonstrated that the level of the endogenous antioxidants, ascorbic acid, and vitamin E are significantly decreased in the ischemic brain (Demopoulos *et al.*, 1982; Yoshida *et al.*, 1982; Pietronigro *et al.*, 1983). However, other studies have demonstrated that although the GSH level is decreased, the level of oxidized glutathione (GSSG) is unchanged during brain ischemia and injury (Agardh and Siesjö, 1981; Cooper *et al.*, 1980). These results have suggested that the decrease in the GSH level during ischemia may reflect only a reduction in the size of the GSH pool (probably owing to the fall in ATP concentration) and may be unrelated to lipid peroxidation (Siesjö, 1981). A third approach to this problem is to measure the lipid peroxidative products including diene conjugates, malondialdehyde

(MDA), and fluorescent MDA in ischemic and injured brains. However, MDA is rapidly metabolized in vivo (Siu and Draper, 1982), and the shortcomings of the method make it unsuitable for lipid peroxidation measurement in the brain in vivo. Furthermore, the rate of lipid degradation in the traumatic injured brain is usually higher than the rate of formation of MDA; thus the availability of the lipid substrates may also be a limiting factor in measuring MDA formation in vivo (Chan et al., 1983c). On the other hand, diene conjugation has been successfully used to study the role of lipid peroxidation following ischemia (Goldberg et al., 1984; Yoshida et al., 1985b). Watson et al. (1984) have demonstrated that diene conjugation takes place in a very small brain sample during both ischemia and reperfusion. A fourth approach is to study the degree of polyunsaturation of membrane phospholipids in the ischemic brain. It has been demonstrated that the release of free fatty acids from vulnerable phospholipids is significantly increased during cerebral ischemia. The levels of arachidonic acid and other free PUFAs are returned to normal following reperfusion and reoxygenation (Yoshida et al., 1980; Rehncrona et al., 1982). The disappearance of PUFAs has been attributed to the peroxidative process of oxygen radicals during reoxygenation. Furthermore, the MDA level is significantly increased in the brain during the recirculation period, but not the ischemic period, suggesting that peroxidative damage occurs during recirculation (Yoshida et al., 1980). Saez et al. (1987) have demonstrated that a brief substrate deprivation cause high mortality of superior cervical ganglion neurons in culture. Pretreatment of cells with SOD reduced the level of O_2^- and neuronal cell death, indicating that superoxide radicals play a role in neuronal death caused by starvation.

3. ROLE OF OXYGEN RADICALS IN BRAIN INJURY AND EDEMA

Evidence for the involvement of oxygen free radicals and lipid peroxidation in brain injury and edema has been accumulating over the last few years. Using a rat model of compression-induced brain edema, Ginsberg's group has demonstrated that supplementation of vitamin E prior to injury ameliorates brain edema and the derangement of cerebral sodium and potassium levels (Yoshida et al., 1983a, 1985a). Furthermore, pretreatment of vitamin E also increases the regional cerebral blood flow (rCBF) in the decompressed and injured cortex (Busto et al., 1984). However, depletion of the dietary intake of vitamin E prior to the compression injury fails to ameliorate rCBF and brain edema. The beneficial effects of vitamin E may be due to its antioxidative and membrane-stabilizing properties, since both free fatty acid release and the level of lipid peroxides are significantly decreased in ischemic tissue homogenates following oxygenation (Yoshida et al., 1985b). These data, although somewhat indirect, indicate that lipid peroxidation is involved in brain injury and that dietary supplementation with the antioxidant vitamin E may have therapeutic value in ameliorating brain edema and injury.

More direct evidence of the involvement of oxygen free radicals has been obtained from the studies of pial arteriolar abnormalities induced by concussive brain injury. It has been demonstrated by Kontos's group that concussive brain injury, induced by fluid percussion in cats, causes sustained relaxation of the smooth muscles of cerebral arterioles and discrete destructive lesions in the endothelium of the cerebral arterioles (Wei *et al.*, 1980). Using a similar animal model equipped with a cranial window, these investigators further observed that vasodilation and a reduced responsiveness to the vasoconstrictive effects of hypocapnia after brain injury are inhibited by topical applications of the free-radical scavenger superoxide dismutase. Pretreatment with free-radical scavengers also inhibits the density of the endothelial lesions in cerebral arterioles (Wei *et al.*, 1981). Although the mechanisms for the formation of oxygen radicals are not clear, it is likely that the released arachidonic acid or bradykinin in injured brain causes the formation of oxygen radicals. Topical application of arachidonic acid (200 µg/ml) or bradykinin (20 µg/ml) on the brain surface equipped with cranial windows in anesthetized cats causes superoxide formation as measured by the reduction of nitroblue tetrazolium (NBT). The levels of superoxide radicals are significantly reduced when either SOD or indomethacin is used, indicating that the superoxide radicals are generated in the course of arachidonate metabolism via the cyclooxygenase pathway (Kontos, 1985; Kontos *et al.*, 1984, 1985; Kamitani *et al.*, 1985). Furthermore, superoxide formation is further reduced by 4,4'-diisothiocyano-2,2'-stilbene disulfonate and phenylglyoxal, two specific inhibitors of anion channels, suggesting that superoxide radicals may be generated either extracellularly or intracellularly (Kontos *et al.*, 1985). However, the intracellularly formed superoxide radicals may cross the membrane of undamaged cells via the anion channel to reach the extracellular space (Kontos and Wei, 1986). These studies have thus clearly established that arachidonic acid-derived superoxide radicals in situ are directly involved in brain injury.

4. ARACHIDONIC ACID CASCADES AND OXYGEN RADICALS IN CEREBRAL ISCHEMIA

It is generally recognized that the level of free PUFAs is very low in the brain and in the spinal cord in situ (Lunt and Rowe, 1968; Bazan *et al.*, 1971; Demediuk *et al.*, 1985; Faden *et al.*, 1987). These PUFAs are usually localized at the C-2 position of the glycerol backbone in membrane phospholipids. It has been demonstrated that free PUFAs, especially arachidonic acid and docosahexaenoic acid, are rapidly released following ischemia, electroconvulsive seizures, and various pathological insults (Bazan, 1970, 1971; Marion and Wolfe, 1979; Gardiner *et al.*, 1981; Tang and Sun, 1982; Yoshida *et al.*, 1982; Chan *et al.*, 1983*c*). The release and accumulation of PUFAs, arachidonic acid in particular, is due to the activation of phospholipase A_2 (Au *et al.*, 1985; Edgar *et al.*, 1982). It has been suggested that phosphatidylinositol-specific phospholipase C is also involved in the formation of diacylglycerols, the metabolic precursors of arachidonic acid (Huang and Sun, 1987; Manning and Sun, 1983). Other inositol phospholipids, including phosphatidylinositol-4-phosphate and phosphatidyl-4,5-bisphosphate, may also be involved in the production of diacylglycerols (Nishizuka, 1984).

Diacylglycerols and water-soluble inositol-1,4,5-triphosphate (IP_3), which formed from the phosphatidylinositol cycle are second messengers for the activation of protein kinase C (Nishizuka, 1986) and Ca^{2+} mobilization (Berridge, 1984), respectively. The processes of receptor-mediated release of second messengers of diacylglycerols and IP_3 are mechanisms underlying the signal transduction. However, their exact role in ischemic neuronal cell death is not clear and requires further elucidation.

Free PUFAs and, again, arachidonic acid in particular, have both physiological and pathological effects on cellular systems. It has been demonstrated that free arachidonic acid readily intercalates into the membrane and produces significant changes in the packing of lipid molecules (Usher *et al.*, 1978; Klausner *et al.*, 1980*a,b*). PUFA-induced membrane fluidity has been associated with the stimulation of chloride transport in corneal epithelium (Schaeffer and Zadunaisky, 1979) and enhances the activities of both membrane-associated adenylate cyclase and guanylate cyclase (Wallach and Pastan, 1976; Anderson and Jaworski, 1977; Asakawa *et al.*, 1978). Furthermore, free arachidonic acid has been postulated as a potential second messenger since it causes Ca^{2+} metabolization (Cheah, 1981) and activates Ca^{2+}-dependent protein kinase C (McPhail *et al.*, 1984).

Arachidonic acid also exerts other neurochemical effects on brain cells. Arachidonic acid at the same concentration as ischemic brain tissue (0.5 mM) significantly inhibited glutamate uptake and Na^+,K^+-ATPase activity in brain slices and synaptosomes (Chan *et al.*, 1983*b*). The inhibition of glutamate uptake by arachidonic acid in primary cell cultures of astrocytes was dose dependent (Yu *et al.*, 1986). Arachidonic acid at 50 μM inhibited 50% of glutamate uptake in astrocytes, suggesting that it plays an important role in the reuptake of extracellular excitotoxin, one of the major protective mechanisms of astrocytes in glutamate-mediated neuronal cell death, by eliminating the extracellular levels of excitotoxins (Figure 1). Incubation of isolated brain mitochondria with arachidonic acid at concentrations relevant to cerebral ischemia caused a dose-dependent increase in substrate-supported (state 4) respiration (i.e., uncoupling) and a concomitant inhibition of substrate-, phosphate-, and ADP-supported (state 3) or dinitrophenol-supported (state 3μ) respiration (Hillered and Chan, 1988*a*). Furthermore, mito-chondrial respiratory activities are enhanced in the ischemic brain when mito-chondrial fatty acids (arachidonic acid in particular) are removed by bovine

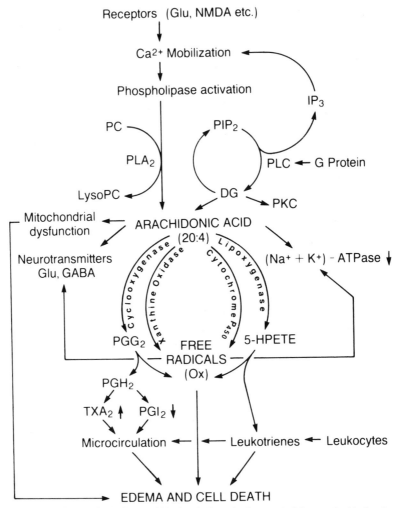

FIGURE 1. Hypothetical scheme of biochemical mechanisms underlying cerebral ischemia.

serum albumin (BSA) during the isolation procedures (Hillered and Chan, 1988*b*). These studies suggest that arachidonic acid plays an important role in mitochondrial dysfunction during cerebral ischemia (Figure 1).

In fact, free fatty acids, exclusively PUFAs, are known potent inducers of cellular (cytotoxic) edema in brain slices (Chan and Fishman, 1978; Chan *et al.*, 1980) and in neuroblastoma and C-6 glioma cells as well as in primary cell culture of astrocytes (Chan and Fishman, 1982; Chan *et al.*, 1988*a*). Intracerebral injection of arachidonic acid and other PUFAs at 0.05 mM causes a breakdown of the blood-brain barrier as indicated by the increased permeability of [^{125}I]BSA and subsequent development of vasogenic brain edema (Chan *et al.*, 1983*a*; Chan and Fishman, 1984).

Since the brain contains very low or negligent amounts of free unesterified arachidonic acid, the high level of arachidonic acid during ischemia and trauma is derived mainly from cellular membranes. Arachidonic acid, once released from membrane phospholipids, is readily metabolized to prostaglandins and thromboxanes via cyclooxygenase or to hydroxy and hydroperoxy fatty acids and leukotrienes via lipoxygenase (Gaudet and Levine, 1979; Ellis *et al.*, 1983; Moskowitz *et al.*, 1984). Prostaglandins and leukotrienes are involved in numerous physiological and pathological functions such as inflammation, membrane permeability, chemotaxis, microcirculating response, receptor binding, platelet aggregation, and hormonal effects (Kuehl and Egan, 1980; Samuelsson, 1983). It has been proposed that a highly reactive oxygen radical species is formed during conversion from prostaglandin G_2 (PGG$_2$) to PGH$_2$ or from 5-hydroperoxyeicosatetraenoic acid (5-HPETE) to leukotriene A_4 (LTA$_4$) (Kuehl and Egan, 1980; Samuelsson *et al.*, 1979). It has also been proposed that superoxide radicals and lipid hydroperoxides could be formed from the cooxidation of xanthine oxidase with arachidonic acid (Fridovich and Porter, 1981). Although the brain parenchyma has a very low level of xanthine oxidase, the much higher level of xanthine oxidase in brain capillaries would make such a cooxidation process possible (Betz, 1985). The hypoxanthine and xanthine which are derived at high levels from the ATP pool during ischemia could be used as substrates for xanthine oxidase. Superoxide radicals and fatty acid peroxides could also be formed from arachidonic acid via the microsomal cytochrome P-450 system (Capdevila *et al.*, 1981, 1982), since the immunohistochemical activities of cytochrome P-450 have been localized in the brain (Kohler *et al.*, 1988). These active oxygen radical species further participate in radical propagation and membrane protein and lipid peroxidation, which are associated with degradation of membrane integrity (Freeman and Crapo, 1982; Mead, 1976). Furthermore, oxygen radicals, derived from the xanthine oxidase/ xanthine system, inhibited synaptosomal neurotransmitter uptake (Braughler, 1985) and Na$^+$,K$^+$-ATPase activity (Braughler *et al.*, 1985; Lo and Betz, 1986). Severe inhibition of mitochondrial respiration is also caused by oxygen radicals (Hillered and Ernster, 1983). These data, when taken together, suggest a possible role for oxygen radicals in ischemic brain injury. Figure 1 shows the hypothetical scheme of biochemical mechanisms underlying brain ischemia and injury.

5. SUPEROXIDE RADICAL FORMATION IN BRAIN SLICES AND PRIMARY CELL CULTURES OF ASTROCYTES

The direct experimental evidence regarding the existence of oxygen free radicals associated with arachidonic acid metabolism in the CNS has been generated mainly from in vitro studies. Our experimental approach to this problem is to investigate the possible formation of oxygen radicals and lipid peroxidation in arachidonic acid-incubated CNS tissues. We have demonstrated that linoleic acid, linolenic acid, and arachidonic acid cause both significant increases in superoxide (O_2^-) formation as measured by the reduction of NBT to nitroblue formazan (NBF) and lipid peroxidation in brain slices as measured by thiobarbituric acid-reactive malondialdehyde (Chan and Fishman, 1980) (Table 1). The increased levels of O_2^- and lipid peroxidation correlate well with the increased level of tissue swelling. Palmitic acid and oleic acid are not effective. Furthermore, 0.1 mM arachidonic acid causes a significant increase in intracellular O_2^- levels in primary cell cultures of astrocytes (Chan et al., 1988a) (Figure 2). The level of MDA is also significantly increased in arachidonic acid-incubated astrocytes. The mechanisms underlying arachidonic acid-induced NBT reduction (or NBF formation) in cultured astrocytes were investigated. Various free-radical scavengers, including tryptophan, histidine, thiourea, vitamin E, catalase, glutathionine peroxidase, and SOD, and other enzyme inhibitors, including allopurinol, indomethacin, monoamine oxidase A and B inhibitors, pargyline, imipramine, and trans-2-phenylcyclopropylamine, were not effective in ameliorating NBT reduction. However, NADH or NADPH stimulated the arachidonate-induced NBF formation by 40 and 33%, respectively. Arachidonic acid alone (without astrocytes) did not induce NBF formation.

The well-described regulator and intermediate of energy metabolism, fructose-1,6-bisphosphate (FBP), is also used extracellularly to protect astrocytes from hypoxic injury (Gregory et al., 1989). Injury of primary cultures resulting from reduced O_2 involves the loss of membrane function and an increase in MDA formation (Yu et al., 1989). Inhibition of this hypoxic injury by FBP may involve the reduction of oxygen radical production.

TABLE 1. Tissue Swelling, Superoxide Radicals, and Lipid Peroxidation in Arachidonic Acid-Incubated Brain Slices[a]

Fatty acid	Swelling (%)	Amount of O_2^- (nmol of NBF/mg of protein)	Amount of MDA (nmol/mg of protein)
Krebs Ringer (control)	11.3 ± 1.0	9.7 ± 0.6	5.3 ± 0.5
Palmitic acid (16:0)	13.0 ± 1.9	10.1 ± 0.5	ND[b]
Oleic acid (18:1)	10.5 ± 2.1	9.0 ± 1.2	6.6 ± 0.9
Linoleic acid (18:2)	25.1 ± 1.1[c]	13.1 ± 1.3[c]	11.2 ± 0.6[c]
Linolenic acid (18:3)	16.4 ± 2.0[c]	14.4 ± 0.9[c]	ND
Arachidonic acid (20:4)	23.2 ± 1.5[c]	12.9 ± 0.7[c]	13.5 ± 0.7[c]

[a]Results are given as mean ± SE.
[b]ND, not determined.
[c]$P < 0.001$, Student's t test.

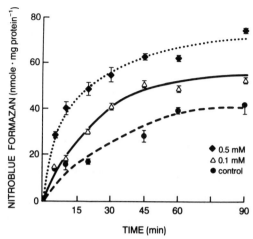

FIGURE 2. Stimulation of NBF formation by 20:4 in intact cultured astrocytes. Cultured astrocytes were incubated with 1.0 mM NBT in the presence of 20:4 (0.1 mM or 0.5 mM) for various times. The extracted NBF was read at 515 nm. Results are means of four different experiments with duplicate assays for each experiment. Vertical bars indicate SD.

6. LIPOSOME-ENTRAPPED SOD AS A TOOL TO STUDY O_2^{-} IN ISCHEMIC BRAIN INJURY

Since superoxide radicals may be involved in ischemia and brain injury, the application of specific free-radical scavengers may identify the superoxide radical reaction in brain tissue. Normally, brain cells and other mammalian cells have their own defense mechanisms against free-radical-induced peroxidation (Freeman and Crapo, 1982). Both enzymatic and nonenzymatic free-radical scavenging systems exist in cellular membranes as well as in cytoplasmic compartments. SOD is a specific scavenger for superoxide radicals, whereas catalase and glutathione peroxidase are specific for the hydrolysis of hydrogen peroxides and other lipid peroxides (Fridovich, 1975; Micheson et al., 1977; Tappel, 1980; Flohe, 1982; Cohen, 1985). The effects of enzymes, especially of SOD, on ischemic and reperfusion injury in the heart, gastrointestinal tract, and lungs have been widely studied (McCord, 1985; Parks and Granger, 1983). However, the beneficial effects of SOD or other antioxidants on cerebral ischemia have not been confirmed. There are many reasons for the ineffectiveness of SOD in ameliorating ischemic brain injury and edema. First, CuZn-SOD, a negatively charged protein with a molecular weight of 31,000 (Steinman, 1982), is almost completely excluded by cerebral endothelial cells and fails to pass through the normal blood-brain barrier. Second, even if the free SOD reaches the extracellular space in the injured brain, it is obvious that the brain cells are also unable to take up the free enzyme, as shown by the studies with both primary neuronal and astrocytic cultures (Chan *et al.*, 1988*a*). Third, the half-life of SOD in plasma is extremely short (about 6 min), as indicated from the pharmacokinetic studies of plasma clearance of SOD which show that SOD is rapidly cleared from the blood (Turrens *et al.*, 1984). Thus, a strategy that could counter these difficulties would be useful for therapeutic approaches. It has been reported by Freeman's group that liposome-entrapped SOD and catalase could counter such difficulties (Turrens *et al.*, 1984; Freeman *et al.*, 1983, 1985). Using liposome-entrapped SOD and catalase, these investigators have successfully inhibited the hyperbaric O_2-induced convulsions in rats, indicating the penetration of liposome-entrapped SOD and catalase into the brain parenchyma (Yusa *et al.*, 1984). Our laboratory has used the liposome-entrapped SOD to study its beneficial effect on the reduction of the level of O_2^- and the level of brain edema in cold-traumatized rat brain (Chan *et al.*, 1983*c*, 1987). Intravenous injection of 10,000 units of liposome-entrapped CuZn-SOD increases the cerebral CuZn-SOD activity twofold at 30 min and maintains it at the same level up to 2 hr following the injection. Furthermore, the brain level of O_2^- is reduced at 1 hr concomitant with the reduction of [^{125}I]BSA-space and edema at the later time points. These data demonstrate that O_2^-, at least in part, plays an important role in blood-brain barrier permeability changes and vasogenic edema following traumatic brain injury.

Using a model of vasogenic brain edema produced by a permanent occlusion of the left middle cerebral artery (MCA) in rats (Tamura *et al.*, 1981), we have studied the possible involvement of O_2^- in the pathogenesis of ischemic edema. The levels of O_2^- (measured by NBF formation) were increased by 222, 420, and 614%, respectively at 1, 4, and 24 hr following MCA occlusion. Liposome-entrapped SOD, when injected 5 min after the MCA occlusion, significantly reduced the degree of edema at 24 hr (Chan *et al.*, 1990). These data indicate that O_2^- plays an important role in the pathogenesis of vasogenic edema in cerebral ischemia.

We have further extended the liposome-entrapped SOD studies into studies of focal cerebral ischemia, by using a method of MCA occlusion with bilateral carotid artery occlusion (Chen *et al.*, 1986). The level of CuZn-SOD activity decreased in a time-dependent fashion in the ischemic infarct and penumbra areas, whereas they were unchanged in the contralateral regions after MCA occlusion. The water content increased significantly only in the infarcted focus (79.2% ± 0.13% before ischemia, 88.8% ± 0.2% after 24 hr of ischemia) but not in the penumbra. Liposome-entrapped CuZn-SOD (10,000 units) when given to the animals 15 min prior to the MCA occlusion, significantly reduced the infarct area, as measured by the staining of mitochondrial dehydrogenase activity with 2,3,5-triphenyltetrazolium chloride (TTC), from 18% ($n = 30$) to 10% ($n = 19$) (Imaizumi *et al.*, 1989). The beneficial effect of liposome SOD on the infarct size suggests that superoxide radicals play a role in ischemic brain injury.

Our data further support the findings of Liu *et al.* (1989). These investigators have studied the beneficial effects and therapeutic potential of polyethylene glycol-conjugated SOD (PEG-SOD) and PEG-catalase on focal cerebral ischemia. They have clearly demonstrated from their carefully controlled, double-blind studies that supplementation with PEG-SOD and PEG-catalase significantly reduced the infarct volume (measured by TTC stain) in the ipsilateral cortex. These studies, together with ours and others, suggest that superoxide radicals are involved in neuronal necrosis following focal cerebral ischemia in rats.

7. LIPOSOME-ENTRAPPED SOD IN PRIMARY CELL CULTURES OF ASTROCYTES

We have demonstrated previously that arachidonic acid, when exposed to primary cell cultures of astrocytes, induced O_2^- formation (Chan *et al.*, 1988a). However, preincubation with CuZn-SOD does not affect the level of O_2^- increased by arachidonic acid. The ineffectiveness of CuZn-SOD is probably due to its inability to be taken up by cultured cells plus the fact that the locus for O_2^- formation is intracellular. These hypotheses have been tested in studies of the uptake of both [125I]CuZn-SOD and fluorescein isothiocyanate (FITC)-conjugated CuZn-SOD into cultured astrocytes, as well as their effects on arachidonic acid-induced O_2^- production. Figure 3 shows the time-dependent uptake of free and liposome-entrapped [125I]SOD in astrocytes. More than 70% of radioactivity was associated with the extensively washed astrocytes at 90 min following the incubation. Free [125I]SOD activity was not associated with astrocytes. Similar uptake studies were performed by using astrocytes with free and liposome-entrapped FITC-conjugated SOD. The uptake of fluorescent SOD at 6 hr following the incubation of cells was demonstrated with liposome-entrapped FITC-conjugated SOD. There was a lack of significant uptake of fluorescent SOD in astrocytes when the free FITC-conjugated SOD was used. These data clearly demonstrate that liposomes facilitate the uptake or transport of SOD into cells. Thus liposome-entrapped SOD could be a useful tool for studying the oxidative mechanisms in ischemic and hypoxic cells. We have further demonstrated that when cultured astrocytes were incubated with liposome-entrapped SOD (100 units/ml), the levels of arachidonic acid (20:4)-induced O_2^- formation and lactic acid release were reduced significantly, whereas empty liposome and free SOD were not effective (Table 2).

8. HUMAN SOD-1 TRANSGENIC MICE: A MODEL FOR STUDYING CEREBRAL ISCHEMIA?

Experimental data accumulated so far clearly point to the likely involvement of oxygen radicals, superoxide radicals in particular, in the pathogenesis of

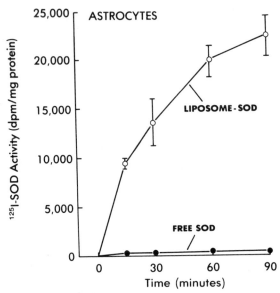

FIGURE 3. Uptake of free and liposome-entrapped [^{125}I]CuZn-SOD into astrocytes. Cultured astrocytes were incubated with 55,000 dpm/dish for both free and liposome-entrapped [^{125}I]CuZn-SOD for various times at 37°C. After the incubation, astrocytes were washed three times with saline phosphate buffer and the cells were solubilized with NaOH and counted for radioactivity. Results are averaged from triplicate assays from two different patches of cells. Values are means ± SD.

TABLE 2. Effects of Liposome-Entrapped CuZn-SOD on 20:4-Induced O_2^- Formation and Lactate Production in Astrocytes[a]

Incubation medium	Amount of NBF (% of control)	Amount of lactate (% of control)
Control	100 ± 16	100 ± 11
20:4	199 ± 15[b]	183 ± 4[b]
+ Empty liposomes	180 ± 17	177 ± 10
+ Free SOD (100 units/dish)	185 ± 13	190 ± 15
+ Liposome-SOD (100 units/dish)	93 ± 9[c]	92 ± 9[c]

[a]Astrocytes were preincubated with empty liposomes, free SOD, or liposome-entrapped SOD in serum-free minimal essential medium for 24 hr prior to the addition of 20:4 (0.1 mM) for another 1 hr. Cell pellets were used for the NBF assay, whereas incubation medium was assayed for lactate content. The control values of NBF and lactate were 54.3 ± 10.4 nmol/mg of protein/hr and 0.35 ± 0.04 μmol/mg of protein/hr, respectively, Values are the means ± SD of three different experiments.
[b]$P < 0.01$ compared with the 20:4 group (analysis of variance).
[c]$P < 0.05$ compared with the 20:4 group (analysis of variance).

vasogenic edema and infarct in focal cerebral ischemia. Although the supplementation of chemically modified SOD (e.g., PEG-SOD) or liposome-entrapped SOD may have therapeutic potential in the improvement of mortality and morbidity outcomes in stroke patients, the beneficial effects of these agents on cerebral ischemia may be indirect, and it may not be able to identify the mechanisms underlying the pathogenesis of ischemic cell injury. In this regard, genetically modified mice with increased CuZn-SOD (SOD-1) activity could be used as an alternative. Human SOD-1 transgenic mice containing a 1.6 to 6.0-fold increase in human SOD-1 activity have been successfully developed (Epstein *et al.*, 1987; Avraham *et al.*, 1988). We have further demonstrated that the primary cell cultures of neurons and astrocytes derived from these human SOD-1 transgenic mice express the increased level of human SOD-1 activity, along with the host CuZn-SOD (Chan *et al.*, 1988*b*, 1991). Thus, these transgenic mice and their derived primary cell cultures of neurons and astrocytes will provide an invaluable tool in the study of the role of superoxide radicals in ischemic brain injury. These experiments are now being carried out in our laboratory (Chan *et al.*, 1988*b*, 1991).

ACKNOWLEDGMENTS

We thank Professor Robert A. Fishman for his constructive criticism and Ms. Dianne Esson for her editorial assistance. This work was supported in part by NIH grants NS-14543 and NS-25372.

REFERENCES

Agardh, C. D., and Siesjö, B. K., 1981, Hypoglycemic brain injury: Phospholipids, free fatty acids, and cyclic nucleotides in the cerebellum of the rat after 30 and 60 minutes of severe insulin-induced hypoglycemia, *J. Cereb. Blood Flow Metab.* **1**:267–275.

Anderson, W. B., and Jaworski, C. J., 1977, Modulation of adenylate cyclase activity of fibroblasts by free fatty acids and phospholipids, *Arch. Biochem. Biophys.* **180**:374–383.

Asakawa, T., Takenoshita, M., Uchida, S., and Tanaka, S., 1978, Activation of guanylate cyclase in synaptic plasma membranes of cerebral cortex by free fatty acids, *J. Neurochem.* **30**:161–166.

Au, A. M., Chan, P. H., and Fishman, R. A., 1985, Stimulation of phospholipase A_2 activity by oxygen-derived free radicals in isolated brain capillaries, *J. Cell. Biochem.* **27**:449–453.

Avraham, K. B., Schickler, M., Sapoznikov, D., Yarom, R., and Groner, Y., 1988, Down's syndrome: Abnormal neuromuscular junction in tongue of transgenic mice with elevated levels of human CuZn-superoxide dismutase, *Cell* **54**:823–829.

Bazan, N. G., 1970, Effects of ischemia and electroconvulsive shock on free fatty acid pool in the brain, *Biochim. Biophys. Acta* **218**:1–10.

Bazan, N. G., 1971, Changes in free fatty acids of the brain by drug-induced convulsions, electroshock and anesthesia, *J. Neurochem.* **18**:1379–1385.

Bazan, N. G., Bazan, H. E. P., Kennedy, W. G., and Joel, C. D., 1971, Regional distribution and rate of production of free fatty acids in rat brain, *J. Neurochem.* **18**:1387–1393.

Berridge, M. J., 1984, Inositol triphosphate and diacylglycerol as second messengers, *Biochem. J.* **220:**345–360.

Betz, A. L., 1985, Identification of hypoxanthine transport and xanthine oxidase activity in brain capillaries, *J. Neurochem.* **44:**574–579.

Boveris, A., and Chance, B., 1973, The mitochondrial generation of hydrogen peroxide, *Biochem. J.* **134:**707–716.

Braughler, J. M., 1985, Lipid peroxidation-induced inhibition of γ-aminobutyric acid uptake in rat brain synaptosomes: Protection by glucocorticoids, *J. Neurochem.* **44:**1282–1288.

Braughler, J. M., Duncan, L. A., and Goodman, T., 1985, Calcium enhances *in vitro* free radical-induced damage to brain synaptosomes, mitochondria, and cultured spinal cord neurons, *J. Neurochem.* **45:**1288–1293.

Busto, R., Yoshida, S., Ginsberg, M. D., Alsonso, O., Smith, D. W., and Goldberg, W. J., 1984, Regional blood flow in compression-induced brain edema in rats: Effect of dietary vitamin E, *Ann. Neurol.* **15:**441–448.

Capdevila, J., Chacos, N., Werringloer, J., Prough, R. A., and Estabrook, R. W., 1981, Liver microsomal cytochrome P-450 and the oxidative metabolism of arachidonic acid, *Proc. Natl. Acad. Sci. USA* **78:**5362–5366.

Capdevila, J., Marnett, L. J., Chacos, N., Prough, R. A., and Estabrook, R. W., 1982, Cytochrome P-450 dependent oxygenation of arachidonic acid to hydroxyicosatetraenoic acids, *Proc. Natl. Acad. Sci. USA* **79:**767–770.

Chan, P. H., 1988, The role of oxygen radicals in brain injury and edema, *in* "Cellular Antioxidant Defense Mechanism," vol. III (C. K. Chow, ed.), pp. 89–109, CRC Press, Boca Raton, Fla.

Chan, P. H., and Fishman, R. A., 1978, Brain edema: Induction in cortical slices by polyunsaturated fatty acids, *Science* **201:**358–360.

Chan, P. H., and Fishman, R. A., 1980, Transient formation of superoxide radicals in polyunsaturated fatty acid-induced brain swelling, *J. Neurochem.* **35:**1004–1007.

Chan, P. H., and Fishman, R. A., 1982, Alterations of membrane integrity and cellular constituents by arachidonic acid in neuroblastoma and glioma cells, *Brain Res.* **248:**151–157.

Chan, P. H., and Fishman, R. A., 1984, The role of arachidonic acid in vasogenic brain edema, *Fed. Proc.* **43:**210–213.

Chan, P. H., Fishman, R. A., Lee, J., and Quan, S., 1980, Arachidonic acid-induced swelling in incubated rat brain cortical slices: Effect of bovine serum albumin, *Neurochem. Res.* **5:**629–640.

Chan, P. H., Fishman, R. A., Caronna, J., Schmidley, J. W., Prioleau, G., and Lee, J., 1983a, Induction of brain edema following intracerebral injection of arachidonic acid, *Ann. Neurol.* **13:**625–632.

Chan, P. H., Kerlan, R., and Fishman, R. A., 1983b, Reductions of gamma-aminobutyric acid and glutamate uptake and (Na$^+$ + K$^+$)-ATPase activity in brain slices and synaptosomes by arachidonic acid, *J. Neurochem.* **40:**309–316.

Chan, P. H., Longar, S., and Fishman, R. A., 1983c, Phospholipid degradation and edema development in cold injured rat brain, *Brain Res.* **227:**329–337.

Chan, P. H., Chen, S. F., and Yu, A. C. H., 1988a, Induction of intracellular superoxide radical formation by arachidonic acid and by polyunsaturated fatty acids in primary astrocytic cultures, *J. Neurochem.* **50:**1185–1193.

Chan, P. H., Yu, A. C. H., Chen, S., Chu, L., and Epstein, C. J., 1988b, Oxidative stress exacerbates cellular damage in primary cultures of astrocytes from human SOD-1 transgenic mice, *J. Cell Biol.* **107:**726a.

Chan, P. H., Yu, A. C. H., and Fishman, R. A., 1988c, Free fatty acids and excitatory neurotransmitter amino acids as determinants of pathological swelling of astrocytes in primary culture, *in* "The Biochemical Pathology of Astrocytes" (M. D. Norenberg, L. Hertz, and A. Schousboe, eds.), pp. 327–355, Alan R. Liss, New York.

Chan, P. H., Longar, S., and Fishman, R. A., 1987, Protective effects of liposome-entrapped superoxide dismutase on post-traumatic brain edema, Ann. Neurol. 21:540–547.

Chan, P. H., Fishman, R. A., Wesley, M. A., and Longar, S., 1990, Pathogenesis of vasogenic edema in focal cerebral ischemia: Role of superoxide radicals, Adv. Neurol. 52:177–183.

Chan, P. H., Yang, G. Y., Chen, S. F., Carlson, E., and Epstein, C. J., 1991, Cold-induced brain edema and infarction are reduced in transgenic mice overexpressing CuZn-superoxide dismutase, Ann. Neurol. 29:482–486.

Cheah, A. M., 1981, Effect of long chain unsaturated fatty acids on the calcium transport of sarcoplasmic reticulum, Biochim. Biophys. Acta 648:113–119.

Chen, S. T., Hsu, C. Y., Hogan, E. L., Maricq, H., and Balentine, J. D., 1986, A model of focal ischemic stroke in the rat: Reproducible extensive cortical infarction, Stroke 17:738–743.

Cohen, G., 1985, Oxidative stress in the nervous system, in "Oxidative Stress" (H. Sies, ed.), pp. 383–402, Academic Press, London.

Cooper, A. J. L., Pulsinelli, W. A., and Duffy, T. E., 1980, Glutathione and ascorbate during ischemia and postischemic reperfusion in rat brain, J. Neurochem. 35:1242–1245.

Demediuk, P., Saunders, R. D., Anderson, D. K., Means, S. E. D., and Horrocks, L. A., 1985, Membrane lipid changes in laminectomized and traumatized cat spinal cord, Proc. Natl. Acad. Sci. USA 82:7071–7075.

Demopoulos, H. B., Flamm, E., Seligman, M., and Pietronigro, D. D., 1982, Oxygen free radicals in central nervous system ischemia and trauma, in "Pathology of Oxygen" (A. P. Autor, ed.), pp. 127–155, Academic Press, New York.

Edgar, A. D., Strosznajder, J., and Horrocks, L. A., 1982, Activation of ethanolamine phospholipase A_2 in brain during ischemia, J. Neurochem. 39:1111–1116.

Ellis, E. F., Wright, K. F., Wei, E. P., and Kontos, H. A., 1983, Cyclooxygenase products of arachidonic acid metabolism in cat cerebral cortex after experimental concussive brain injury, J. Neurochem. 37:892–896.

Epstein, C. J., Avraham, K. B., Lovett, M., Smith, S., Elroy-Stein, O., Rotman, G., Bry, C., and Groner, Y., 1987, Transgenic mice with increased Cu/Zn-superoxide dismutase activity: Animal model of dosage effects in Down syndrome, Proc. Natl. Acad. Sci. USA 84:8044–8048.

Faden, A. I., Chan, P. H., and Longar, S., 1987, Alterations in lipid metabolism, $Na^+ + K^+$-ATPase activity, and tissue water content of spinal cord following experimental traumatic injury, J. Neurochem. 48:1809–1816.

Flamm, E. S., Demopoulos, H. B., Seligman, M. L., Poser, R. G., and Ransohoff, J., 1978, Free radicals in cerebral ischemia, Stroke 9:445–447.

Flohe, L., 1982, Glutathione peroxidase brought into focus, in "Free Radicals in Biology," vol. 5 (W. A. Pryor, ed.), pp. 223–254, Academic Press, New York.

Freeman, B. A., and Crapo, J. D., 1982, Biology of disease. Free radicals and tissue injury, Lab. Invest. 47:412–426.

Freeman, B. A., Young, S. L., and Crapo, J. D., 1983, Liposome-mediated augmentation of superoxide dismutase in endothelial cells prevents oxygen injury, J. Biol. Chem. 258:12534–12542.

Freeman, B. A., Turrens, J. F., Mirza, Z., Crapo, J. D., and Young, S. L., 1985, Modulation of oxidant lung injury by using liposome-entrapped superoxide dismutase and catalase, Fed. Proc. 44:2591–2595.

Fridovich, I., 1975, Superoxide dismutase, Annu. Rev. Biochem. 44:147–159.

Fridovich, I., 1986, Biological effects of the superoxide radical, Arch. Biochem. Biophys. 274:1–11.

Fridovich, S. E., and Porter, N. A., 1981, Oxidation of arachidonic acid in micelles by superoxide and hydrogen peroxide, J. Biol. Chem. 256:260–265.

Gardiner, M., Nilsson, B., Rehncrona, S., and Siesjö, B. K., 1981, Free fatty acids in the rat brain in moderate and severe hypoxia, J. Neurochem. 36:1500–1505.

Gaudet, R. J., and Levine, L., 1979, Transient cerebral ischemia and brain prostaglandins, *Biochem. Biophys. Res. Commun.* **86**:893–901.

Goldberg, W. J., Watson, B. D., Busto, R., Kurchner, H., Santiso, M., and Ginsberg, M. D., 1984, Concurrent measurement of $(Na^+ + K^+)$-ATPase activity and lipid peroxides in rat brain following reversible global ischemia, *Neurochem. Res.* **9**:1737–1747.

Gregory, G. A., Yu, A. C. H., and Chan, P. H., 1989, Fructose-1,6-bisphosphate protects astrocytes from hypoxic damage, *J. Cereb. Blood Flow Metab.* **9**:29–34.

Hillered, L., and Chan, P. H., 1988a, Effects of arachidonic acid on respiratory activities in isolated brain mitochondria, *J. Neurosci. Res.* **19**:94–100.

Hillered, L., and Chan, P. H., 1988b, Role of arachidonic acid and other fatty acids in mitochondrial dysfunction in brain ischemia, *J. Neurosci. Res.* **20**:451–456.

Hillered, L., and Ernster, L., 1983, Respiratory activity of isolated rat brain mitochondria following *in vitro* exposure to oxygen radicals, *J. Cereb. Blood Flow Metab.* **3**:207– 214.

Huang, S. F.-L., and Sun. G. Y., 1987, Acidic phospholipids, diacylglycerols, and free fatty acids in gerbil brain: A comparison of ischemic changes resulting from carotid ligation and decapitation, *J. Neurosci. Res.* **17**:162–167.

Imaizumi, S., Woolworth, V., Fishman, R. A., and Chan, P. H., 1989, Superoxide dismutase activities and their role in focal cerebral ischemia, *J. Cerebral Blood Flow Metab.* **9**:5217.

Kamitani, T., Little, M. H., and Ellis, E. F., 1985, Evidence for a possible role of brain kallikreinkinin system in the modulation of the cerebral circulation, *Circ. Res.* **57**:545–552.

Klausner, R. D., Bhalla, D. K., Dragsten, P., Hoover, R. L., and Karnovsky, M. J., 1980a, Model for capping derived from inhibition of surface receptor capping by free fatty acids, *Proc. Natl. Acad. Sci. USA* **77**:437–441.

Klausner, R. D., Kleinfield, A. M., Hoover, R. L., and Karnovsky, M. J., 1980b, Lipid domains in membranes. Evidence derived from structural perturbations induced by free fatty acids and lifetime heterogeneity analysis, *J. Biol. Chem.* **255**:1286–1296.

Kogure, K., Watson, B. D., Busto, R., and Abe, K., 1982, Potentiation of lipid peroxides by ischemia in rat brain, *Neurochem. Res.* **7**:437–454.

Kohler, C., Eriksson, L. G., Hansson, T., Warner, M., and Ake-Gustafsson, J., 1988, Immunohisto-chemical localization of cytochrome P-450 in the rat brain, *Neurosci. Lett.* **84**:109–114.

Kontos, H. A., 1985, Oxygen radicals in cerebral vascular injury, *Circ. Res.* **57**:508–516.

Kontos, H. A., and Wei, E. P., 1986, Superoxide production in experimental brain injury, *J. Neurosurg.* **64**:803–807.

Kontos, H. A., Wei, E. P., Povlishock, J. T., and Christman, C. W., 1984, Oxygen radicals mediate the cerebral arteriolar dilation from arachidonate and bradykinin in cats, *Circ. Res.* **55**:295–303.

Kontos, H. A., Wei, E. P., Ellis, E. F., Jenkins, L. W., Povlishock, J. T., Rowe, G. T., and Hess, M. L., 1985, Appearance of superoxide anion radical in cerebral extracellular space during increased prostaglandin synthesis in cats, *Circ. Res.* **57**:142–151.

Kuehl, F. A., and Egan, R. N., 1980, Prostaglandins, arachidonic acid, and inflammation, *Science* **210**:978–984.

Liu, T. H., Beckman, J. S., Freeman, B. A., Hogan, E. L., and Hsu, C. Y., 1989, Polyethylene glycol-conjugated superoxide dismutase and catalase reduce ischemic brain injury, *Am. J. Physiol.* **256**:H589–H593.

Lo, W. D., and Betz, A. L., 1986, Oxygen free-radical reduction of brain capillary rubidium uptake, *J. Neurochem.* **46**:394–398.

Lunt, G. G., and Rowe, C. E., 1968, The production of unesterified fatty acid in brain, *Biochim. Biophys. Acta* **152**:681–693.

Manning, R., and Sun, G. Y., 1983, Detergent effects on the phosphatidylinositol-specific phospholipase C in rat brain synaptosomes, *J. Neurochem.* **41**:1735–1743.

Marion, J., and Wolfe, L. S., 1979, Origin of the arachidonic acid released post-mortem in rat forebrain, *Biochim. Biophys. Acta* **54**:25–32.

McCord, J. M., 1985, Oxygen-derived free radicals in postischemic tissue injury, *N. Engl. J. Med.* **312**: 159–163.

McPhail, L. C., Clayton, C. C., and Snyderman, R., 1984, A potential second messenger role for unsaturated fatty acids: Activation of Ca^{2+}-dependent protein kinase, *Science* **224**:622–625.

Mead, J. F., 1976, Free radical mechanisms of lipid damage and consequences for cellular membranes, *in* "Free Radicals in Biology" (W. A. Pryor, ed.), pp. 51–68, Academic Press, New York.

Micheson, A. M., McCord, J. M., and Fridovich, I., 1977, "Superoxide and Superoxide Dismutases," Academic Press, London.

Moskowitz, M. A., Kiwak, K. J., Herkimin, K., and Levine, L., 1984, Synthesis of compounds with properties of leukotrienes C_4 and D_4 in gerbil brains after ischemia and reperfusion, *Science* **224**: 886–889.

Nishizuka, Y., 1984, Turnover of inositol phospholipids and signal transduction, *Science* **225**:1365–1370.

Nishizuka, Y., 1986, Studies and perspectives of protein kinase C, *Science* **233**:305–312.

Parks, D. A., and Granger, D. N., 1983, Oxygen-derived radicals and ischemia-induced tissue injury, *in* "Oxy Radicals and Their Scavenger Systems" (R. A. Greenwald and G. Cohen, eds.), pp. 135–144, Elsevier, Amsterdam.

Pietronigro, D. D., Horsepian, M., Demopoulos, H. B., and Flamm, E. S., 1983, Loss of ascorbic acid from injured feline spinal cord, *J. Neurochem.* **41**:1072–1076.

Rehncrona, S., Westerberg, E., Akesson, B., and Siesjö, B. K., 1982, Brain cortical fatty acids and phospholipids during and following complete and severe incomplete ischemia, *J. Neurochem.* **38**:84–93.

Saez, J. C., Kessler, J. A., Bennett, M. V. L., and Spray, D., 1987, Superoxide dismutase protects cultured neurons against death by starvation, *Proc. Natl. Acad. Sci. USA* **84**:3056–3059.

Samuelsson, B., 1983, Leukotrienes: Mediators of immediate hypersensitivity reactions and inflammation, *Science* **220**:568–575.

Samuelsson, B., Hammarstrom, S., and Borgeat, P., 1979, Pathway of arachidonic acid metabolism, *Adv. Inflamm. Res.* **1**:405–411.

Schaeffer, B. E., and Zadunaisky, J. A., 1979, Stimulation of chloride transport by fatty acids in corneal epithelium and relation to changes in membrane fluidity, *Biochim. Biophys. Acta* **556**: 131–143.

Siesjö, B. K., 1981, Cell damage in the brain: A speculative synthesis, *J. Cereb. Blood Flow Metab.* **1**: 155–185.

Siu, G. M., and Draper, H. H., 1982, Metabolism of malondialdehyde *in vivo* and *in vitro*, *Lipids* **17**: 349–355.

Steinman, H. M., 1982, Superoxide dismutase: protein chemistry and structure-function relationships, *in* "Superoxide Dismutase," vol. 1 (L. W. Oberley, ed.), pp. 12–68, CRC Press, Boca Raton, Fla.

Tamura, A., Graham, D. I., McCullock, J., and Teasdale, G. M., 1981, Focal cerebral ischemia in the rat. 1. Description of technique and early neuropathological consequences following middle cerebral artery occlusion, *J. Cereb. Blood Flow Metab.* **1**:53–60.

Tang, W., and Sun,G. Y., 1982, Factors affecting the free fatty acids in rat brain cortex, *Neurochem. Int.* **4**:269–273.

Tappel, A. L., 1980, Measurement of and protection from *in vivo* lipid peroxidation, *in* "Free Radicals in Biology," vol. 4 (W. A. Pryor, ed.), pp. 1–47, Academic Press, New York.

Turrens, J. F., Crapo, J. D., and Freeman, B. A., 1984, Protection against oxygen toxicity by intravenous injection of liposome-entrapped catalase and superoxide dismutase, *J. Clin. Invest.* **73**:87–95.

Usher, J. R., Epand, R. M., and Papahadjopoulos, D., 1978, The effect of free fatty acids on the thermotropic phase transition of dimyristoyl glycerophosphocholine, *Chem. Phys. Lipids* **22:** 245–253.

Wallach, D., and Pastan, I., 1976, Stimulation of guanylate cyclase of fibroblasts and free fatty acids, *J. Biol. Chem.* **251:**5802–5809.

Watson, B. D., Busto, R., Goldberg, W. J., Santiso, M., Yoshida, S., and Ginsberg, M. D., 1984, Lipid peroxidation *in vivo* induced by reversible global ischemia in rat brain, *J. Neurochem.* **42:** 268–274.

Wei, E. P., Dietrich, W. D., Povlishock, J. T., Navari, R. M., and Kontos, H. A., 1980, Functional morphological and metabolic abnormalities of the cerebral microcirculation after concussive brain injury in cats, *Circ. Res.* **46:**37–47.

Wei, E. P., Ellison, M. D., Kontos, H. A., and Povlishock, J. T., 1981, O_2 radicals in arachidonate-induced increased blood-brain barrier permeability to proteins, *Am. J. Physiol.* H693–H699.

Yoshida, S., Inoh, S., Asano, T., Sano, K., Kubota, J., Shimazaki, H., and Meta, N., 1980, Effect of transient ischemia on free fatty acids and phospholipids in the gerbil brain, *J. Neurosurg.* **53:** 323–331.

Yoshida, S., Abe, K., Busto, R., Watson, B. D., Kogure, K., and Ginsberg, M. D., 1982, Influence of transient ischemia on lipid-soluble antioxidants, free fatty acids and energy metabolites in rat brain, *Brain Res.* **245:**307–316.

Yoshida, S., Busto, R., Ginsberg, M. D., Abe, L., Martinez, E., Watson, B. P., and Scheinberg, P., 1983*a*, Compression-induced brain edema: Modification by prior depletion and supplementation of vitamin E, *Neurology* **33:**166–172.

Yoshida, S., Inoh, S., Asano, T., Sano, K., Shimasaki, H., and Ueta, N., 1983*b*, Brain free fatty acids, edema, and mortality in gerbils subjected to transient, bilateral ischemia, and effect of barbiturate anesthesia, *J. Neurochem.* **40:**1278–1286.

Yoshida, S., Busto, R., Abe, K., Santiso, M., and Ginsberg, M. D., 1985*a*, Compression-induced brain edema in rats: Effect of dietary vitamin E on membrane damage in the brain, *Neurology* **35:** 126–130.

Yoshida, S., Busto, R., Watson, B. D., Santiso, M., and Ginsberg, M. D., 1985*b*, Postischemic cerebral lipid peroxidation *in vitro*: Modification by dietary vitamin E, *J. Neurochem.* **44:**1593–1601.

Yu, A. C. H., Chan, P. H., and Fishman, R. A., 1986, Effects of arachidonic acid on glutamate and GABA uptake in primary cultures of rat cerebral cortical astrocytes and neurons, *J. Neurochem.* **47:**1181–1189.

Yu, A. C. H., Gregory, G. A., and Chan, P. H., 1989, Hypoxia-induced dysfunctions and injury of astrocytes in primary cell cultures, *J. Cereb. Blood Flow Metab.* **9:**20–28.

Yusa, T., Crapo, J. D., and Freeman, B. A., 1984, Liposome-mediated augmentation of brain SOD and catalase inhibits CNS O_2 toxicity, *J. Appl. Physiol.* **57:**1674–1681.

BIOCHEMICAL FACTORS AND MECHANISMS OF SECONDARY BRAIN DAMAGE IN CEREBRAL ISCHEMIA AND TRAUMA

A. BAETHMANN and O. KEMPSKI

1. INTRODUCTION

A distinction between primary and secondary manifestations of brain damage from acute insults, such as trauma, or ischemia is not only of scientific interest but also of the highest clinical significance. After all, prevention of secondary brain damage in patients with severe head injury or cerebral ischemia is the ultimate purpose of treatment, including the measures of emergency care. It can be

A. BAETHMANN and O. KEMPSKI • *Institute for Surgical Research, Klinikum Grosshadern, Ludwig Maximilians University, 8000 München 70, and Institute of Neurosurgical Pathophysiology, University of Mainz, 6500 Mainz, Germany.*

Neurochemical Correlates of Cerebral Ischemia, Volume 7 of *Advances in Neurochemistry*, edited by Nicolas G. Bazan, Pierre Braquet, and Myron D. Ginsberg. Plenum Press, New York, 1992.

assumed that the secondary sequelae of head injury are as important for the outcome as the primary insult is. Therefore, it is obvious that development of more effective forms of treatment requires a better understanding of the mechanisms underlying secondary brain damage. Manifestations of secondary brain damage can be defined on a neuropathological or pathophysiological basis. They have a wide spectrum reaching from macroscopic phenomena, such as brain swelling, to subtle processes, such as cytotoxic cell damage from distinct molecular mechanisms. This chapter is a summary of recent concepts and findings.

2. SECONDARY BRAIN DAMAGE IN SEVERE HEAD INJURY AND CEREBRAL ISCHEMIA

Figure 1 is a model illustrating schematically the primary and secondary forms of brain damage in head injury. The most important manifestations of primary damage are (1) destruction of brain tissue causing necrosis, such as the contusion focus; (2) disruption of blood vessels leading to epidural, subdural, or intracerebral bleeding; and (3) shearing and tearing of nerve fibers in the white matter (the diffuse axonal injury). The intracranial primary lesions give rise to secondary brain damage. Formation of an intracranial mass from haemorrhage or edema is particularly threatening because it may induce intracranial hypertension with its disastrous consequences. Secondary brain damage in severe head injury also has extracranial causes related to impairment of the cardiovascular and pulmonary function. Patients with severe head injury quite frequently also have peripheral insults which lead to arterial hypotension from blood loss and circulatory shock. Moreover, they may suffer from respiratory disturbances, e.g., from an aspiration. Secondary brain damage resulting from extracranial causes is particularly frequent in patients with a fatal outcome (Graham et al., 1978).

Whereas identification of the secondary sequelae from severe head injury is rather straightforward (Figure 1), differentiation of primary and secondary damage in cerebral ischemia is less obvious. The gross pathophysiology resulting from an intracranial mass, such as edema or haemorrhage, is similar to that in severe head injury, underlining the predominant role of intracranial hypertension. However, whereas the increase of intracranial pressure is a major determinant in severe head injury, its significance is not clearly understood in global or focal forms of cerebral ischemia. Nevertheless, evidence is available that early death from cerebral infarction with ischemic brain edema and intracranial mass shift is related to intracranial hypertension (Shaw et al., 1959).

Hence, ischemic brain edema can be considered a major manifestation of secondary brain damage, evolving from focal cerebral ischemia around the ischemic tissue necrosis. It is an entity which relates to the penumbral zone according to the concept of Astrup et al. (1977) and Symon (1986). The penumbra

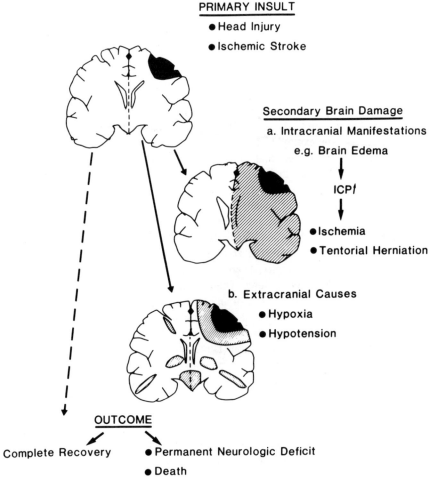

PRIMARY INSULT
- Head Injury
- Ischemic Stroke

Secondary Brain Damage
a. Intracranial Manifestations
   e.g. Brain Edema
   ↓
   ICP↑
   ↓
- Ischemia
- Tentorial Herniation

b. Extracranial Causes
   - Hypoxia
   - Hypotension

OUTCOME

Complete Recovery   • Permanent Neurologic Deficit
                     • Death

FIGURE 1. Formation of secondary brain damage from a primary process as in head injury or focal ischemia. If the primary lesion is limited, recovery may follow. However, focal ischemic or traumatic insults of the brain are frequently associated with intra- and extracranial complications leading to the formation of secondary brain damage. Major intracranial manifestations of secondary brain damage are brain edema and hemorrhage causing intracranial hypertension and, eventually, tentorial herniation. Important extracranial causes of secondary brain damage are arterial hypoxia from ventilatory failure and arterial hypotension from hemorrhagic shock, such as occur in polytraumatized patients. (From Baethmann, 1987*b*.)

is an area around an ischemic focus with preservation of residual blood flow too low to maintain functional activity yet above the threshold causing infarction. Measurements of blood flow and of ion activities have provided further characterization. The penumbral zone may suffer occasionally from extracellular K^+ transients, i.e., reversible increases of the K^+ concentration (Branston et al., 1977). It is clinically relevant as an area that is probably amenable to salvage by effective treatment, although identification and assessment of its extension in a patient might be difficult.

Another secondary phenomenon of cerebral ischemia is delayed neuronal death in selectively vulnerable areas of the brain after short periods of cerebral circulatory arrest. The CA1 sector of the hippocampus and layers III and V of the cerebral cortex, for example, are selectively vulnerable areas. The secondary nature of the delayed neuronal death from global ischemia is supported by observations that it can be therapeutically prevented. Effective measures are Ca^{2+} channel antagonists, glutamate receptor-antagonists or glutamate-dependent channel blockers, or creation of lesions in the glutamatergic afferences of the selectively vulnerable cells (Deshpande and Wieloch, 1985; Gill et al., 1987; Onodera et al., 1986; Simon et al., 1984; Wieloch et al., 1985). Furthermore, it might be assumed that formation of border zone infarction between supply territories of large cerebral arteries from global cerebral ischemia is a manifestation of secondary damage. The underlying hemodynamic mechanisms are not understood.

It is not clear whether the size of an ischemic infarction is finite or whether it does subsequently increase. Recent experimental findings on reduction of infarct size from a standard ischemic insult by the glutamate-dependent channel blocker MK-801 support the latter conclusion (Duverger et al., 1987; Park et al., 1988). Generally, identification of damage as primary or secondary might be facilitated by its reversibility in response to therapeutic measures ranging from improvement or preservation of flow to specific forms of antagonism of cytotoxic mediator mechanisms.

The complexity of the many simultaneous pathophysiological events in damaged brain tissue requires approaches to disentangle relevant processes from epiphenomena. This aspect is considered in greater detail below in the discussion on mechanisms of cell swelling and damage in cerebral ischemia.

The concept of mediators of secondary brain damage in trauma and cerebral ischemia is particularly fruitful for our understanding of both the underlying pathophysiology and the development of therapeutic guidelines. The discovery of the effects of an intracellular influx of Ca^{2+} ions on cell function and cell viability or of the neurotoxic potential of glutamate may serve as an example. However, recent advances in this field notwithstanding, it is a safe assumption that marked improvements in the clinical outcome of cerebral ischemia and head injury are already possible. Effective organization and implementation of prehospital emergency care can be viewed as the most efficient currently available method of prevention of secondary brain damage. Obviously, delays, failures, and omissions in emergency treatment cannot be repaired later by even the most advanced and sophisticated treatment available in the hospital (Baethmann, 1987a).

3. MEDIATOR COMPOUNDS IN SECONDARY BRAIN DAMAGE

Acute formation of a traumatic or ischemic brain tissue necrosis with opening of the blood-brain barrier providing for entrance of intravascular material into the cerebral parenchyma, hemorrhage, coagulation, etc., are processes suggestive of formation and involvement of active mediator compounds enhancing damage to the primarily injured tissue. The situation is appropriately characterized by Mayer and Westbrook (1987a) ". . .in essence, the brain is loaded with the seeds of its own destruction. . . ." Evidence supporting a mediator role is particularly convincing for the excitatory amino acid glutamate, arachidonic acid and its metabolites, and the kallikrein-kinin system. In addition, functional impairment and structural damage can be expected from the derangements of tissue homeostasis leading to increased extracellular K^+ concentrations or to the development of tissue acidosis. Owing to the potentially unlimited number of active substances which may be liberated in brain tissue under these circumstances, strict guidelines for identification are required. This laboratory suggests the following (Baethmann, 1978):

- Induction of cerebral damage by a compound, e.g., vasogenic or cytotoxic edema, opening of the blood-brain barrier, necrosis of nerve or glial cells, disturbances of the microcirculation and vasomotor control, among others.
- Formation or release of the compound in brain tissue in relationship to the severity of the insult.
- Prevention or attenuation of brain damage by specific inhibition of release or function of a mediator candidate.

Only a limited number of compounds have met the above requirements and been identified as mediators of secondary brain damage. Most often, evidence has been obtained that a substance causes brain damage in one way or the other and that it is released in damage brain tissue or into compartments, respectively, where it is normally not present. Reduction of tissue damage by specific antagonization of the release or pathological function of a mediator compound is clinically the most important requirement. Table 1 summarizes the state of the art for identification of mediator compounds according to these specifications. All requirements are met in the case of the kallikrein-kinin system and glutamate, whereas the degree of identification of arachidonic acid is less comprehensive. This may be attributed to the fact that suppression of the formation of arachidonic acid in the acutely damaged brain is difficult. Nevertheless, findings on effects of administra-

TABLE 1. Current Level of Evidence for Identification of Potent Factors
as Mediators of Secondary Brain Damage

	Level of evidence for a role as mediator		
Factor	Level 1 (Induction of damage)	Level 2 (Induction of damage + evidence of release)	Level 3 (Induction of damage + evidence of release + specific therapeutic inhibition)
Kallikrein-kinin-system	+	+	+
Arachidonic acid	+	+	(+)
Glutamate	+	+	+
Serotonin	+	+	?
Prostaglandins, free radicals, etc.	+	+	?

tion of glucocorticosteroids on acute cerebral lesions support the contention that damage is reduced in association with reduction of the release of arachidonic acid (Politi *et al.*, 1985).

3.1. Kallikrein-Kinin System

The active principles of the kallikrein-kinin system are the peptides brady-kinin and kallidin, which consist of 9 and 10 amino acids, respectively. Kinins are formed in acute processes such as inflammation, coagulation, and trauma and are rapidly degraded again by potent enzymes present in all tissues. All components of the kallikrein-kinin system, including its inhibitors, occur in a complex structural association in the intravascular compartment (Erdös, 1979; Frey *et al.*, 1968). Kinins are released if the proteolytic enzyme kallikrein is activated from inactive prokallikrein. Coagulation leading to release of Hageman factor is highly effective in triggering the kallikrein-kinin cascade. Brain tissue contains the components of the kallikrein-kinin system, however, at a lower level than in the intravascular compartment (Clark, 1979). Hyperemia and swelling as classical symptoms of inflammation can be attributed to a release of kinins on account of their potency to cause vasodilation and extravasation (Frey *et al.*, 1968). These properties are also relevant to the formation of vasogenic brain edema. Besides, kinins are powerful pain-inducing compounds.

This laboratory has been involved in experimental studies on a mediator function of kinins in secondary brain damage. It was shown that cerebral administration of bradykinin causes a marked increase of the water content in the cerebral cortex, caudate nucleus, and periventricular white matter (Unterberg and Baethmann, 1984). In vivo fluorescence microscopy of the cerebral surface during superfusion with bradykinin demonstrated selective opening of the blood-brain barrier to a low-molecular-weight indicator (Na^+ fluorescein, MW 376), whereas high-molecular-weight indicators such as fluorescein isothiocyanate (FITC)-dextran (MW ca. 20,000) were not found to enter the cerebral parenchyma from the intravascular space. Simultaneously, bradykinin caused marked dilation of cerebral arterioles and constriction of cerebral venules (Unterberg et al., 1984). Dilation of cerebral arterioles and opening of the blood-brain barrier by kinins might be attributable to an interaction with B_2-kininergic receptors of the cerebral vasculature (Wahl et al., 1988).

In fulfillment of another requirement, release of kinins was demonstrated to occur in acutely damaged brain with vasogenic edema. Formation of kinins was quantified by measurements of consumption of the kininogen precursor, which was extravasating from the intravascular space into the focal lesion and perifocal parenchyma (Maier-Hauff et al., 1984a). Kinins were found not only in acute necrotic brain tissue but also in the surrounding edematous areas. Within 7 hr after the insult, approximately 600 ng/g fresh weight of brain tissue was liberated in the necrosis, while ca. 200 ng/g was formed in perifocal edema. Additional development of cerebral ischemia due to a malignant increase of the intracranial pressure led to a marked enhancement of the formation of kinins in edematous perifocal brain, indicative of a relationship between the extent of mediator formation and the severity of brain damage. Under the latter circumstances, kinin concentrations of 10^{-7} to 10^{-6} M accumulated in the interstitial fluid (Maier-Hauff et al., 1984a). This might be sufficient to induce vasomotor changes as well as an increase in blood-brain barrier dysfunction, enhancing edema formation.

Final evidence for a mediator role of the kallikrein-kinin system was obtained in studies on its inhibition in animals with an acute cerebral lesion. When the polyvalent proteinase inhibitor aprotinin (Inhibin; Thiemann, Inc.) was used, the extent of hemispheric brain swelling resulting from a standardized focal trauma was significantly reduced (Unterberg et al., 1986). The therapeutic reduction of hemispheric brain swelling by aprotinin appeared to require continuous infusion over a period of 24 hr after trauma and a higher dose than is usually administered. Another inhibitor of the kallikrein-kinin system (soybean trypsin inhibitor) was only marginally effective in inhibiting formation of brain swelling from the standard lesion (Unterberg et al., 1986). Taken together, the currently available evidence on induction of cerebral damage, assessment of formation and, finally, therapeutically useful inhibition of brain edema can be considered complete now under all practical circumstances for identifying the kallikrein-kinin system as a mediator of secondary brain damage. Validation of these findings in patients with an acute cerebral lesion causing vasogenic brain edema thus appears promising.

3.2. Glutamate

A pathophysiological role of glutamate in acute brain damage has been suspected for many years. Previous observations of Van Harreveld (1959, 1972) and Van Harreveld and Fifkova (1973) have indicated that the compound is involved in the phenomenon of spreading depression and ischemic cell swelling. Glutamate has received widespread attention as a mediator of secondary brain damage only during recent years. A role of glutamate in the formation of cytotoxic brain edema could be confirmed in experiments performed in our laboratory on cerebral administration of the amino acid by ventriculocisternal perfusion (Kempski, 1982a; Rothenfusser, 1982). Measurements of cerebral water content and electrical tissue impedance revealed an intracellular accumulation of edema fluid. In vitro studies with C-6 glioma cells provided additional evidence for the cell swelling-inducing properties of glutamate, even when low concentrations are used (Kempski et al., 1982). Systemic administration of glutamate in newborn animals before maturation of the blood-brain barrier resulted in the development of neurodegenerative disorders (Lucas and Newhouse, 1957; Olney and Sharpe, 1969).

A wealth of data has been reported concerning cell biological and molecular details of the powerful physiological and pathophysiological functions of glutamate. The findings indicate a central role of the amino acid in phenomena such as long-term potentiation, formation of memory, epilepsy, and delayed neuronal death from ischemia (Baudry and Lynch, 1980; Chapman et al., 1987; Gill et al., 1987; Kauer et al., 1988; Simon et al., 1984; Van Harreveld and Fifkova, 1975). In studies on characterization of the cellular binding of glutamate, different receptor types, for example the N-methyl-D-aspartate (NMDA) receptor, were discovered. NMDA receptor-ligand interactions appear to play a predominant role not only in synaptic transmission but also in the manifestations of excitotoxic cell damage (Fonnum, 1984; Garthwaite and Garthwaite, 1987; Mayer and Westbrook, 1987a,b; Rothman and Olney, 1987). These studies have yielded valuable information on antagonization of glutamate effects concerning the glutamate NMDA receptor proper and on glutamate-dependent channel blockers, e.g., by opiate agonists (Chapman et al., 1987; Choi, 1987; Meldrum et al., 1987). This area of research is clinically highly relevant, since it was shown that administration of glutamate receptor antagonists or glutamate-dependent channel blockers or inhibition of glutamatergic excitation by dissection of afferent fibers is protective against nerve cell damage from ischemia, hypoglycemia, or epilepsia (Chapman et al., 1987; Gill et al., 1987; Meldrum et al., 1987; Olney et al., 1986; Onodera et al., 1986).

These findings, in association with its damaging potential (see above), have rendered glutamate a likely candidate as a mediator of secondary brain damage. Final evidence for its identification concerning release under pathological conditions is difficult to obtain. Glutamate is also present in brain tissue in high concentrations under normal conditions, albeit almost exclusively in the intracellular compartment. Therefore, evidence for release of glutamate requires assessment of its extracellular accumulation.

Various methods, such as in vitro superfusion of brain slices, push-pull perfusion of the living brain in vivo, microfiber dialysis, and interstitial fluid drainage in vasogenic brain edema, have been used for this purpose (Baethmann *et al.*, 1989). Findings on interstitial fluid drainage in animals with vasogenic brain edema from a focal lesion are demonstrated in Figure 2, indicative of a marked release of the amino acid in perifocal edematous brain surrounding a focus of tissue necrosis. As a reference of the normal extracellular concentration, glutamate levels found in control cerebrospinal fluid (CSF) prior to trauma were used. As seen in Figure 2, vasogenic edema fluid had about 10 to 15 times the glutamate concentration of normal CSF. When intracranial hypertension developed from vasogenic edema, resulting in cerebral ischemia, the glutamate concentrations of edema fluid were dramatically increased, e.g., up to 1500 μmol/liter (Baethmann *et al.*, 1989). This is 100 to 150 times the concentration found under normal conditions in the extracellular compartment (Benveniste *et al.*, 1984; Kim *et al.*, 1983; Perry *et al.*, 1975). Development of cerebral ischemia under these conditions was indicated not only by the decrease of the cerebral perfusion pressure (< 40 mmHg for 30 min or longer) but also by the appearance of an isoelectric electroencephalogram (EEG) and an ischemia pattern of labile energy metabolites of nontraumatized brain tissue (Baethmann *et al.*, 1989). The abnormal extracellular glutamate concentrations found in perifocal edematous tissue with and without additional ischemia were within the range required to induce secondary damage, such as cell swelling.

As to the secondary cellular messenger mechanisms induced by an extracellular accumulation of glutamate in brain tissue, recent findings so far limited to the developing central nervous system (CNS) suggest an involvement of the phosphatidylinositol pathway (Nicoletti *et al.*, 1986; Weiss *et al.*, 1988). An association of cytotoxic glutamate effects with this important system would provide for a functional connection between the transmitter and the arachidonic acid cascade. Experimental findings suggest that the early release of arachidonic acid in the brain after induction of circulatory arrest is attributable to a receptor-dependent activation of the phosphatidylinositol pathway with stimulation of phospholipase C as the central enzymatic step (Ikeda *et al.*, 1986). A relationship between glutamate and arachidonic acid would be a pertinent example of mutual stimulation of mediator systems in acute brain damage, indicating activation of a complex network rather than of a single factor (see below).

3.3. Arachidonic Acid

Damage of brain tissue brought about by release of free fatty acids, particularly arachidonic acid, has been assumed for many years. Experiments conducted

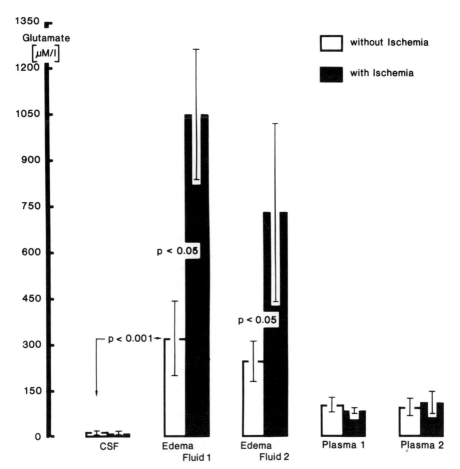

FIGURE 2. Glutamate concentrations (mean ± SEM) in CSF (control), edema fluid, and plasma of experimental animals with focal cold injury of the brain. Edema fluid was obtained by interstitial fluid drainage by the method of Gazendam *et al.* (1979) within 140 min after trauma (edema fluid 1) and up to 7 hr (edema fluid 2). Animals with vasogenic edema causing malignant intracranial hypertension (ischemia) are distinguished from animals with a moderate rise of intracranial pressure (without ischemia). Focal injury without additional ischemia raised interstitial glutamate concentrations up to 10 to 20 times the level found in normal CSF prior to trauma. Additional development of cerebral ischemia led to a further increase in the glutamate concentration in the interstitial edema fluid to 100 to 150 times the normal extracellular concentration. CSF was sampled prior to trauma and used as a reference of the interstitial glutamate concentration under control conditions. (From Baethmann *et al.*, 1989.)

by Sato *et al*. (1969) indicated that fatty acids played a role in the disturbances of metabolism evolving in damaged brain tissue. Incubation of brain slices in medium containing lipids which were extracted from cerebral tissue led to accelerated fluid uptake in vitro from the incubation medium as compared with that in tissue incubated without cerebral lipids. More direct evidence was obtained by the studies of Chan and Fishman (1978), who used incubation of brain tissue slices in vitro to compare the edema-inducing properties of various free fatty acids including the highly unsaturated compounds arachidonic acid and linolenic acid. Furthermore, another requirement is met in many studies demonstrating activation of lipolysis and release of arachidonic acid under conditions such as cerebral ischemia, convulsions, trauma, and hypoglycemia (Baethmann *et al*., 1989; Bazan and Rakowski, 1970; Bazan and Rodriguez de Turco, 1980; Chan *et al*., 1983; Gardiner *et al*., 1981; Siesjö and Wieloch, 1986).

It is continuously asked whether a given pathological mechanism resulting from release of arachidonic acid in damaged brain is attributable to the compound itself or to its potent metabolites (the eicosanoids and free radicals among others). This question cannot be answered in general terms but only on the basis of the specific phenomenon induced by activation of the arachidonic acid cascade. Usually inhibition of an activating enzyme is employed for that purpose.

Studies may be mentioned in this context (Kontos *et al*., 1980) which indicate that inhibition of cyclooxygenase by indomethacin to prevent formation of prostaglandins is associated with attenuation of damage to the cerebrovascular system by administration of arachidonic acid. This is in contrast to the findings in our laboratory that opening of the blood-brain barrier to intravenously administered FITC-dextran (MW 62,000) by superfusion of the exposed brain with arachidonic acid could not be prevented by indomethacin or by a dual-pathway inhibitor (BW 755 C), which antagonizes both the lipoxygenase and cyclooxygenase pathways (Unterberg *et al*., 1987). In these studies, administration of arachidonic acid to the brain by superfusion resulted in gross opening of the blood-brain barrier as compared with a selective enhancement of permeability when superfusing the brain with bradykinin (Unterberg *et al*., 1984). However, both bradykinin and arachidonic acid were found to initiate opening of the barrier in the postcapillary venules. Furthermore, evidence was provided that arachidonic acid and other free fatty acids accumulate in the extracellular compartment of perifocal edematous brain tissue. However, contrary to the respective findings with glutamate, the level of most of the fatty acids accumulating in the interstitial vasogenic edema fluid after a cold lesion did not exceed concurrent levels found in the plasma compartment (Baethmann *et al*., 1989). Arachidonic acid was an exception (Figure 3).

Respective concentrations of arachidonic acid exceeded the simultaneously measured plasma levels by a factor of 2. This indicates that accumulation of the fatty acid in the extracellular edema fluid can be attributed not only to transport of

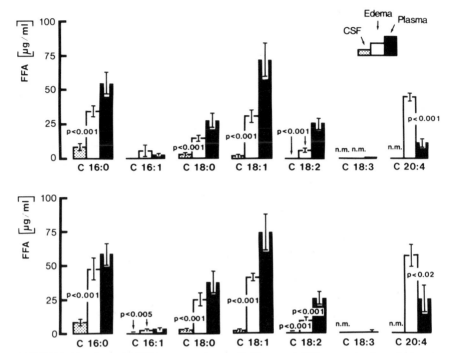

FIGURE 3. Free fatty acid (FFA) concentrations studied in normal CSF, vasogenic edema fluid, and plasma of experimental animals with focal cold injury of the brain. Fatty acid concentrations in animals with additional ischemia are shown at the top, and those in animals without additional ischemia are shown at the bottom. Levels of all fatty acid species were increased in vasogenic edema fluid as compared with normal CSF (used as reference of normal interstitial fluid). In contrast to the findings for glutamate, the free fatty acid levels in edema fluid did not exceed those in concurrently drawn plasma samples. Therefore, their increase in edema fluid might be attributed to transport into the cerebral parenchyma from the intravascular compartment secondary to the breakdown of the blood–brain barrier. Arachidonic acid ($C_{20:4}$) was an exception. Its concentrations were significantly higher in the vasogenic edema fluid than in simultaneously studied plasma samples, indicating release from the cerebral parenchyma rather than mere passive uptake from the intravascular compartment. Some fatty acids were not measurable (n.m.) in CSF or edema fluid. (From Baethmann *et al.*, 1989.)

the compound from the intravascular compartment into the edematous parenchyma, but also to a release from damaged brain tissue. Unlike activation of the kallikrein-kinin system or accumulation of glutamate in the edema fluid, additional development of cerebral ischemia from intracranial hypertension was not found to enhance the release of arachidonic acid into the vasogenic edema fluid, at least up to 7 hr after trauma (Baethmann *et al.*, 1989).

Studies conducted in patients with acute or subacute cerebral insults in cooperation with the Department of Neurosurgery, Ludwig Maximilians University, also demonstrated a release of fatty acids into CSF. Patients with lumbar disk herniation served as controls. In patients with severe head injury or spontaneous cerebral hemorrhage, levels of diverse fatty acids, such as $C_{16:0}$ (palmitic acid), $C_{18:0}$ (stearic acid), and $C_{18:1}$ (oleic acid) were increased compared with the levels in the control group, whereas the arachidonic acid levels remained unchanged (Maier-Hauff *et al.*, 1984*b*). The levels of these fatty acids were also significantly increased in the intravascular compartment under the same conditions and in patients with hydrocephalus.

The understanding concerning arachidonic acid as a pathophysiologically relevant mediator compound in secondary brain damage is rendered difficult by various circumstances. One is that the compound might be active only if it is not bound to proteins. Thus, only release into a compartment with a low protein concentration might be pathophysiologically relevant, whereas accumulation in the cytosol or in the intravascular compartment might be less damaging owing to the abundant presence of proteins. Similar considerations might apply with regard to the formation of the arachidonic acid cascade metabolites, particularly of free radicals. Normally, powerful defense mechanisms against the adverse effects of an overwhelming release of free radicals are available in the cells. Observations in this laboratory, using xanthine oxidase/hypoxanthine as a potent free radical-generating system (Unterberg *et al.*, 1988), provided marginal evidence at best for a pathophysiological function of these short-lived substances. The discussion of whether arachidonic acid itself or its many metabolites in acute lesions, such as ischemia or trauma, are the principal agents causing damage on a parenchymal or cellular level might be academic. Arachidonic acid is required for the production of the numerous prostanoids and of other metabolites, making inhibition of the release of arachidonic acid a superior therapeutic approach to the inhibition of the secondary metabolic pathways.

4. MOLECULAR MECHANISMS OF NERVE AND GLIAL SWELLING

Formation of intracellular (cytotoxic) brain edema involves a multitude of complex mechanisms, which we are just beginning to understand. Manifestations of cytotoxic brain edema as occur in focal or global forms of cerebral ischemia or intoxications (Kempski, 1986) may induce extensive brain swelling with an increase in the intracranial pressure and its deleterious consequences. Obviously, sensitive and effective mechanisms for control of the cell volume are necessary for normal brain function. Little attention has been paid so far to the mechanisms adjusting cell volume under physiological conditions. Maintenance of a normal cell volume is thought to obey the so-called Gibbs-Donnan equilibrium (Macknight and Leaf, 1977), which in essence reflects a steady state between a passive leak of Na^+ ions into the cell along their concentration gradient and an active extrusion afforded by the energy-dependent Na^+ pump (Na^+, K^+-ATPase). This view, however, ignores the requirement of volume-sensing mechanisms that constantly inform the cell about its actual volume so that volume-regulatory processes may be activated when necessary. Besides, experimental evidence indicates that the Gibbs-Donnan equilibrium as a basic concept of cell volume control is too simple: inhibition of the active sodium pump by ouabain or induction of complete energy failure in vitro does not suffice to induce swelling of glial cells (Kempski *et al.*, 1987, 1988*b*).

Thus, failure of cell volume regulation on the basis of the pump-leak model may not be adequate to explain cytotoxic brain edema evolving under various pathophysiological conditions. Moreover, given our increasing understanding of the underlying complexity, involving specific membrane proteins, receptors, channels, and ion transporters, much more sophisticated interactions can be expected. Attempts to elucidate the mechanisms in vivo by using whole-animal preparations are challenged by the problem that many pathophysiologically significant or epiphenomenal parameters are simultaneously changing and, thus, hard to control. Therefore, in vitro models are increasingly used either with brain tissue slices or with defined cells for the analysis of specific cell-damaging mechanisms including cell swelling. Obviously, such a procedure allows for better control of the experimental conditions than is possible in vivo.

4.1. Mechanisms of Cell Swelling: General Considerations

Changes of the cell volume in essence result from changes of the intracellular concentration of osmotically active material. Alterations of intracellular osmotic concentrations can be induced by (1) an increase in the membrane permeability for Na^+ ions, causing a downhill influx along the electrochemical gradient; (2) changes of membrane ion pumps including the Na^+,K^+-ATPase, which control intracellular electrolytes, or activation of the Na^+/H^+-antiporter by intracellular acidosis; (3) disturbances of energy metabolism fueling active ion pumps; and (4) generation of osmotically active solutes in the cytosol ("idiogenic osmoles"), e.g., by breakdown of macromolecules, dephosphorylation, or dissociation of cations and anions from macromolecular structures.

Understanding of cell swelling is complicated not only by the fact that more than one mechanism is involved, but also because the above-mentioned processes may have to act together. Consequently, an increase in the membrane permeability to Na^+ ions may be compensated by the active Na^+ pump. Alternatively, inhibition of the active Na^+ pump may cause cell swelling only if the resulting accumulation of Na^+ ions in the cell exceeds the depletion of intracellular K^+ ions. An example is given by ouabain, which causes glial swelling in the cerebral cortex in vivo (Lowe, 1978) but not in vitro (Kempski *et al.*, 1988*b*). Inhibition of the Na^+ pump by ouabain in vitro led to a loss of intracellular K^+ ions with a near-equimolar gain of Na^+ ions. Consequently, the net sum of Na^+ and K^+ ions in the cell remained unchanged. Apparently the Na^+ permeability of the glial cell membranes remained low in these in vitro studies, whereas in vivo secondary effects, such as a release of transmitters or of K^+ ions into the interstitial compartment, cannot be excluded as the ultimate cause of cell swelling in cerebral cortex. Actually, Lowe (1978) concluded that ". . .changes in the chemical milieu surrounding the glial process . . ." might be responsible for the glial swelling by ouabain in vivo.

4.2. Mediators of Cytotoxic Brain Edema

The concept of mediator compounds (see above) may also apply to the pathogenesis of cytotoxic brain edema. Ample evidence is provided by the results of in vitro studies. Isolated retinas incubated in a comparatively large extracellular compartment were found to tolerate anoxia and substrate deprivation for extensive periods without damage or cell swelling, whereas the same conditions caused an uptake of water and a decrease in cell viability, if the extracellular/intracellular volume ratio was markedly restricted (Ames and Nesbett, 1983a,b,c). In addition, swelling of retinas was significantly enhanced if the tissue had been incubated in a medium which was conditioned by previous anoxic incubation of other retinas. The findings suggest that nervous tissue may tolerate even extended periods of anoxia without swelling, provided that the extracellular compartment is large. Corresponding observations were made in our laboratory by using suspensions of C-6 glioma cells under strictly controlled conditions (Kempski et al., 1987). The cell volume was assessed by flow cytometry, allowing detection of subtle changes. The glial cells did not swell during 2 hr of exposure to complete anoxia with and without inhibition of glycolysis by iodoacetate. Nevertheless, as occurred after exposure to ouabain, the glial cells were markedly depleted of K^+ ions while accumulating Na^+ ions. Recently, the absence of glial swelling from hypoxia or anoxia in vitro for more than 12 hr has been confirmed (Yu et al., 1989). These observations lend support to the contention that cell swelling evolving early after ischemia in vivo is caused by release of swelling-inducing compounds which rapidly accumulate in the comparatively small extracellular compartment in the brain, while energy failure per se may not suffice to induce ischemic cell swelling. According to our studies based on experiments with C-6 glioma cells or primary cultured astrocytes in vitro, the following factors and mediator mechanisms are suggested (Figure 4): (1) increase in concentration of extracellular K^+, (2) activation of lipolysis leading to accumulation of arachidonic acid, (3) release of glutamate into the extracellular compartment, and (4) development of acidosis.

Figure 5 is a synthesis of the various processes involved in ischemic cell swelling. The significance of acidosis and of the extracellular release of glutamate is discussed below.

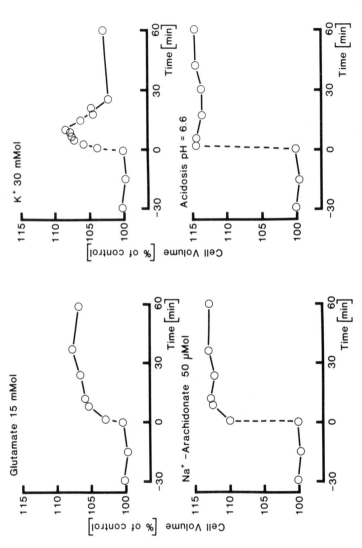

FIGURE 4. Volume changes in C-6 glioma single-cell suspensions during exposure with putative mediators of cytotoxic brain edema. The glial cells were suspended in an incubation chamber, oxygen was supplied, and continuous measurements of pH, pO_2, and temperature were made. The cell volume was assessed by flow cytometry (Metricell). Glutamate or arachidonate was added at the concentrations given in the figure. Furthermore, K^+ concentrations of 30 mM or acidosis of pH 6.6 by addition of sulfuric acid were also studied. The osmolality of the medium was not changed during testing of the cell volume response (given as percentage of control values).

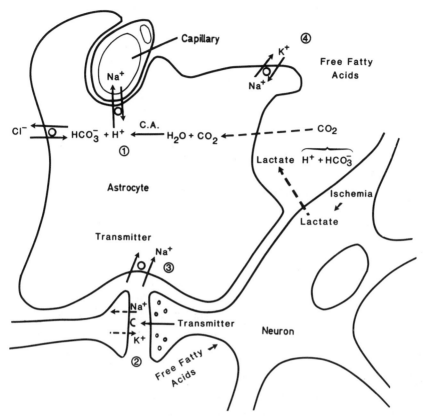

FIGURE 5. Synthesis of mechanisms causing swelling of nerve and glial cells from anoxia or ischemia. Swelling may result from (1) acidosis by activation of the Na^+/H^+-antiporter (see Figure 6); (2) release of glutamate, increasing Na^+ permeability of postsynaptic membranes and of glial cells; (3) uptake of glutamate together with Na^+ ions into glial cells, causing an increase in the intracellular osmotic concentration; and (4) perturbation of membrane integrity by free fatty acids, leading to an increased influx of ions and water into the cell. A specific role of lactate produced during ischemia might also be considered. (From Kempski, 1986.)

4.3. Acidosis

Development of anaerobic glycolysis in ischemic brain tissue, causing accumulation of lactic acid and, hence, acidosis, can be considered to promote ischemic brain damage (Siesjö, 1988). One minute after onset of ischemia, lactate levels may increase to 8 mmol/kg (FG), possibly more than doubling within the subsequent few minutes, particularly at blood glucose levels exceeding the normal range (Siesjö, 1988). Both a decrease in brain tissue pH and increased concentrations of lactate anions may be involved in the formation of cell swelling and brain tissue damage. Kraig *et al.* (1987) found an extracellular pH threshold of 5.3 at and below which brain tissue necrosis ensued after injection of lactic acid into the cerebral parenchyma in rats. This laboratory found the cell viability of C-6 glioma cells in vitro to decrease if the pH fell below 5.6.

Exposure of glial cells in vitro was studied to elucidate the mechanisms of acidosis-induced cell swelling. Acidosis was induced by addition of either sulfuric or lactic acid to medium buffered with bicarbonate. Marked differences between sulfuric and lactic acid were found in their potency to induce cell swelling. With sulfuric acid an increase in cell volume was observed once the pH of the medium fell below 6.8. With further increasing acidosis, the cell volume increased in a pH-independent manner up to 115% of the normal cell size (Kempski *et al.*, 1986, 1988*a*). The glial swelling was significantly more pronounced when lactic acid was used for acidification. With the latter, at pH 4.2, cell volume reached nearly 200% of normal and appeared to increase in an acidosis-dependent manner (Staub *et al.*, 1989, 1990).

Additional experiments with inhibitors of ion pumps and exchange mechanisms (Kempski *et al.*, 1988*a*) led to the following concept of acidosis-induced glial swelling (Figure 6). Extracellular buffering of H^+ ions with bicarbonate causes release of CO_2 which easily diffuses into the cells. CO_2 is hydrated inside the cell, forming carbonic acid (this reaction is catalyzed by carbonic anhydrase). Carbonic anhydrase is found only in glial cells and erythrocytes. Carbonic acid rapidly dissociates into H^+ and HCO_3^- ions, leading to intracellular acidosis. Acidosis activates pH-controlling mechanisms in the cell, such as the Na^+/H^+ and Cl^-/HCO_3^- antiporters, resulting in an elimination of H^+ ions from the intracellular compartment. Thus, Na^+ and Cl^- ions accumulate in the intracellular space as the ultimate mechanism of acidosis-induced cell swelling. Besides, the extracellular accumulation of lactic acid itself is a potent mechanism of cell swelling. The acid enters the cell from the extracellular space in its protonated, hydrophobic form, where it immediately dissociates again. Lactate anions, however, become trapped inside the cell as a result of the low membrane permeability of the polar molecule. Accumulation of lactate in the intracellular compartment may further increase the osmotic concentration as an additional factor of cell swelling. Besides, the H^+ ions dissociating from the lactic acid molecules are exchanged for Na^+ ions by activation of the transmembrane Na^+-H^+ shuttle, leading to further increase of the intracellular Na^+ concentration.

4.4. Glutamate

Glutamate is a ubiquitous amino acid which, in the brain, accumulates almost exclusively in the intracellular compartment, reaching concentrations of up to 15 mmol/kg of cell water. The extracellular concentrations are lower by approx-

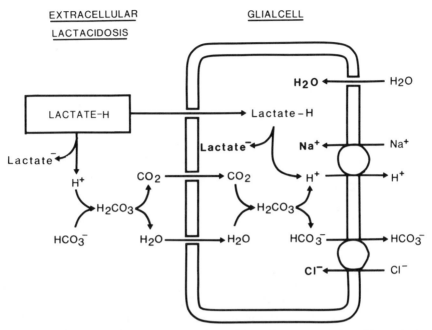

FIGURE 6. Specific mechanisms of lactic acid in glial swelling. Accumulation of lactate in the extracellular space, requiring buffering with bicarbonate, causes formation of H_2CO_3 and subsequently CO_2 and water. CO_2 diffuses into the cell, forming H_2CO_3 (catalyzed by carbonic anhydrase). H_2CO_3 dissociates rapidly into H^+ and HCO_3^-, which are subsequently eliminated from the intracellular compartment by specific exchange mechanisms. As a consequence, Na^+ and Cl^- ions accumulate in the cell, causing cell swelling. A futile cycle may develop with further influx of CO_2 and elimination of H^+ and HCO_3^-, causing further accumulation of Na^+ and Cl^- inside the cell. Lactic acid in protonated form enters the cell from the extracellular compartment, where it dissociates into H^+ and lactate ions. Lactate anions become trapped in the cell, whereas H^+ ions are eliminated by the Na^+/H^+-antiporter. (From Staub *et al.*, 1990.)

imately three orders of magnitude. As well as having a key role in the intermediary metabolism, glutamate is a principal excitatory neurotransmitter in the cerebral cortex and hippocampus. Different glutamate receptor types have been localized on the surface of dendrites. According to their specific agonists, kainate, quisqualate and NMDA receptors can be distinguished (Mayer and Westbrook, 1987*b*; Watkins, 1981). Under pathological conditions two mechanisms might be responsible for both cell swelling and damage of neurons. (1) Activation of glutamate receptors causes opening of Na^+ channels and consequently influx of Na^+ ions together with Cl^- ions and water as a mechanism of dendritic swelling (Mayer and Westbrook, 1987*a*; Rothman and Olney, 1987). (2) Activation of the NMDA receptor causes opening of large channels, permitting entrance not only of Na$^+$ but also of Ca^{2+} ions into the cell (Mayer and Westbrook, 1987a; Rothman and Olney, 1987; Zanotto and Heinemann, 1983). The large channels are blocked under physiological conditions by Mg^{2+} ions (Reynolds and Miller, 1988).

An uncontrolled influx of Ca^{2+} ions following prolonged stimulation of the NMDA receptor by glutamate is considered to mediate the death of nerve cells (Choi, 1985; Rothman and Olney, 1986) in selectively vulnerable areas by ischemia or epilepsia. This hypothesis is supported by in vivo as well as in vitro observations that glutamate receptor antagonists or glutamate receptor-dependent channel blockers selectively protect vulnerable nerve cells against ischemia or anoxia (see above).

The normal brain is able to protect itself against excitotoxic damage. Glutamate accumulating in the extracellular compartment is rapidly taken up by nerve and glial cells. Drejer *et al.* (1982) found K_m values for the uptake of glutamate of 34 to 82 μM in cultivated nerve and glial cells obtained from different regions of the brain. High-affinity uptake sites for glutamate were discovered on glial cells many years ago (Benjamin and Quastel, 1976; Henn *et al.*, 1974). Transport of glutamate into glial cells occurs against a concentration gradient of 1:1000 and is therefore energy dependent. The intracellular uptake of glutamate from the extracellular compartment is fueled by a simultaneous downhill influx of Na$^+$ ions into the cell. The stoichiometric coupling ratio between the glutamate molecules and Na$^+$ ions has a range of 1:1 to 1:3 (Barbour *et al.*, 1988; Drejer *et al.*, 1982).

Glutamate is amidated in the glial cells to glutamine (this is catalyzed by glutamine synthetase). Formation of glutamine and intracellular uptake of glutamate are ATP-consuming steps, which may fail under conditions of energy failure as in cerebral ischemia. Glutamine accumulating in the glial cells may eventually be released and taken up by nerve cell endings. There, glutamine is converted back to glutamate or to γ-aminobutyrate (GABA) (Hertz, 1979; Shank and Aprison, 1981).

Coupling of the glial uptake of glutamate with an intracellular accumulation of Na$^+$ ions might be considered a major mechanism of glial swelling under adverse conditions, such as ischemia or epilepsy associated with an excessive release of glutamate from nerve cells. Glial swelling could be verified in studies in this laboratory in which C-6 glioma cells (Figure 4) (Kempski *et al.*, 1982) or primary cultured astrocytes (G.-H. Schneider, personal communication) were used. Exposure of glial cells in vitro to glutamate was found to induce cell swelling in a dose-dependent manner.

The increase in cell volume in experiments with a glutamate concentration of 5 mM was in the order of 120% during a 2-hr exposure. However, cell swelling could even be elicited with glutamate concentrations as low as 0.05 mM. At moderate glutamate levels, normalization of the cell size followed a cellular clearance of glutamate. The dependence of the intracellular accumulation of glutamate on the transmembrane Na^+ gradient was ascertained by preincubation with ouabain. Under these conditions, associated with a breakdown of the extracellular to intracellular Na^+ concentration gradient (see above), glutamate failed to induce glial swelling. As with ouabain, energy deprivation has also been reported to cause a breakdown of the intracellular to extracellular glutamate gradient in astrocytes (Kauppinen *et al.*, 1988).

Taken together, glial swelling caused by an extracellular increase of glutamate may not indicate failure of the glial function or irreversible cell damage, but rather an important homeostatic control capacity. However, under borderline conditions such as ischemia, glial cells may be unable to clear the extracellular space from glutamate once the extracellular to intracellular Na^+ gradient is abolished. Then a further increase in the extracellular glutamate concentration can be expected, with its deleterious consequences for the survival of nerve cells. Therefore, glutamate antagonists designed to prevent excitotoxic damage of neurons should not interfere with the high-affinity uptake systems of the glial cells.

5. CONCLUSIONS AND OUTLOOK

It might be an oversimplification to expect activation of one mediator compound or system alone to be responsible for the variety of adverse effects occurring in traumatic or ischemic brain tissue. Thus, the pathophysiological potential of each of the above-mentioned mediator compounds notwithstanding, complex interactions and mutual stimulation of different mediator systems must be assumed. Evidence indicative of an interacting mediator network is available. For example, kinins have been found to cause a release of glutamate or of arachidonic acid, and, conversely, arachidonic acid has been found to induce formation of kinins. Moreover, an extracellular accumulation of glutamate causes not only further release of the amino acid from the intracellular compartment but also enhancement of intracellular acidosis. Finally, it has been reported that the extracellular clearance of glutamate is impaired by increased levels of arachidonic acid (cf. Baethmann *et al.*, 1989). These findings provide the basis for a vicious cycle of mediator activation in a positive-feedback manner.

Activation of a mediator network rather than of an individual factor renders specific treatment more complicated than prevention of a single compound. Therefore, pathophysiological research must identify the earliest activation processes, the "bottleneck" of activation of the network, where specific inhibitory methods still are effective. The kallikrein-kinin cascade or the enhanced release of glutamate might be considered such a bottleneck. These precautions and reservations on the therapeutic chances of effective inhibition of mediator activation notwithstanding, current evidence on therapeutic benefits of inhibition of mediator compounds which effectively interfere with the development of secondary brain damage from trauma or ischemia justifies further expectations.

ACKNOWLEDGMENTS

The technical and secretarial assistance of H. Fuderer, U. Goerke, I. Juna, and H. Kleylein is gratefully acknowledged. The work described in this report was supported by grant Ba 452 from the Deutsche Forschungsgemeinschaft.

REFERENCES

Ames, A., and Nesbett, F. B., 1983a, Pathophysiology of ischemic cell death. I. Time of onset of irreversible damage; importance of different components of the ischemic insult, *Stroke* **14:** 219–226.

Ames, A., and Nesbett, F. B., 1983b, Pathophysiology of ischemic cell death. II. Changes in plasma membrane permeability and cell volume, *Stroke* **14:**227–233.

Ames, A., and Nesbett, F. B., 1983c, Pathophysiology of ischemic cell death. III. Role of extracellular factors, *Stroke* **14:**233–240.

Astrup, J., Symon, L., Branston, N. M., and Lassen, N. A., 1977, Cortical evoked potential and extracellular K^+ and H^+ at critical levels of brain ischemia, *Stroke* **8:**51–57.

Baethmann, A., 1978, Pathophysiological and pathochemical aspects of cerebral edema, *Neurosurg. Rev.* **1:**85–100.

Baethmann, A., 1987a, Organversagen nach Trauma—der zerebrale Sekundärschaden, *Melsunger Med. Mittlg.* **59:**53–61.

Baethmann, A., 1987b, Mechanisms of secondary brain damage, *in* "Traumatic Brain Edema" (F. Cohadon, A. Baethmann, K. G. Go, and J. D. Miller, eds.), Fidia Research Series, vol. 8, pp. 81–97, Liviana Press, Padua, Italy.

Baethmann, A., Maier-Hauff, K., Schürer, L., Lange, M., Guggenbichler, C., Vogt, W., Jacob, K., and Kempski, O., 1989, Release of glutamate and of free fatty acids in vasogenic brain edema, *J. Neurosurg.* **70:**578–591.

Barbour, B., Brew, H., and Attwell, D., 1988, Electrogenic glutamate uptake in glial cells is activated by intracellular potassium, *Nature* **335:**433–435.

Baudry, M., and Lynch, G., 1980, Hypothesis regarding the cellular mechanisms responsible for long-term synaptic potentiation in the hippocampus, *Exp. Neurol.* **68:**202–204.

Bazan, N. G., and Rakowski, H., 1970, Increased levels of brain free fatty acids after electroconvulsive shock, *Life Sci.* **9:**501–507.

Bazan, N. G., and Rodriguez de Turco, E. B., 1980, Membrane lipids in the pathogenesis of brain edema. Phospholipids and arachidonic acid, the earliest membrane components changed at the onset of ischemia, *Adv. Neurol.* **28:**197–205.

Benjamin, A. M., and Quastel, J. H., 1976, Cerebral uptakes and exchange diffusion in vitro of L- and D-glutamates, *J. Neurochem* **26:**431–441.

Benveniste, H., Drejer, J., Schousboe, A., and Diemer, N. H., 1984, Elevation of the extracellular concentrations of glutamate and aspartate in rat hippocampus during transient cerebral ischemia monitored by intracerebral microdialysis, *J. Neurochem.* **43:**1369–1374.

Branston, N. M., Strong, A. J., and Symon, L., 1977, Extracellular potassium activity, evoked potential and tissue blood flow, *J. Neurol. Sci.* **32:**305–321.

Chan, P. H., and Fishman, R. A., 1978, Brain edema: Induction in cortical slices by polyunsaturated fatty acids, *Science* **201**:358–360.

Chan, P. H., Longar, S., and Fishman, R. A., 1983, Phospholipid degradation and edema development in cold-injured rat brain, *Brain Res.* **227**:329–337.

Chapman, A. G., Engelsen, B., and Meldrum, B. S., 1987, 2-Amino-7-phosphonoheptanoic acid inhibits insulin-induced convulsions and striatal aspartate accumulation in rats with frontal cortical ablation, *J. Neurochem.* **49**:121–127.

Choi, D. W., 1985, Glutamate neurotoxicity in cortical cell cultures is calcium dependent, *Neurosci. Lett.* **58**:293–297.

Choi, D. W., 1987, Dextrorphan and dextromethorphan attenuate glutamate neurotoxicity, *Brain Res.* **403**:333–336.

Clark, W. G., 1979, Kinins and the peripheral and central nervous systems, *in* "Bradykinin, Kallidin, and Kallikrein" (E. G. Erdös, ed.), Handbook of Experimental Pharmacology, vol. 25, pp. 311–356, Springer-Verlag, Berlin.

Deshpande, J., and Wieloch, T., 1985, Amelioration of ischemic brain damage by postischemic treatment with flunarizine, *Neurol. Res.* **7**:27–29.

Drejer, J., Larsson, O. M., and Schousboe, A., 1982, Characterization of L-glutamate uptake into and release from astrocytes and neurons cultured from different brain regions, *Exp. Brain Res.* **47**: 259–269.

Duverger, D., Benavides, J., Cudennec, A., MacKenzie, E. T., Scatton, B., Seylaz, J., and Verecchia, C., 1987, A glutamate antagonist reduces infarction size following focal cerebral ischaemia independently of vascular and metabolic changes, *J. Cereb. Blood Flow Metab.* **7**(Suppl. 1):S144.

Erdös, E. G. (ed.), 1979, "Bradykinin, Kallidin and Kallikrein," Handbook of Experimental Pharmacology, vol. 25, Supplement, Springer-Verlag, Berlin.

Fonnum, F., 1984, Glutamate: A neurotransmitter in mammalian brain, *J. Neurochem.* **42**:1–11.

Frey, E. K., Kraut, H., Werle, E., Vogel, R., Zickgraf-Rüdel, G., and Trautschold, I. (eds), 1968, "Das Kallikrein-Kinin-System und seine Inhibitoren," F. Enke Verlag, Stuttgart, Germany.

Gardiner, M., Nilsson, B., Rehncrona, S., and Siesjö, B. K., 1981, Free fatty acids in the rat brain in moderate and severe hypoxia, *J. Neurochem.* **36**:1500–1505.

Garthwaite, G., and Garthwaite, J., 1987, Receptor-linked ionic channels mediate N-methyl-D-aspartate neurotoxicity in rat cerebellar slices, *Neurosci. Lett.* **83**:241–246.

Gazendam, M. D., Go, K. G., Van Zonten, A. K., 1979, Composition of isolated edema fluid in cold-induced brain edema, *J. Neurosurg.* **51**:70–77.

Gill, R., Foster, C., Iversen, L., and Woodruff, G. N., 1987, Ischaemia-induced degeneration of hippocampal neurones in gerbils is prevented by systemic administration of MK-801, *J. Cereb. Blood Flow Metab.* **7**(Suppl. 1):S153.

Graham, D. I., Adams, J. H., and Doyle, D., 1978, Ischemic brain damage in fatal non-missile head injuries, *J. Neurol. Sci.* **39**:213–234.

Henn, F. A., Goldstein, M. N., and Hamberger, A., 1974, Uptake of the neurotransmitter candidate glutamate by glia, *Nature* **249**:663–664.

Hertz, L., 1979, Functional interactions between neurons and astrocytes. I. Turnover and metabolism of putative amino acid transmitters, *Prog. Neurobiol.* **13**:277–323.

Ikeda, M., Yoshida, S., Busto, R., Santiso, M., and Ginsberg, M. D., 1986, Polyphosphoinositides as a probable source of brain free fatty acids accumulated at the onset of ischemia, *J. Neurochem.* **47**: 123–132.

Kauer, J. A., Malenka, R. C., and Nicoll, R. A., 1988, NMDA application potentiates synaptic transmission in the hippocampus, *Nature* **334**:250–252.

Kauppinen, R. A., Enkvist, K., Holopainen, I., and Akerman, K. E. O., 1988, Glucose deprivation depolarizes plasma membrane of cultured astrocytes and collapses transmembrane potassium and glutamate gradients, *Neuroscience* **26**:283–289.

Kempski, O., 1982, "Die Lokalisation des Glutamat-induzierten Hirnödems," Dissertation, Ludwig-Maximilians-University, Munich, Germany.

Kempski, O., 1986, Cell swelling mechanisms in brain, *NATO ASI Ser. A: Life Sci.* **115**:203–220.

Kempski, O., Gross, U., and Baethmann, A., 1982, An in-vitro model of cytotoxic brain edema: Cell volume and metabolism of cultivated glial and nerve cells, *Adv. Neurosurg.* **10**:254–258.

Kempski, O., Baethmann, A., Neu, A., Staub, F., 1986, Analysis of molecular mechanisms causing ischemic cell swelling in-vitro, in "Pharmacology of Cerebral Ischemia" (J. Krieglstein, ed.), pp. 131–139, Elsevier, Amsterdam.

Kempski, O., Zimmer, M., Neu, A., von Rosen, F., Jansen, M., and Baethmann, A., 1987, Control of glial cell volume in anoxia. In vitro studies on ischemic cell swelling, *Stroke* **18**:623–628.

Kempski, O., Staub, F., Jansen, M., Schödel, F., and Baethmann, A., 1988a, Glial swelling during extracellular acidosis in-vitro, *Stroke* **19**:385–392.

Kempski, O., Staub, F., von Rosen, F., Zimmer, Neu, A., and Baethmann, A., 1988b, Molecular mechanisms of glial swelling in-vitro, *Neurochem. Pathol.* **9**:109–126.

Kim, J. S., Claus, D., and Kornhuber, H. H., 1983, Cerebral glutamate, neuroleptic drugs and schizophrenia: Increase of cerebrospinal fluid glutamate levels and decrease of striate body glutamate levels following sulpiride treatment in rats, *Eur. Neurol.* **22**:367–370.

Kontos, H. A., Wei, E. P., Povlishock, J. T., Dietrich, W. D., Magiera, C. J., and Ellis, E. F., 1980, Cerebral arteriolar damage by arachidonic acid and prostaglandin G_2, *Science* **209**:1242–1245.

Kraig, R. P., Petito, C. K., Plum, F., and Pulsinelli, W. A., 1987, Hydrogen ions kill brain at concentrations reached in ischemia, *J. Cereb. Blood Flow Metab.* **7**:379–386.

Lowe, D. A., 1978, Morphological changes in the cat cerebral cortex produced by superfusion of ouabain, *Brain Res.* **148**:347–363.

Lucas, D. R., and Newhouse, J. P., 1957, The toxic effect of sodium l-glutamate on the inner layers of the retina, *AMA Arch. Ophthalmol.* **58**:193–201.

Macknight, A. D. C., 1984, Cellular response to injury, in "Edema" (N. Staub and Taylor, eds.), pp. 489–520, Raven Press, New York.

Macknight, A. D. C., and Leaf, A., 1977, Regulation of cellular volume, *Physiol. Rev.* **37**:510–573.

Maier-Hauff, K., Baethmann, A., Lange, M., Schürer, L., and Unterberg, A., 1984a, The kallikrein-kinin system as mediator in vasogenic brain edema. 2. Studies on kinin formation in focal and perifocal brain tissue, *J. Neurosurg.* **61**:97–106.

Maier-Hauff, K., Baethmann, A., Vogt, W., Jacob, K., and Marguth, F., 1984b, Mediator compounds in CSF of neurosurgical patients with raised intracranial pressure, *Adv. Neurosurg.* **12**:302–306.

Mayer, M. L., and Westbrook, G. L., 1987a, Cellular mechanisms underlying excitotoxicity, *Trends Neurosci.* **10**:59–61.

Mayer, M. L., and Westbrook, G. L., 1987b, The physiology of excitatory amino acids in the vertebrate central nervous system, *Prog. Neurobiol.* **28**:197–276.

Meldrum, B. S., Evans, M. C., Swan, J. H., and Simon, R. P., 1987, Protection against hypoxic-ischemic brain damage with excitatory amino acid antagonists, *Med. Biol.* **65**:153–157.

Nicoletti, F., Wroblewski, J. T., Novelli, A., Alho, H., Guidotti, A., and Costa, E., 1986, The activation of inositol phospholipid metabolism as a signal-transducing system for excitatory amino acids in primary cultures of cerebellar granule cells, *J. Neurosci.* **6**:1905–1911.

Olney, J. W., and Sharpe, L. G., 1969, Brain lesions in an infant rhesus monkey treated with monosodium glutamate, *Science* **166**:386–388.

Olney, J. W., Price, M. T., Fuller, T. A., Labruyere, J., Samson, K., Carpenter, M., and Mahan, K., 1986, The anti-excitotoxic effects of certain anesthetics, analgetics and sedative-hypnotics, *Neurosci. Lett.* **68**:29–34.

Onodera, H., Sato, G., and Kogure, K., 1986, Lesions to Schaffer collaterals prevent ischemic death of CA1 pyramidal cells, *Neurosci. Lett.* **68**:169–174.

Park, C. K., Nehls, D. G., Graham, D. I., Teasdale, G. M., and McCulloch, J., 1988, Focal cerebral ischaemia in the cat: Treatment with the glutamate antagonist MK-801 after induction of ischaemia, *J. Cereb. Blood Flow Metab.* **8**:757–762.

Perry, T. L., Hansen, S., and Kennedy, J., 1975, CSF amino acids and plasma-CSF amino acid ratios in adults, *J. Neurochem.* **24**:587–589.

Politi, L. E., Rodriguez de Turco, E. B., and Bazan, N. G., 1985, Dexamethasone effect on free fatty acid and diacylglycerol accumulation during experimental induced vasogenic brain edema, *Neurochem. Pathol.* **3**:249–269.

Reynolds, I. J., and Miller, R. J., 1988, Multiple sites for the regulation of the N-methyl-D-aspartate receptor, *Mol. Pharmacol.* **33**:581–584.

Rothenfusser, W., 1982, Die Bedeutung von Glutamat als Hirnödemfaktor, Dissertation, Ludwig-Maximilians-University, Munich, Germany.

Rothman, S. M., and Olney, J. W., 1986, Glutamate and the pathophysiology of hypoxic-ischemic brain damage, *Ann. Neurol.* **19**:105–111.

Rothman, S. M., and Olney, J. W., 1987, Excitotoxicity and the NMDA receptor, *Trends Neurosci.* **10**: 299–302.

Sato, K., Yamaguchi, M., Mullan, S., Evans, J. P., and Ishii, S., 1969, Brain edema: A study of biochemical and structural alterations, *Arch. Neurol.* **21**:413–424.

Shank, R. P., and Aprison, M. H., 1981, Present status and significance of the glutamine cycle in neural tissues, *Life Sci.* **28**:837–842.

Shaw, C. M., Alvord, E. C., and Berry, R. G., 1959, Swelling of the brain following ischemic infarction with arterial occlusion, *Arch. Neurol.* **1**:161–177.

Siesjö, B. K., 1988, Mechanisms of ischemic brain damage, *Crit. Care Med.* **16**:954–963.

Siesjö, B. K., and Wieloch, T., 1986, Epileptic brain damage: Pathophysiology and neurochemical pathology, *Adv. Neurol.* **44**:813–847.

Simon, R. P., Swan, J. H., Griffiths, T., and Meldrum, B. S., 1984, Blockade of N-methyl-D-aspartate receptors may protect against ischaemic damage in the brain, *Science* **226**:850–852.

Staub, F., Baethmann, A., Peters, J., and Kempski, O., 1990, Effects of lactacidosis on volume and viability of glial cells, *Acta Neurochir.* (Suppl. 51), 3–6.

Staub, F., Baethmann, A., Peters, G., Weigt, H., and Kempski, O., 1990, Effects of lactacidosis on glial cell volume and viability, *J. Cereb. Blood Flow Metab.* **10**:866–876.

Symon, L., 1986, Progression and irreversibility in brain ischaemia, *NATO ASI Ser. A: Life Sci.* **115**: 221–237.

Unterberg, A., and Baethmann, A., 1984, The kallikrein-kinin system as mediator in vasogenic brain edema. 1. Cerebral exposure to bradykinin and plasma, *J. Neurosurg.* **61**:87–96.

Unterberg, A., Wahl, M., and Baethmann, A., 1984, Effects of bradykinin on permeability and diameter of pial vessels in vivo, *J. Cereb. Blood Flow Metab.* **4**:574–585.

Unterberg, A., Dautermann, C., Baethmann, A., and Müller-Esterl, W., 1986, The kallikrein-kinin system as mediator in vasogenic brain edema. 3. Inhibition of the kallikrein-kinin system in traumatic brain swelling, *J. Neurosurg.* **64**:269–276.

Unterberg, A., Wahl, M., Hammersen, F., and Baethmann, A., 1987, Permeability and vasomotor response of cerebral vessels during exposure to arachidonic acid, *Acta Neuropathol.* **73**:209–219.

Unterberg, A., Wahl, M., and Baethmann, A., 1988, Effects of free radicals on permeability and vasomotor response of cerebral vessels, *Acta Neuropathol.* **76**:238–244.

Van Harreveld, A., 1959, Compounds in brain extracts causing spreading depression of cerebral cortical activity and contraction of crustacean muscle, *J. Neurochem.* **3**:300–315.

Van Harreveld, A., 1972, The extracellular space in the vertebrate central nervous system, *in* "The Structure and Function of Nervous Tissue IV" (G. H. Bourne, ed.), pp. 447–511, Academic Press, New York.

Van Harreveld, A., and Fifkova, E., 1973, Mechanisms involved in spreading depression, *J. Neurobiol.* **4**:375–387.

Van Harreveld, A., and Fifkova, E., 1975, A mechanism for potentiation and short term memory, *Proc. K. Ned. Akad. Wet. Ser. C.* **78**:21–24.

Wahl, M., Unterberg, A., Baethmann, A., and Schilling, L., 1988, Mediators of blood-brain barrier dysfunction and formation of vasogenic brain edema, *J. Cereb. Blood Flow Metab.* **8**:621–634.

Watkins, J. C., 1981, Pharmacology of excitatory amino acid receptors, *in* "Glutamate: Transmitter in the Central Nervous System" (G. Roberts, A. Storm-Mathisen, and R. Johnston, eds.), pp. 1–24, John Wiley & Sons, New York.

Weiss, S., Schmidt, B. H., Sebben, M., Kemp, D. E., Bockaert, J., and Sladeczek, F., 1988, Neurotransmitter-induced inositol phosphate formation in neurons in primary culture, *J. Neurochem.* **50**:1425–1433.

Wieloch, T., Lindvall, O., Blomqvist, P., and Gage, F. H., 1985, Evidence for amelioration of ischaemic neuronal damage in the hippocampal formation by lesions of the perforant pathway, *Neurol. Res.* **7**:24–26.

Yu, A. C. H., Gregory, G. A., and Chan, P. H., 1989, Hypoxia-induced dysfunctions and injury of astrocytes in primary cell cultures, *J. Cereb. Blood Flow Metab.* **9**:20–28.

Zanotto, L., and Heinemann, U., 1983, Aspartate and glutamate induced reductions in extracellular free calcium and sodium concentration in area CA1 of "in vitro" hippocampal slices of rats, *Neurosci. Lett.* **35**:79–84.

MODULATORS OF NEURAL CELL SIGNALING AND TRIGGERING OF GENE EXPRESSION FOLLOWING CEREBRAL ISCHEMIA

NICOLAS G. BAZAN

1. INTRODUCTION

Changes in brain lipids are a well-known correlate of cerebral ischemia involving free fatty acids, especially free arachidonic and docosahexaenoic acids, which reflects phospholipase A_2 activation (Bazan, 1970). An additional early correlate in ischemia is the activation of phospholipase C, since diacylglycerols also accumulate (Bazan, 1970; Aveldano and Bazan, 1975a). The predominant fatty

NICOLAS G. BAZAN • LSU Eye Center and Neuroscience Center, LSU Medical Center School of Medicine, New Orleans, Louisiana.

Neurochemical Correlates of Cerebral Ischemia, Volume 7 of Advances in Neurochemistry, edited by Nicolas G. Bazan, Pierre Braquet, and Myron D. Ginsberg. Plenum Press, New York, 1992.

acid of the diacylglycerol pool that accumulates is 1-stearoyl-2-arachidonoyl sn-glycerol, as it is in the inositol lipids (phosphatidylinositol, phosphatidylinositol 4'-phosphate, and phosphatidylinositol 4'5'-bisphosphate). Therefore this neurochemical correlate of ischemia reflects inositol lipid degradation (Aveldano and Bazan, 1975a; Ikeda *et al.*, 1986) and has been postulated to be linked to synaptic vulnerability under these conditions (Aveldano and Bazan, 1975a).

Because both neurochemical correlates, phospholipase A$_2$ and C activation, occur at about the same time, and also because arachidonic and stearic acids are the two fatty acids whose profiles change the most in both free fatty acids and diacylglycerols, several alternative interpretations should be considered, e.g., the sites of these changes and the possible relationships between these lipid pools (1) phospholipase A$_2$ and phospholipase C are enzymes activated either in the same or in different synapses; and (2) the two enzymes may be activated at different sites (phospholipase C in the postsynaptic membrane, through a receptor-mediated event, and phospholipase A$_2$ in the presynaptic membrane), and although there is no compelling evidence, the enzymes may be in the reverse order or in both pre- and postsynaptic membranes. It has been proposed, however, that this neurochemical correlate probably occurs predominantly in the same synaptic structures, or very close ones, since diacylglycerol degradation follows its accumulation, and at the same time, the same free fatty acids are generated, as if a diacylglycerol lipase were also being activated (Aveldano and Bazan, 1975a).

One of the polyunsaturated fatty acids whose concentration increases in the free fatty acid pool, docosahexaenoic acid, probably derives from phospholipase A$_2$ activation, as does a large proportion of the free arachidonic acid. It is of interest to single out docosahexaenoic acid because it is heavily concentrated in membrane phospholipids of the nervous system, particularly in synapses (Bazan, 1989a). At the same time, few changes occur in docosahexaenoate of inositol lipids, which supports the contention that the free docosahexaenoic acid is derived through the degradation of a membrane phospholipid that is distinct from the inositol lipids and through phospholipase A$_2$ (Bazan, 1970; Aveldano and Bazan, 1975a). Other experimental approaches have also added support for a major role of phospholipase A$_2$ in brain ischemia (see, e.g., Cendella *et al.*, 1975; Edgar *et al.*, 1982; Horrocks *et al.*, 1985). Ischemia-induced free fatty acid accumulation prevailed in gray matter compared with white matter (Bazan, 1971), occurred only to a very small extent in the brains of newborn rats (Bazan *et al.*, 1971), and lacked ischemic sensitivity in the brains of adult toads (Aveldano and Bazan, 1975b). Since newborn mammals and adult poikilothermic animals (e.g., toads, snakes, and frogs) are known to survive prolonged periods of anoxia, it was suggested that phospholipase A$_2$ activation is linked to the onset of brain damage (Aveldano and Bazan, 1975b; Bazan *et al.*, 1976).

The lipid neurochemical correlate of cerebral ischemia involves changes in pool size and composition of certain lipids that are exceedingly small when compared with their counterparts that are esterified in membrane phospholipids (as in the fatty acids) or that are part of inositol lipids (as in the diacylglycerol). This further supports the view that the lipid neurochemical correlate of ischemia involves selective pools of membrane phospholipids hydrolyzed through an overactivation of receptor-mediated processes with major consequences for excitable membrane functioning (Bazan, 1989a).

Convulsions also enhance brain free fatty acid and diacylglycerol levels through anoxia-independent mechanisms (Bazan, 1970; Siesjö et al., 1982; Bazan et al., 1982; Rodriguez de Turco and Bazan, 1983), which strongly suggests that neurotransmitters released upon stimulation trigger lipid changes in excitable membranes and/or that an enhanced intracellular calcium concentration has indirectly brought about the changes in lipids. In support of this hypothesis, a marked inhibition of lipid changes was observed in mice depleted of biogenic amines by pretreatment with α-methyl-p-tyrosine, a competitive inhibitor of the rate-limiting step of catecholamine biosynthesis (Aveldano de Caldironi and Bazan, 1979), which is further evidence for the involvement of neurotransmitters in the lipid changes. The synaptic location of these events was ascertained by demonstration of enhanced free polyunsaturated fatty acids in synaptosomes isolated from rats undergoing bicuculline-induced status epilepticus (Birkle and Bazan, 1987). Since the phospholipases activated by ischemia are believed to be components of neural cell signal transduction, convulsions apparently transiently activate those events (Bazan, 1970; Bazan and Rakowski, 1970; Aveldano de Caldironi and Bazan, 1979). Hence, excitable membranes are a central target for ischemia and may give rise to events underlying neural vulnerability in ischemic conditions (Aveldano and Bazan, 1975a; Rothman, 1983; Kass and Lipton, 1982; Choi, 1990). Figure 1 depicts an outline of receptor-mediated events altered in ischemia that lead to changes in the amount and nature of second messengers (e.g., arachidonic acid, diacylglycerol, and other messengers).

Reperfusion of an ischemic area of the brain, either experimentally or after stroke, brings a surge of oxygen, which, among other effects, activates the enzyme-mediate oxygenation pathways of arachidonic acid (arachidonic acid cascade; e.g., formation of prostaglandins, hydroxyeicosatetraenoic acids, and leukotrienes), as well as nonenzymatic peroxidation of lipids (free-radical generation). These arachidonic acid metabolites are biologically active (and some do play a role in the responses of tissues to injury); therefore, if the phospholipase A_2 activation in brain ischemia is large and sustained, the availability of free arachidonic acid may lead to accumulation of metabolites that will in turn play a major role in brain damage.

In this chapter, a review of work on lipid correlates of brain ischemia, as well as studies on platelet-activating factor (PAF) under ischemic conditions from the author's laboratories, is provided. In addition, recent studies on the possible effect of lipid mediators altered during ischemia on gene expression are discussed.

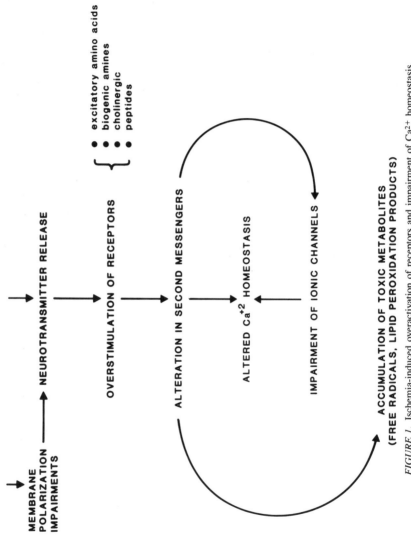

FIGURE 1. Ischemia-induced overactivation of receptors and impairment of Ca^{2+} homeostasis.

2. NEW LIPID CORRELATES OF CEREBRAL ISCHEMIA

PAF (1-O-alkyl-2-acetyl-sn-glycero-3-phosphocholine), a lipid mediator involved in inflammation and immune responses, also accumulates during cerebral ischemia (Bazan, 1989a). The exploration of the role of PAF in cerebral ischemia began with the idea that phospholipase A_2 activation (reviewed above) may be linked at least in part to the synthesis of PAF (Panetta et al., 1987; Birkle et al., 1988; Gilboe et al., 1989, 1990; Bazan, 1989b; Squinto et al., 1989). The basis for this idea is the fact that the membrane phospholipid precursor of PAF contains arachidonoyl and docosahexaenoyl chains at C-2. A phospholipase A_2 releases arachidonic acid from the precursor, generating lyso-PAF, prior to the introduction of acetate into the C-2 position, which gives rise to PAF (Figure 2). PAF is one of several lipid mediators that may be generated at the plasma membrane (Figure 3) through the pathways of remodeling (as after tissue injury, inflammation, or other acute conditions) or de novo synthesis (Figure 4). Phospholipase A_2 activation occurs during the former pathway; this enzyme is also activated in the brain during ischemia.

The hypothesis of the involvement of PAF in ischemic damage was based on the determinations that PAF receptor antagonists protect the brain from damage during ischemia and reperfusion (Panetta et al., 1987) and that a decreased accumulation of free polyunsaturated fatty acids occurs when these compounds are systemically administered during ischemia or convulsions (Panetta et al., 1987; Birkle et al., 1988).

Specific PAF-binding sites in the cerebral cortex have been located both in synaptic membranes and intracellular membranes. The latter contain two binding sites, one of which is the highest-affinity PAF-binding site reported to date for any membrane or cell (Marcheselli et al., 1990).

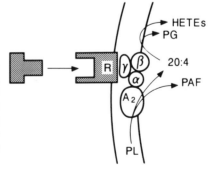

FIGURE 2. Activation of phospholipase A_2 by binding of an agonist to a receptor. This enzyme degrades membrane phospholipids, producing PAF (with prior formation of lyso-PAF) and arachidonic acid (20:4). Free arachidonic acid oxygenation leads to other lipid mediators, including prostaglandins (PG) and hydroxyeicosatetraenoic acids (HETEs). (From Bazan, 1990.)

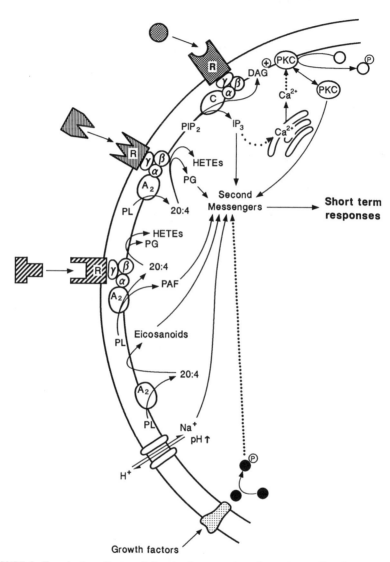

FIGURE 3. Transduction of extracellular signals across the cell membrane. Signaling molecules (ligands) that bind to membrane receptors activate phospholipases, which in turn release lipid mediators (or second messengers) and precursors of them, including free arachidonic acid, eicosanoids, PAF, prostaglandins, hydroxyeicosatetraenoic acids (HETEs), and IP_3. These messengers elicit or contribute to the intracellular effects (particularly short-term) of the agonist. (From Bazan, 1990.)

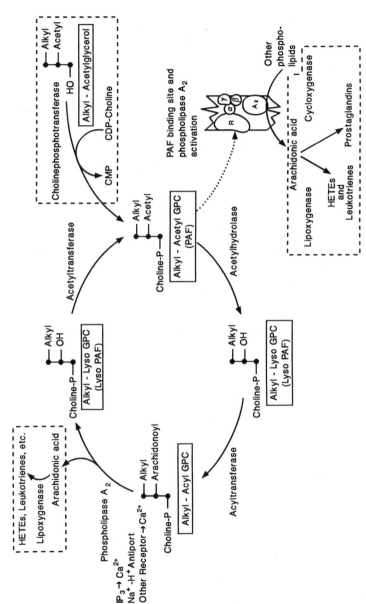

FIGURE 4. Synthesis of PAF: Two major pathways are involved. One leads from alkyl-acyl-GPC to lyso-PAF then to PAF through reactions catalyzed by a phospholipase A_2 and acetyltransferase, respectively. This pathway comprises a cycle through acetylhydrolase and acyltransferase. The major feature of this pathway is that it is mainly plasma membrane bound, Ca^{2+} sensitive, and activated in inflammatory conditions, ischemia, and immunologic challenge. The other pathway, catalyzed by cholinephosphotransferase, is located in the endoplasmic reticulum and is Ca^{2+} insensitive. This figure also indicates that the released arachidonic acid, either during the initial step or after PAF formation, by its action on a receptor, may lead to an activation of the arachidonic acid cascade. (From Bazan, 1990.)

3. CHANGES IN LIPID MEDIATORS IN THE BRAIN DURING ISCHEMIA AND TRANSCRIPTIONAL ACTIVATION OF GENES

One of the central issues in cell signal transduction is the nature of the mechanisms through which extracellular information is communicated to genes, triggering long-term responses such as cellular differentiation, long-term synaptic potentiation, and synaptic plasticity changes. This issue is particularly important in terms of the responses of the brain to ischemic insults, since, in addition to the synaptic circuits that are irreversibly damaged, others may be retrieved and regenerated. Such mechanisms might either facilitate recovery of damaged circuits or activate circuits that would then cope with functions left unattended by those that have been irreversibly impaired. Figure 5 outlines the two major fates of brain cells after ischemia, one leading to permanent damage and the other to recovery. We have been exploring the possibility that some of the lipid mediators accumulated during ischemia could play a role in the communication between plasma membrane signaling and genetic events. We have hypothesized that PAF may exert transcription-regulating functions because (1) it is often retained in cells upon formation, as in the retina after neurotransmitter-induced synthesis (Bussolino *et al.*, 1986); (2) when PAF is added to cells in culture, it promotes the transcriptional activation of immediate-early genes (Squinto *et al.*, 1989); and (3) there are very high-affinity PAF-binding sites located in intracellular membranes (Marcheselli *et al.*, 1990).

Figure 6 shows that second messengers, either directly or by way of third messengers, may activate the expression first of proto-oncogenes and then of gene cascades, leading to the synthesis of ion channels, G-proteins, or receptors (among other proteins) engaged in long-term responses. This coupling, by way of messengers generated rapidly during injury, or subsequent events and the triggering of gene expression, may underlie recovery of function. Transcription of the immediate-early gene c-*fos* is activated after ischemia (Panetta *et al.*, 1987; Birkle *et al.*, 1988); PAF is a transcriptional activator of c-*fos* and c-*jun* in neuroblastoma cells (Squinto *et al.*, 1989) and has subsequently been shown to enhance the expression of other genes, such as calcyclin (unpublished data).

Functional recovery after ischemia may result from interactions of growth factors, cofactors of growth factors (e.g. GM-1), and other, as yet undefined, events. Neurotrophic factors are currently being identified, and to a great extent their role in repair is not yet well defined. Some injured cells may be able to repair dendrites and axons by activating growth cone formation and path-finding processes, leading to the establishment of new synapses. In the trigeminal sensory endings of the cornea, damage triggers increases in GAP-43 mRNA in the trigeminal ganglion (Tao *et al.*, 1990; H. E. P. Bazan *et al.*, 1990; Bazan and Bazan, 1990). Synaptic circuitry may also be reestablished by "turning on" neurons that are not committed to performing a given function, but may become "reassigned" after ischemic damage has irreversibly impaired the original neurons.

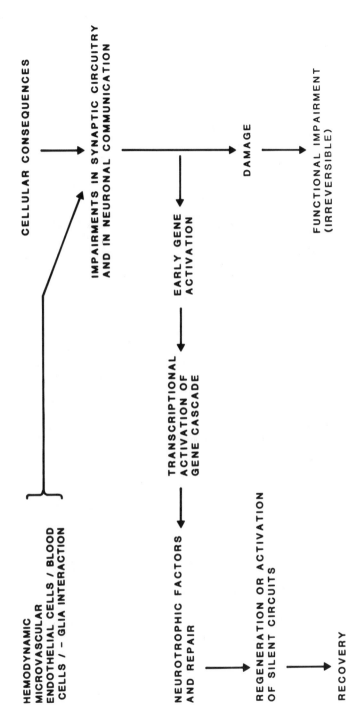

FIGURE 5. Ischemia-induced alterations in excitable membranes lead to impairments in synaptic circuitry. Some cells may be irreversibly damaged, while others either may recover or may be activated from silent circuits to replace lost cells. Signals that trigger gene expression may be engaged in these repair reactions.

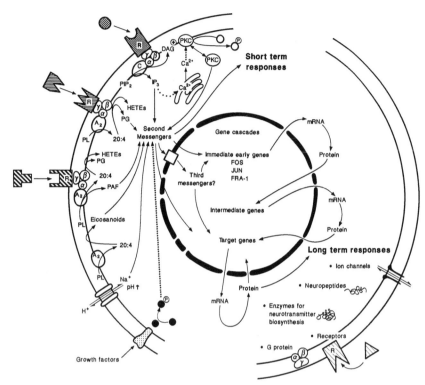

FIGURE 6. Gene activation results in long-term responses to cell signaling systems. Messengers in the nucleus carry the signal from the cytoplasm to the genome. Immediate-early genes that are activated encode gene products that are regulatory molecules for still other genes whose expression comprises the long-term response to neural stimulation. (From Bazan, 1990.)

The inositol lipid cell signal transduction system, acting through the second messengers diacylglycerol and inositol trisphosphate (IP_3), is a prime candidate for modulator of the consequences of ischemia for brain function. This is mainly due to the Ca^{2+}-ionizing ability of IP_3, to the protein kinase C-modulating role of diacylglycerol, and to the feedback "cross-talk" between the branches of the bifurcating signal pathway that spans the plasma membrane, as exemplified by phosphorylation of ion channels and other functionally important proteins.

The targets of cerebral ischemia in membranes are phospholipids with polyunsaturated fatty acyl chains (arachidonic acid and docosahexaenoic acid). Both are derived from essential fatty acids and are easily lost from neural tissue (Bazan, 1989b), especially after ischemia. Neural tissue preferentially uses docosahexaenoic acid instead of other fatty acids of the linolenic acid series, and the liver is the site of the conversion of dietary linolenic acid into docosahexaenoic acid; the transport of this acid as phospholipids of lipoproteins to the brain then resupplies neural membranes. A signaling system following cerebral ischemia has been postulated to trigger the resupply of docosahexaenoic acid from the liver (Gilboe *et al.*, 1989). A similar mechanism may operate for functionally important arachidonic acid-containing phospholipids. The modulation of repair and regeneration may therefore require the rebuilding of critical signaling molecules in excitable membranes by replenishment of essential fatty acids.

ACKNOWLEDGMENT

This work was supported by U.S. Public Health Service grant NS23002 from the National Institute of Neurological Diseases and Stroke.

REFERENCES

Aveldano, M. I., and Bazan, N. G., 1979*a*, Rapid production of diacylglycerols enriched in arachidonate and stearate during early brain ischemia, *J. Neurochem.* **25**:919–920.

Aveldano, M. I., and Bazan, N. G., 1975*b*, Differential lipid deacylation during brain ischemia in a homeotherm and a poikilotherm. Content and composition of free fatty acids and triacylglycerols, *Brain Res.* **100**:99–110.

Aveldano de Caldironi, M. I., and Bazan, N. G., 1979, Alpha-methyl-p-tyrosine inhibits the production of free arachidonic acid and diacylglycerols in brain after a single electroconvulsive shock, *Neurochem. Res.* **4**:213–221.

Bazan, H. E. P., Martin, R. E., Tao, Y., and Bazan, N. G., 1990, Trigeminal neurons respond to injury of their sensory terminals in cornea by increasing levels of GAP-43 (growth associated protein-43) protein and mRNA, *Soc. Neurosci.* **16**:164.

Bazan, N. G., 1970, Effects of ischemia and electroconvulsive shock on free fatty acid pool in the brain, *Biochim. Biophys. Acta* **218**:1–10.

Bazan, N. G., 1971, Free fatty acid production in cerebral white and grey matter of the squirrel monkey, *Lipids* **6**:211–212.

Bazan, N. G., 1989*a*, Lipid-derived metabolites as possible retina messengers; Arachidonic acid, leukotrienes, docosanoids, and platelet-activating factor, *in* "Extracellular and Intracellular Messengers in the Vertebrate Retina Neurobiology" (D. Redburn and H. Pasantes Morales, eds.), pp. 269–300, Alan R. Liss, New York.

Bazan, N. G., 1989*b*, Ginkgolide B (BN 52021) decreases brain phospholipase A_2 activated by ischemia or electroconvulsive shock, *in* "Ginkgolide—Chemistry, Biology, Pharmacology and Clinical Perspectives," vol. II (P. Braquet, ed.), pp. 629–637, J. R. Prous Science, Barcelona, Spain.

Bazan, N. G., 1990, Neuronal cell transduction and second messengers in cerebral ischemia, *in* "Pharmacology of Cerebral Ischemia" (J. Krieglstein and H. Oberpichler, eds.), pp. 391–398, Wissenschaftliche Verlagsgesellschaft, Stuttgart, Germany.

Bazan, N. G., and Bazan, H. E. P., 1990, Ocular responses to inflammation and the triggering of wound healing: Lipid mediators, proto-oncogenes, gene expression and neuromodulation, *in* "New Trends in Lipid Mediators Research. Lipid Mediators in Eye Inflammation," vol. 5 (N. G. Bazan, ed.), pp. 168–180, Karger, Basel, Switzerland.

Bazan, N. G., and Rakowski, H., 1970, Increased levels of brain free fatty acids after electroconvulsive shock, *Life Sci.* **9**:501–507.

Bazan, N. D., Bazan, H. E. P., Kennedy, W. G., and Joel, C. D., 1971, Regional distribution and rate of production of free fatty acids in rat brain, *J. Neurochem.* **18**:1387–1393.

Bazan, N. G., Ilincheta de Boschero, M. G., Giusto, N. M., and Bazan, H. E. P., 1976, De novo glycerolipid biosynthesis in the toad and cattle retina. Redirecting of the pathway by propranolol and phentolamine, *in* "Function and Metabolism of Phospholipids in the Central and Peripheral Nervous System," vol. 72 (G. Porcellati, L. Amaducci, and C. Galli, eds.), pp. 139–148, Plenum Press, New York.

Bazan, N. G., Morelli de Liberti, S. M., and Rodriguez de Turco, E. B., 1982, Arachidonic acid and arachidonoyl-diglycerides increase in rat cerebrum during bicuculline-induced status epilepticus, *Neurochem. Res.* **7**:839–843.

Birkle, D. L., and Bazan, N. G., 1987, Effect of bicuculline-induced status epilepticus on prostaglandins and hydroxyeicosatetraenoic acids in rat brain subcellular fractions, *J. Neurochem.* **48**:1768–1778.

Birkle, D. L., Kurian, P., Braquet, P., and Bazan, N. G., 1988, The platelet-activating factor antagonist BN 52021 decreases accumulation of free polyunsaturated fatty acid in mouse brain during ischemia and electroconvulsive shock, *J. Neurochem.* **51**:1900–1905.

Bussolino, F., Gremo, F., Tetta, C., Pescarmona, G. P., and Camussi, G., 1986, Production of platelet-activating factor by chick retina, *J. Biol. Chem.* **261**:16502–16508.

Cendella, R. J., Galli, C., and Paoletti, R., 1975, Brain free fatty acid levels in rats sacrificed by decapitation versus focused microwave irradiation, *Lipids* **10**:290–293.

Choi, D. W., 1990, Cerebral hypoxia: Some new approaches and unanswered questions, *J. Neurosci.* **10**:2493–2501.

Edgar, A. D., Strosznajder, J., and Horrocks, L. A., 1982, Activation of ethanolamine phospholipase A_2 in brain during ischemia, *J. Neurochem.* **39**:1111–1116.

Gilboe, D. D., Fitzpatrick, J. H., Jr., Kintner, D., Emoto, S. E., Bazan, N. G., and Braquet, P., 1989, Biochemical changes in normoxic and post-ischemic brain tissue following treatment with BN 52021, *in* "Ginkgolide—Chemistry, Biology, Pharmacology and Clinical Perspectives," vol. II (P. Braquet, ed.), pp. 639–648, J. R. Prous Science, Barcelona, Spain.

Gilboe, D. D., Kinter, D., Fitzpatrick, J. H., Jr., Emoto, S. E., Esanu, A., Braquet, P. G., and Bazan, N. G., 1991, Recovery of postischemic brain metabolism and function following treatment with a free radical scavenger and platelet-activating factor antagonists, *J. Neurochem.* **56**:311–319.

Horrocks, L. A., Harder, H., Nakagawa, Y., Yeo, Y., Birkle, D., and Bazan, N. G., 1985, Turnover of polyunsaturated fatty acids in different molecular species, *Trans. Am. Soc. Neurochem.* **16**:154.

Ikeda, M. S., Yoshida, R., Busto, M., Santiso, M., and Ginsberg, M., 1986, Polyphosphoinositides as a probable source of brain free fatty acid accumulated at the onset of ischemia, *J. Neurochem.* **47**:123–132.

Kass, I. S., and Lipton, P., 1982, Mechanisms involved in irreversible anoxic damage to the *in vivo* rat hippocampal slice, *J. Physiol.* **332**:459–472.

Marcheselli, V. L., Rossowska, M., Domingo, M. T., Braquet, P., and Bazan, N. G., 1990, Distinct platelet-activating factor binding sites in synaptic endings and in intracellular membranes of rat cerebral cortex, *J. Biol. Chem.* **265**:9140–9145.

Panetta, T., Marcheselli, V. L., Braquet, P., Spinnewyn, B., and Bazan, N. G., 1987, Effects of a platelet-activating factor antagonist (BN 52021) on free fatty acids, diacylglycerols, polyphosphoinositides and blood flow in the gerbil brain: Inhibition of ischemia-reperfusion induced cerebral injury, *Biochem. Biophys. Res. Commun.* **149**:580–587.

Rodriguez de Turco, E. B., and Bazan, N. G., 1983, Changes in free fatty acids and diglycerides in mouse brain at birth and during anoxia, *J. Neurochem.* **41**:794–800.

Rothman, S. M., 1983, Synaptic activity mediates death of hypoxic neurons, *Science* **220:**536–537.

Siesjö, B. K., Ingvar, M., and Westberg, A., 1982, The influences of bicuculline-induced seizures on free fatty acid concentration in cerebral cortex, hippocampus and cerebellum, *J. Neurochem.* **39:** 796–802.

Squinto, S. P., Block, A. L., Braquet, P., and Bazan, N. G., 1989, Platelet-activating factor stimulates a Fos/Jun/AP-1 transcriptional signaling system in human neuroblastoma cells, *J. Neurosci. Res.* **24:**558–566.

Tao, Y., Allan, G., Bazan, H. E. P., Lin, N., and Bazan, N. G., 1990, Corneal wound healing triggers an increase in growth-associated protein (GAP-43) mRNA in the trigeminal ganglia, *Suppl. Invest. Ophthalmol. Vis. Sci.* **31:**55.

CELLULAR AND METABOLIC SIGNIFICANCE OF CELLULAR ACID-BASE SHIFTS IN HUMAN STROKE

K. M. A. WELCH, STEVEN R. LEVINE, G. B. MARTIN, and J. A. HELPERN

1. INTRODUCTION

Stroke is most often due to the occlusion of a single intracranial artery, resulting in incomplete focal ischemia. This has an immediate deleterious effect upon cerebral energy metabolism and dependent processes (Lowry and Passonneau, 1964). There is a rapid decrease of high-energy phosphate intermediates, a shift toward

K. M. A. WELCH and STEVEN R. LEVINE • Center for Stroke Research, Department of Neurology, Henry Ford Hospital and Health Science Center, Detroit, Michigan. G. B. MARTIN • Department of Emergency Medicine, Henry Ford Hospital and Health Science Center, Detroit, Michigan. J. A. HELPERN • Center for Stroke Research, Department of Neurology, Henry Ford Hospital and Health Science Center, Detroit, Michigan, and Department of Physics, Oakland University, Rochester, Michigan.

Neurochemical Correlates of Cerebral Ischemia, Volume 7 of *Advances in Neurochemistry*, edited by Nicolas G. Bazan, Pierre Braquet, and Myron D. Ginsberg. Plenum Press, New York, 1992.

reduction of mitochondrial respiratory chain metabolites, increased lactic acid, and acidosis in the ischemic focus (Goldberg *et al.*, 1966; Michenfelder and Theye, 1970). Most investigators have considered that acidosis causes or contributes in a major way to cellular damage in ischemic brain (for a review, see Welch and Barkley [1986]). In recent clinical studies of acute focal ischemic stroke, using the capability of ^{31}P nuclear magnetic resonance spectroscopy (NMRS) to dynamically measure the brain intracellular pH, we observed a transition from acidosis to alkalosis in ischemic brain as early as 18 hr after the onset of stroke (Levine *et al.*, 1987). Positron emission tomography (PET) has corroborated the finding of alkalosis in clinical studies of subacute and late focal ischemic stroke (Syrota *et al.*, 1985; Hakim *et al.*, 1987). A rapid transition from acidosis to alkalosis has also been observed in experimental stroke models of either focal or global complete or incomplete ischemia, with or without reperfusion (Kogure *et al.*, 1980; Mabe *et al.*, 1983; Paschen *et al.*, 1985; Yoshida *et al.*, 1985). In this chapter we explore in clinical patients with cerebral ischemia (1) the significance of brain acidosis and (2) the currently unknown mechanisms and meaning of what we have termed the acid-to-base pH "flip-flop."

The particular mechanisms whereby increased $[H^+]$ is toxic to neural or glial cells are uncertain and probably diverse. We will focus on those that can be assessed by in vivo NMRS techniques. ^{31}P NMRS can measure both brain high-energy phosphate and brain pH, thus permitting the hypothesis to be tested that low pH may prevent recovery of energy phosphates (Welsh *et al.*, 1980; Siesjö, 1981). A second possible toxic mechanism involves the enhancement of membrane breakdown by free-radical reactions at low pH (Siesjö, 1985*a*). ^{31}P NMRS can also measure phosphomonoesters and phosphodiesters in the brain. This provides a gross index of membrane phospholipid turnover (Pettegrew *et al.*, 1987) and, therefore, offers a means of indirectly testing this free-radical hypothesis. A third mechanism is loss of cellular volume control, a distinct accompaniment of brain acidosis perhaps related to glial buffering (Siesjö, 1985*b*; Kraig *et al.*, 1986). NMR imaging can monitor shifts in position in brain water and, together with ^{31}P NMRS, can test this hypothesis (Horikawa *et al.*, 1986).

^{31}P NMRS using surface coils allows sequential and near-simultaneous measurement of phosphorus metabolites and pH in animals and humans (Ackerman *et al.*, 1980; Behar *et al.*, 1983). Considerable experimental literature describing the use of this technique in acute stroke models has now accrued to document deterioration of high-energy phosphates as well as acidosis. Human studies have been infrequent, mostly limited to neonatal hypoxic-ischemic injury (Hope *et al.*, 1984). Adult clinical ^{31}P NMRS studies of chronic stroke have reported cerebral alkalosis without substantial changes in high-energy phosphates (Bottomley *et al.*, 1986; Welch *et al.*, 1985). With the exception of our own, no serial studies of acute stroke have been available in the literature. Methodological problems, now mostly surmounted, together with difficulties in studying seriously sick patients with this complex technology, probably account for the current dearth of studies.

2. METHODS

2.1. Bruker/Oxford Research Systems 80-MHz TMR Spectrometer

The magnet is a 1.9-T (80-MHz), 60-cm horizontal-bore topical magnetic resonance (TMR) magnet. It is the only whole-body TMR magnet in operation today and is equipped with a Bruker Biospec I console (Bruker Instruments, Billerica, Mass.). Data are transferred to a Sun Microsystems 3/180 computer, where they are archived and processed by using NMR-1 software (New Methods Research, Inc., Syracuse, N.Y.).

2.2. Topical Magnetic Resonance

The problem of primary concern with the application of in vivo NMRS is confirmation of the locus of signal. One of the first techniques developed to approach the problem of isolation of the signal sources was TMR (Gordon *et al.*, 1980, 1982). In TMR, nonlinear magnetic field gradients are superimposed on the main static homogeneous field of the magnet, generating a spherical region of magnetic field (commonly called the profiled field) within which the magnetic field is very homogeneous. Everywhere outside the homogeneous spherical region, the magnetic field is extremely inhomogeneous. Since high-resolution NMR signals can be obtained only from regions of magnetic fields that are highly homogeneous, the tissue lying within the sphere generates high-resolution NMR signals and the tissue lying outside the sphere (in the inhomogeneous field) generates excessively broadened NMR signals. The technique results in a composite of a high-resolution spectrum superimposed on an inhomogeneously broadened spectrum. The broad "hump," which results from the edges of the profiled field, can then be removed by using deconvolution computer programs, and the resulting high-resolution spectrum can be analyzed.

The center of the profiled field is fixed at the center of the bore of the magnet. The size of the profiled field can be adjusted by adjusting the current in room-temperature high-order shim coils (mostly Z^4). In the system used in our laboratory for human studies, the profiled field can be adjusted from a minimum of 4 cm diameter spherical volume (dsv) to 10 cm dsv in 1-cm increments.

2.3. Topical Magnetic Resonance with ¹H Image Viewfinding

In the application of TMR in the Department of Neurology at Henry Ford Hospital, we use ¹H NMR imaging prior to spectroscopy to verify the proper location of the profiled field within the tissue region of spectroscopic interest. This approach is possible since ^{1}H NMR imaging is less stringent with regard to static magnetic field homogeneity requirements. Hence, although the largest profiled field in our magnet is 10 cm dsv for spectroscopy, imaging is possible up to a size of 20 cm dsv.

For human studies, the subject's head is placed inside a ^{1}H imaging head coil which is constructed in such a way as to incorporate a large surface coil for ^{31}P spectroscopy. The surface coil is placed on the scalp over the region of spectroscopic interest. A thin tube of water (doped with $CuSO_4$) around the outside of the surface coil provides markers in the ^{1}H image to verify the positioning of the surface coil. The subject is then placed inside the magnet, and the first image is obtained. From this image, measurements in frequency are converted to distances in centimeters; if necessary, the subject is repositioned inside the bore of the magnet until the region of spectroscopic interest coincides with the center of the profiled field. Once the subject is appropriately positioned, the surface coil is used to obtain ^{31}P spectra.

2.4. Signal Acquisition

The need for good signal/noise ratio (S/N) to reduce error in the signal area measurements must be weighed against the errors incurred with partial saturation. Acquisition rates which are less than approximately $5 \times T_1$ of the slowest-relaxing nuclei result in some saturation of the resonance signals. Knowledge of the amount of saturation at the given sampling rate (aside from any changes in T_1 which may occur during the experiment) is all that is necessary to obtain meaningful and interpretable data. This problem can be avoided by choosing rates of signal acquisition which result in fully relaxed spectra (i.e., ca. one transient per 10 sec for in vivo ^{31}P) at the expense of S/N (within the same time frame of data acquisition). Given the constraints of the need for good S/N, datum point sampling rate, and experimental time in the magnet in a clinical setting, it is unrealistic to obtain fully relaxed spectra. For human brain studies performed to date, we have used a recycle time of 1.512 sec. Individual resonant peak areas are not corrected for partial saturation.

All ^{31}P spectra for both human and animal studies are acquired by using a straightforward pulse-acquisition-delay experiment. Typically, spectra are obtained with a spectral width of 4 kHz, and 4k datum points, resulting in a signal acquisition time of 0.512 sec. For human studies a recycle delay of 1.0 sec is used, resulting in a total interpulse interval of 1.512 sec. Spectra are zero-filled to 8k data points before processing. The volume of tissue from which the spectra are obtained is approximately 33 ml (this is with a profiled field of 4 cm dsv) and requires the summation of approximately 512 transients for good S/N.

2.5. Spectral Analysis

2.5.1. pH Measurement

One of the more significant contributions ^{31}P NMRS has offered to the field of physiology is the ability to provide a noninvasive accurate measure of [H^+]. For the most part, this is accomplished by measuring the relative frequency shift of the inorganic phosphate (P_i) resonance signal (Moon and Richards, 1973). This frequency shift is pH dependent because the constant rate for the equilibrium:

$$H^+ + HPO_4^{2-} \rightleftharpoons H_2PO_4^-$$

is fast on the NMR time scale, so that both forms of phosphate give rise to only one resonance signal (an average of the two forms of phosphate). The frequency of this averaged resonance signal depends on the position of this equilibrium, which, in turn, depends on [H^+]. Therefore, a measure of the resonant frequency of P_i (relative to some frequency reference point) is a measure of pH. Typically this reference point is taken from the frequency of phosphocreatine (PCr). The formula used to calculate the pH of brain from the chemical shifts of the ^{31}P spectrum is (Petroff *et al.*, 1985) as follows:

$$pH = 6.77 + \log \left[\frac{\delta_{P_i} - 3.29}{5.58 - \delta_{P_i}} \right]$$

Using the chemical shift of the P_i peak to measure pH can give erroneous results because of the influence of large variations in ionic strength (Gadian *et al.*, 1979), metal ion binding (Jacobson and Cohen, 1981), and temperature. In addition, the binding of P_i to macromolecules (e.g., proteins) can affect the chemical shift of P_i. An additional problem exists in the uncertainty of the relative distribution of the P_i within various intracellular compartments. In the brain, where the intracellular compartment is large compared with vascular and extracellular compartments (Fishman, 1973), the observed pH probably reflects intracellular hydrogen ion concentrations (Gadian, 1982). Varying the ionic strength and Mg^{2+} ion concentration can affect the pK_a of P_i. Roberts *et al.* (1981) observed that a change from 0.1 to 0.5 in ionic strength caused a displacement of the titration curve over a pH range of 4 to 8. This displacement is due to the lowering of the phosphate pK_a.

2.5.2. Metabolic Data

Readily identifiable resonances in the in vivo ^{31}P spectra are commonly labeled: phosphomonoesters (PME), P_i, phosphodiesters (PDE), PCr, and the γ-, α-, and β-phosphates of ATP (Gadian, 1982). However, the peaks commonly labeled ATP are more accurately described as ionized ends, esterified ends, and middles. The ionized-ends region contains resonances from the γ-phosphate of nucleoside triphosphates and the β-phosphate of nucleoside diphosphates. In the mammalian brain, the predominant contributors to the nucleoside triphosphate and nucleoside diphosphate resonances are ATP and ADP (Pettegrew *et al.*, 1986), respectively. The esterified-ends region contains resonances from the α-phosphate of nucleoside triphosphates, the α-phosphate of nucleoside diphosphates, the NADs, and the uridine diphosphosugars (galactose, glucose, and mannose). In adult mammalian brain the predominant contribution to the esterified-ends region is made by α-ATP and α-ADP. The only resonance that contributes to the middle region is the β-phosphate of nucleoside triphosphates.

Existing methodology for resonance signal quantitation of in vivo ^{31}P NMR spectra consists of computer programs for curve fitting, computer integration, triangulation by hand, and peak height measurements. All four techniques suffer various limitations. The most significant problem common to all is definition of the baseline of the spectrum. This is a particularly difficult problem when dealing with in vivo ^{31}P spectra since almost all such spectra include a broad-frequency component resulting from immobilized phosphates. Typically this broad-frequency component is removed from the flame ionization detector (FID) prior to exponential weighting and subsequent Fourier transformation, by using a computer-drive operator-dependent convolution difference or profile correction routine. Basically, all baseline correction procedures involve a filtering process. The parameters selected to define the amount of filtering are adjusted empirically to produce as flat a baseline as possible without introducing distortion. Because of the subjectivity of this process, all of these techniques contain an unknown amount of bias.

In the present studies, triangulation by hand was performed by drawing a "best-fit" straight line through the noise of the baseline of the spectrum. Triangles were then drawn over the individual peaks and areas were calculated. Sources of error include estimation of baselines and apex angles for poorly resolved peaks. The contribution of each of the seven identified resonance signals in the ^{31}P NMR spectra is reported as the mole percent of the total phosphate signal. The major problem with analysis of the ^{31}P spectra involves the P_i peak, which is not well resolved in normal subjects and can, therefore, be difficult to quantitate.

2.5.3. Bioenergetic Ratios

^{31}P NMRS is currently the only available technique for monitoring the adenylate energy status of tissue in vivo. Also, it offers an advantage over biochemical techniques that require freeze-inactivation of the brain, which induces energetic breakdown during the process, so that measurements are probably more physiological. However, the NMR method is inherently insensitive, detecting only millimolar concentrations, and unless some system of internal standardization is used, the spectral peaks cannot be strictly quantitated. Bioenergetic

ratios can be obtained from spectra which may be adequate to characterize the energetic state of the tissue.

From the equation (Atkinson, 1968)

$$\frac{[ATP]}{[ADP][P_i]}(phosphorylation\ ratio) = \frac{[PCr]K_{eq}[H^+]}{[P_i][Creatine]}$$

it can be seen that the PCr/P_i ratio is an approximate measure of the phosphorylation potential of the tissue when the creatine kinase (CK) reaction is at equilibrium (Atkinson, 1968). The extent to which the steady state of the CK reaction differs from the equilibrium condition is a subject of controversy (Nunnally and Hollis, 1979). The inference of actual ATP synthesis rate from the PCr/P_i ratio is problematic if either the V_{max} of the CK reaction or the pH changes (Shoubridge et al., 1982). Nevertheless, if ATP synthesis decreases, the PCr/P_i ratio should decrease, as expected in situations of insufficient energy production such as ischemia. On the other hand, the PCr/P_i ratio decreases during increased metabolic activity (e.g., epilepsy) (Prichard et al., 1983). An accompanying increase in the cerebral metabolic rate of oxygen (CMRO$_2$) would differentiate the PCr/P_i decrease of metabolic stimulation from that of impaired energy production. In our stroke studies we must assume that a low PCr/P_i reflects impaired energy production, since CMRO$_2$ was not measured. This ratio has been used effectively by others (Mayevsky et al., 1988). Nevertheless, the PCr/P_i ratio is not an exact measure of the phosphorylation potential, but experience has shown it to be an adequate monitor or estimate of the phosphorylation potential in anoxic ischemia (Prichard et al., 1983; Radda, 1986).

2.5.4. Phospholipids

Contributing to the PME region are, primarily, phosphocholine, phosphoethanolamine, and α-glycerophosphate. Less prominent contributions come from hexose 6-phosphates, triose phosphates, pentose phosphates, P_i, anomeric sugar phosphates, and several other uncharacterized signals. Contributing to the PDE region are glycerophosphodiesters (primarily glycerol 3-phosphoethanolamine and glycerol 3-phosphocholine), a broad resonance from phosphorylated glycolipids and glycoproteins, and several uncharacterized resonances (Pettegrew et al., 1987).

The phospholipid composition of the adult human cerebral cortex gray matter is 37% phosphatidylethanolamine, 35% phosphatidylcholine, 13% phosphatidylserine, 11% sphingomyelin, and 4% phosphatidylinositol (Kwee and Nakada, 1988). The components of the PME peak are found only in the anabolic pathway of 89% of the phospholipids and are found in the anabolic (phosphocholine) as well as catabolic (phosphoethanolamine and phosphocholine) pathways of 11% (sphingomyelin). Therefore, to a first approximation, the PMR resonance may reflect phospholipid anabolic activity (Pettegrew et al., 1987). The PDE components are found only in catabolic pathways. The PME/PDE ratio, therefore, may reasonably be considered an index of phospholipid turnover reflecting the ratio of anabolic precursors to the catabolic breakdown products of phospholipid metabolism. The PMEs are an essential component of neuronal and mitochondrial membranes and are involved in membrane transport processes. We will explore the use of this ratio as a marker of altered membrane function in the ischemic brain.

3. ACUTE FOCAL CORTICAL ISCHEMIA

Disturbances of brain acid-base status are important in the mechanisms of ischemic neuronal damage for the following reasons: (1) the pH may control local cerebral blood flow and tissue oxygen delivery (Kuschinsky and Wahl, 1978); (2) there is a pH dependence of membrane transfer mechanisms (Choi and Abramson, 1978; Lund-Anderson, 1979; Siesjö, 1978; Wanke et al., 1979); (3) intracellular hydrogen ion concentration controls the activity of cytoplasmic enzymes, particularly those involved in glycolysis (Siesjö, 1978); and (4) ATP production in mitochondria may be pH linked (Mitchell, 1961). Regulation of $[H^+]$ is severely stressed by ischemia. The crucial acid-base event in the ischemic brain is caused by deterioration of energy status and the ensuing stimulation of anaerobic glycolysis to preserve ATP synthesis at the cost of lactic acid accumulation and CO_2 entrapment which, together with a relatively minor contribution from ATP hydrolysis, seems primarily responsible for tissue acidosis (Siesjö, 1985a,b).

In our studies of focal cortical ischemia we first completed a series of nine patients, comprising eight with established stroke and one with transient ischemia who underwent intense serial study. Figure 1 displays the serial ^{31}P NMR spectra from a patient studied six times within 1 month, the earliest being 18 hr after the ictus (spectra from only four occasions are shown). The pH was acidotic (6.74) acutely shifting to alkalotic values (7.20 to 7.26) subacutely. Intermediate and late pH values returned to within normal limits. The PCr/P_i ratio was reduced acutely with gradual recovery to normal within 1 month. There was incomplete recovery of neurological deficit. Figure 2 illustrates a typical series of spectra obtained in a patient studied subacutely and on separate occasions over a 2 month interval. Alkalotic pH values were obtained at the first time of study. Obliteration of the PCr and ATP peaks with increase of P_i was seen at this time and then gradually recovered, somewhat variably, toward the normal spectral characteristics of the opposite hemisphere. Recovery of neurological deficit consistently lagged behind recovery of cerebral high-energy phosphates. The PME value in both cases appeared decreased but recovered over time.

Student's t-tests were used to compare normal controls separately with the stroke hemisphere and contralateral hemisphere of stroke patients at three time

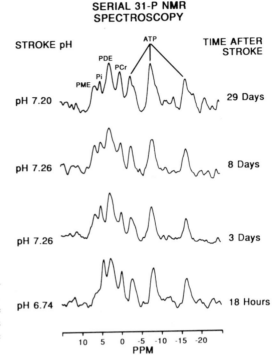

SERIAL 31-P NMR
SPECTROSCOPY

STROKE pH

TIME AFTER
STROKE

pH 7.20 — 29 Days

pH 7.26 — 8 Days

pH 7.26 — 3 Days

pH 6.74 — 18 Hours

10 5 0 -5 -10 -15 -20
PPM

FIGURE 1. Serial ^{31}P NMRS of patient taken from the ischemic focus. The P_i is elevated compared with the PCr peak acutely. The ischemic focus pH is acidotic acutely and alkalotic subacutely.

points. The mean of the PCr/P_i ratios in six patients studied over time was significantly reduced in the ischemic focus during the subacute period (2 to 3 days after onset, $P < 0.002$ compared with normal controls), but recovered to control values in the ischemic focus 7 to 9 days after onset despite persistent neurological deficit and prominent evidence for infarction on the NMR and computed tomography (CT) scans. This is consistent with the concept that, although deterioration of high-energy phosphate metabolism is initially responsible for neuronal dysfunction, other factors probably play a more important role in causing cell death. Apart from partial recovery of some neurons, the return of measurable adenine metabolites could also originate from glial cells, which are relatively more resistant to ischemia, or macrophages that infiltrate the infarct. Diaschisis might, in part, explain a strong trend ($P < 0.09$) toward lower PCr/P_i ratios measured in the contralateral hemisphere 10 days after stroke onset.

Whereas the pH was acidic in the ischemic focus of patients studied acutely, by the time patients were studied in the subacute and intermediate periods (Figure 3) the pH was alkalotic compared with that in the contralateral hemisphere and to normal controls. Alkalotic shifts were seen after 24 hr from stroke onset, but were

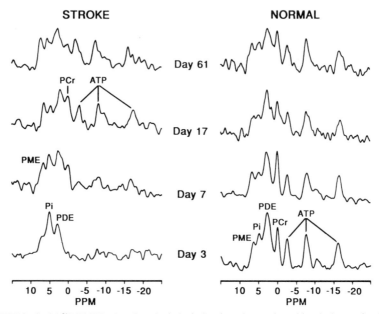

FIGURE 2. Serial ^{31}P NMRS taken from both the ischemic and contralateral hemispheres of a single patient during four study times over a 2-month period. PCr and ATP were depleted initially, with gradual return of signal. The P_i was initially elevated with a return toward values of the contralateral hemisphere.

present even earlier on the basis of heterogeneity of infarct pH obtained in one patient at 18 hr (Levine *et al.*, 1988*a*) and in a patient with transient ischemia (7.09 ischemic region versus 6.95 nonischemic). Spectra in this patient were obtained from the fronto-temporal cortex within 24 hr of the onset of symptoms when the patient was asymptomatic.

Figure 4 shows ^{31}P NMRS and cerebral pH determination in the ischemic hemisphere and the homologous region of the contralateral hemisphere in a patient studied first on day 4 and again on days 5 and 6 after stroke. Serial serum glucose data are also provided. Throughout the course of study the serial spectra and pH measurements obtained from the homologous regions of the opposite nonischemic hemisphere were unchanged. In contrast, neither high-energy phosphates, PMEs, nor PDEs were detected in the serial spectra obtained from the infarct center. The sole spectral peak identified was P_i. Serial examinations failed to show recovery of the high-energy phosphates, PME, or PDE components of the spectra. The pH was markedly acidotic (6.14 to 6.20) as long as the serum glucose levels were high (325 to 450 mg/dl) but, after serum glucose levels were corrected (93 mg/dl) at day 6, did not differ from that in the contralateral hemisphere (7.06). Although this

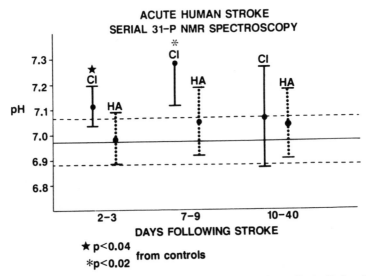

ACUTE HUMAN STROKE
SERIAL 31-P NMR SPECTROSCOPY

FIGURE 3. ³¹P NMRS. Mean brain intracellular pH data ± 1 SD are shown. Cerebral infarct (CI) pH was more alkalotic than controls during the periods 2 to 3 days and 7 to 9 days following stroke, reaching maximum alkalotic values during the 7 to 9 days following stroke. The cerebral infarct pH returned to levels not significantly different from controls by days 10 to 40 after stroke. HA, contralateral hemisphere.

could coincide with a shift toward eventual alkalosis similar to that observed in stable or recovering patients, this patient died within hours of the last measurement. Furthermore, the total absence of high-energy phosphate peaks and severe acidosis persisted well beyond the much earlier return of high-energy phosphate levels and time of alkalotic shifts observed in the normoglycemic stroke patient (Levine *et al.*, 1988*b*).

From these preliminary cases, at some time point in the progression of focal ischemia, there appeared to be a reversal or "flip-flop" in pH from the more immediate acidosis to a latent alkalosis. Acidosis appeared closely linked to deterioration of energy metabolism. Systemic hyperglycemia appeared to be associated with more severe and prolonged cerebral acidosis.

Because of these encouraging findings, we proceeded to investigate a second, larger series of a total 44 patients with hemispheric focal ischemia (Table 1). In accord with our preliminary findings of dynamic shifts in brain pH over time, patients were separated into acidotic, alkalotic, and normal pH groups. The normal group was defined as having a pH within 1 standard deviation of the controls. If a significant difference among groups was detected by analysis of variance, each patient group was compared with the control group by using

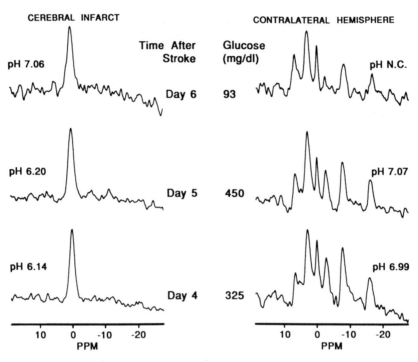

FIGURE 4. Serial ^{31}P NMRS of cerebral infarct (CI) and contralateral hemisphere of a hyperglycemic patient with acute MCA territory infarct. The serial spectra obtained from the homologous regions of the opposite noninfarcted hemisphere were normal, as was the brain pH throughout the course of study. In contrast, high-energy phosphates were not seen in the ischemic infarct. The only spectral peak in the infarct center was P_i. Serial examination failed to show recovery of the high energy-phosphates, PME, or PDE compounds of the spectra. The pH was markedly acidotic as long as the serum glucose levels were high but normalized as the glucose levels decreased to normal.

Dunnett's test. Owing to heterogeneous variances, the analysis was performed on the ranks of the data except for PCr/P_i and PME/PDE. That variability in pH and brain energetics exists during the early stages of stroke is not unexpected in view of the variability in clinical neurological deficit and frequent systemic complications.

When the ischemic brain was acidotic, a highly significant elevation of P_i was noted with a decrease in ATP but no change in PCr (Table 1). The PCr/P_i ratio was reduced as a function of the high P_i. Problematically, either acid shifts or ischemic metabolism should lead to a PCr decrease. Differential recovery rates for the high-energy phosphates or the effect of free divalent cations such as Mg^{2+} might explain

TABLE 1. Relationships of pH Changes to Energy and Phospholipid Metabolism Ratios

Ratio	Value in			
	Control (<6.91) (n = 3)	Acid (n = 9–10)	Normal (>7.07) (n = 11–13)	Alkalotic (n = 19–21)
PCr/P$_i$[a]	2.2 (0.5)	0.8 (0.9)[b]	1.7 (0.8)	1.7 (0.9)
PCr/TP[a]	13.1 (2.1)	10.1 (6.5)	14.3 (3.1)	13.7 (3.2)
P$_i$/TP[a]	6.2 (1.0)	39.5 (38.4)[b]	9.3 (2.4)[b]	10.5 (7.4)[b]
β-ATP/TP[a]	11.1 (1.5)	7.3 (4.5)[b]	9.4 (2.2)	10.5 (2.5)
PME/TP[a]	9.1 (3.1)	7.4 (5.2)	11.0 (3.2)	8.9 (2.3)
PDE/TP[a]	29.2 (1.9)	22.4 (13.0)	29.4 (3.1)	27.9 (3.5)
PME/PDE[a]	0.3 (0.1)	0.3 (0.1)	0.4 (0.1)	0.3 (0.1)

[a]Values in parentheses indicate S.D.
[b]Different from controls ($P < 0.05$).

this discrepancy. Alternatively, the inhomogeneity of the ischemic groups in the acute stages of progressing stroke and the wide range of PCr values could have made it difficult to achieve statistical significance of PCr fall; a number of patients studied with acidosis showed obliterated or small PCr spectral peaks (Figure 4). In support of this, when the brain was acidotic there were near-significant correlations of pH with reduction of PCr/P$_i$ and PCr/TP and significant relationships to Pi/TP increase (Table 2). As the pH normalized and progressed into relative alkalosis, P$_i$ remained elevated in ischemic brain but ATP and PCr/P$_i$ recovered. Also, there were also strong correlations between the degree of acidity and levels of both PME and PDE (Table 2). Taken together, the findings support a relationship between ischemic acidosis and impaired recovery of energy metabolism together with breakdown of membrane phospholipids.

When serial pH measurements were correlated with a gross scale of neurologic deficit (0 = normal, I = mild, II = moderate, III = severe), at the final

TABLE 2. Correlations of Acidosis to Energy and Phospholipid Metabolism

Ratio	Correlation coefficient	n	Two-tailed P value[a]
PCr/P$_i$	0.61	9	>0.08
PCr/TP	0.59	10	>0.07
P$_i$/TP	−0.70	9	<0.04
β-ATP/TP	0.48	10	>0.15
PME/TP	0.81	9	<0.01
PDE/T	0.88	9	<0.002
PME/PDE	−0.11	7	>0.81

[a]No significance was found within normal, control, or alkalotic groups.

spectroscopic assessment (7 to 30 days after onset) there was a negative trend for the degree of acidosis versus deficit ($n = 28$, $r = 0.204$, $P = 0.29$) but a significant positive correlation with the degree of alkalosis ($n = 28$, $r = 0.383$, $P = 0.44$). These data support the hypothesis that the greater the alkalosis subsequent to acidosis, the worse is the neurological outcome. There is also indirect support for the hypothesis that an alkalotic pH is perhaps more due to metabolic paralysis, cell death, cerebral edema, or all three, than to active cell buffering.

Such prevailing findings of ischemic cerebral alkalosis as stroke progresses deserves in-depth discussion. Kogure *et al.* (1980) observed that after cerebral embolism in the rat, a permanent decrease of cerebral blood flow (CBF) in the ischemic focus, although at first associated with acidosis and lactic acid accumulation, later resulted in alkalosis despite persistence of ischemia and high tissue lactate. ATP was depleted in the same region, but there was hyperoxidation of the mitochondrial electron transport system, which suggested to the authors either a flow/metabolism uncoupling or ATP consumption. After temporary middle cerebral artery (MCA) occlusion in the cat, Paschen *et al.* (1985) found regions of alkalosis associated with complete or partial ATP loss, despite reperfusion. A regional block in the glycolytic pathway was demonstrated in the same regions, attributed by the authors as possibly due to a decrease of NAD$^+$. Mabe *et al.* (1983) found transient alkalosis 60 min into reperfusion after 15 min of transient forebrain ischemia. Reperfusion alkalosis could be seen even after 5 min of transient ischemia and persisted for as long as 90 min after the moment of recirculation at times when lactate levels were still above control values. Using a similar model, Yoshida *et al.* (1985) found postischemic alkalosis to be present 4 hr after reperfusion and to be more pronounced after complete than incomplete ischemia. Metabolic recovery was more impaired in regions of greater alkalosis, leading the authors to speculate that severe tissue alkalosis might be a physico-chemical marker of advanced tissue injury.

PET studies in a small number of patients have documented alkalosis in the subacute (within 48 hr) (Hakim *et al.*, 1987) and later (10 to 14 days) (Syrota *et al.*, 1985) stages after stroke. Hakim *et al.* (1987) measured alkaline pH values only in reperfused brain regions. Of interest, these pH shifts correlated with a regional increase in the glucose/oxygen ratio, suggesting ongoing anaerobic glucose metabolism. This is something of a paradox, since anaerobic metabolism should generate lactic acid and a lowered tissue pH and raises the issue that alkalotic pH may be related to intrinsic cellular buffering against lactic acid accumulation or else other factors such as edema. In a separate study, alkaline pH values measured 10 to 19 days after acute stroke (Syrota *et al.*, 1985) failed to correlate with CBF, extracellular water, or CMRO$_2$ but did correlate with reduced oxygen extraction fraction (OEF), suggesting a relationship to luxury perfusion or tissue metabolic paralysis.

On the basis of the studies cited above, as well as our own, in the dynamic process of deterioration or recovery that takes place over hours or days, there appears to be a dramatic, relatively rapid switch from the potentially damaging tissue acidosis to an alkaline pH. This may persist for days after a stroke. The mechanism and meaning of this "flip-flop" to alkalosis are unknown and most certainly multifactorial. Intracellular alkalosis of the magnitude that has been observed occurs in very few other conditions (Pelligrino and Siesjö, 1981; McMillan and Siesjö, 1983). Cellular buffering mechanisms, ATP resynthesis, and temperature effects are causal considerations, the first being probably of most importance and the last unlikely in the reperfused brain. Reduced cellular production of acid metabolites and CO_2 as a result of complete or partially impaired metabolic function in ischemic or infarcted brain in the presence of luxury reperfusion may lead to lower $[H^+]_i$ accumulation than usual, producing a relative alkalosis. Such a mechanism for alkalosis was proposed by Syrota et al. (1985) on the basis of their PET measurements, which showed an indirect correlation between decreased OEF (metabolic impairment) and pH. Reperfusion alkalosis was also observed by Hakim et al. (1987). However, this was observed at a time when anaerobic metabolism was stimulated; alkalosis is a well-established stimulus to glycolysis. Mabe et al. (1983) postulated that with the resumption of tissue circulation and ATP synthesis, lactic acidosis can be buffered in part by active energy-consuming efflux of protons from cells. Lactate production is compensated for only partly by its oxidation when other pH-buffering mechanisms are active. After ischemia, a transient overcompensation and alkalotic pH may result during reperfusion. The greater the lactic acid accumulation or pH fall during ischemia, the more pronounced and protracted this overcompensation is likely to be. Siesjö (1985b) has argued that the most likely buffering mechanism brought into play under these circumstances includes an energy-consuming electrosilent Na^+/H^+ antiport system with H^+ extrusion in exchange for Na^+. Many cells also contain an electroneutral Cl^-/HCO_3^- antiport. The linkage of these two antiport systems could cause increased intracellular NaCl and alkaline pH. This pH regulation to alkalotic levels occurs at the expense of cell volume control. Alkaline pH shifts in ischemic brain might therefore be a marker of cellular edema.

There is increasing evidence that glia, which occupy one-third of the cellular element of the neocortex, behave differently from neurons in pH and volume regulation (Plum et al., 1985; Siesjö, 1985b; Kempski et al., 1988; Kraig et al., 1985; Kraig, 1989). Glial cells also possess antiport systems that can be activated by acidosis with an increase in cell volume and alkalinization. Glia can become alkaline during ischemia, thus confirming them as a major source of bicarbonate to the ischemic brain under normoglycemic conditions (Kraig et al., 1985). Noticeably under hyperglycemic conditions, the glial buffering capacity is more rapidly exhausted and infarction is more pronounced (Kraig, 1989). During reperfusion, glial acidosis, not alkalosis, was observed at a time of expected glial swelling (Kraig, 1989).

Because of the potential multifactorial causes of ischemic alkalosis, it is difficult to identify one mechanism as predominant in an in vivo investigation. Metabolic paralysis, cell death, and intracellular edema formation with equilibration of intracellular and extracellular HCO_3^- are most probably the major mechanisms in focal ischemic infarction in theory distinguishable by lack of high-energy phosphate recovery. From our studies, it is notable that some recovery of high-energy phosphates occurs in the majority of patients with ischemic alkalosis. This energy resynthesis could in fact be from other cellular elements such as endothelial new growth, macrophage invasion, and glial proliferation rather than neuronal recovery. For these reasons it will also be difficult to determine the activity of glial buffering mechanisms which produce intracellular alkalosis but which require ATP and intact membranes for effective functioning of the antiport systems. This does not detract from the significance of alkalosis as an event in ischemic progression or from attempts to identify the events with which it is associated. We hypothesize that, independent of mechanism, the acid-to-base shift in ischemic brain is a salutary event which could signify either the beginning of recovery or, more probably, cellular irrecoverability and, as such, may be a distinct marker of a particular stage in stroke evolution. Thus it has the potential to indicate a therapeutic window for cell protection as well as serve as a prognostic index.

3.1. Glucose Effects on pH in Focal Ischemia

It has been proposed that the severity of acidosis in the ischemic brain is dependent on the blood glucose concentration and brain glucose and glycogen stores, which, in turn, on the basis of experimental and clinical evidence, may dictate the neurological outcome (for a review, see Welch and Barkley [1986]). When glucose delivery to the brain is continued as a result of incomplete ischemia or during reflow, there is apparent further stimulation of glycolytic activity, which provides more metabolic acids at a time when the cell is already stressed to compensate for decreased pH. Myers and Yamaguchi (1976) were able to produce irreversible neurological deficit in the Rhesus monkey when lactate levels exceeded 25 μmol/g. Starvation of the animals increased their resistance to ischemia. As a corollary to these studies, pretreatment of cats with glucose prior to complete ischemia dramatically impaired the restitution of CBF and energy metabolism during the postischemic period; this has been attributed in part to tissue lactic acidosis (Chopp et al., 1987). On the other hand, hypoglycemia markedly attenuates ischemic brain acidosis, reduces infarct size, and decreases the ischemic neurological deficit (Chopp et al., 1988; Nedergaard and Diemer, 1989).

The clinical literature has suggested that neurological outcome is worsened by high systemic blood glucose levels at the time of hospital administration for stroke (Asplund *et al.*, 1980; Melamed, 1976; Pulsinelli *et al.*, 1980). This appears to be limited to nonlacunar anterior circulation infarcts (Mohr *et al.*, 1985; Adams *et al.*, 1988; Berger and Hakim, 1986; Cox and Lorains, 1986). Furthermore, it appears that blood glucose at the time of stroke onset, rather than a history of diabetes, is the critical factor (Cox and Lorains, 1986). Only one PET study, reported in abstract form, has correlated cerebral metabolic data with hyperglycemia and poor outcome (Nencini *et al.*, 1988). To date no studies have examined the value of controlling glucose levels in preventing progression of stroke, probably because of difficulty in using euglycemic techniques in clinical patients and the absence, heretofore, of methods for dynamically monitoring brain acidosis and its effects on energy metabolism. Accordingly, we examined the relationship of systemic glucose levels to energy metabolism.

Our patient group with acute focal cortical ischemia described above was studied. We found a significant negative correlation of blood glucose with brain pH (Table 3). Subgroup analysis of the acidotic and normal pH groups or both groups combined revealed additional significant negative correlations. There was, however, no correlation of blood glucose with pH in the alkalotic group. Furthermore, the hyperglycemic group (glucose > 145 mg%) showed a significant negative correlation with systemic glucose with pH, but the normoglycemic group did not. In the hyperglycemic group, but not in the normoglycemic group, there was a near-significant positive correlation between pH and the PCr/P_i ratio, but strongly significant relationships with P_i, PCr, and β-ATP; these data indicate an adverse influence of pH on energy metabolism (Table 4). In addition, strong correlations were found with PME and PDE; these data suggest that acidosis promotes phospholipid breakdown. Some of these relationships (P_1, PCr, β-ATP, PME, and PDE) were maintained in normoglycemic patients but at less significant levels.

Thus, we now have metabolic data in clinical patients to support the concept

TABLE 3. Correlation Coefficients
of Blood Glucose with Brain pH

Group	n	Correlation coefficient	Two-tailed P value
Total patients	28	−0.64	<0.001
Acidotic	10	−0.82	<0.004
Normal pH	5	−0.96	<0.001
Alkalotic	13	−0.11	>0.71
Hyperglycemic	10	−0.76	<0.02
Normoglycemic	18	−0.30	>0.22

TABLE 4. Relationship of pH with Energy and Phospholipid
Metabolism in Hyperglycemia and Normoglycemia

Parameter	High glucose ($n = 12$)		Low glucose ($n = 22$)	
	r	P value	r	P value
Glucose	−0.76	<0.02	−0.30	>0.22
PCr/P$_1$	0.62	>0.07	0.33	>0.21
P$_1$/TP	−0.84	<0.005	−0.62	<0.02
PCr/TP	0.66	<0.04	0.49	<0.05
β-ATP/TP	0.67	<0.04	0.47	<0.05
PME/TP	0.76	<0.02	0.43	>0.08
PDE/TP	0.83	<0.006	0.50	<0.04

that high systemic glucose levels contribute to brain acidosis and poor neurological outcome. These preliminary findings, although positive and encouraging, require the use of more subjects and more sophisticated techniques of volume localization in a more rapid time of total study. Regional measures through the ischemic focus should add further rewarding information.

4. ACUTE GLOBAL CEREBRAL ISCHEMIA

Cerebral acidosis plays an important role in the energy failure and poor neurological outcome after global ischemia in animal models and is profoundly influenced by systemic glucose levels (Welsh et al., 1980; Chopp et al., 1987, 1988). The common clinical problem of cardiac arrest and resuscitation provides the human model of complete global cerebral ischemia and reperfusion, the histopathology and metabolic features of which differ from focal ischemia (Petito, 1987; Siesjö et al., 1987). Unfortunately, despite the prevalent and serious clinical problem of anoxic ischemic encephalopathy after cardiac resuscitation, there is to date complete absence of any information on cerebral pH and energy metabolism in this condition. Nevertheless, we have now had the opportunity to compare and contrast the findings of acidosis and the acid-to-base pH "flip-flop" in focal ischemia with complete cerebral ischemia by studying patients after cardiac arrest.

To date, five patients (Mean age 70.5 ± 7 years) with severe postischemic anoxic encephalopathy after resuscitation have been studied. All were comatose and given artificial respiration. Initial spectroscopy was performed at 18 ± 4 hr and repeated at 67 ± 19 hr. The mean Glasgow coma scale was 3.6 ± 1.3 at the time of first spectroscopy. The mean serum glucose was 349 ± 107 mg/dl initially after resuscitation and 278 ± 107 and 184 ± 62 mg/dl at the times of initial and repeat spectroscopy, respectively. Arterial blood pH at the times of study was 7.46 ± 0.07 and 7.42 ± 0.07, respectively.

Of 18 pH readings from differing cortical regions in the five patients, 4 were less than 6.95 (mean 6.35 ± 0.10), 6 were normal (6.95 to 7.07), and 8 were greater than 7.07 (mean 7.16 ± 0.03). This alkalotic shift was already evident on initial spectroscopy. Every patient had at least one area of abnormal pH (alkalosis or acidosis or both). One patient with severe acidosis was clinically and electrophysiologically brain dead (Figure 5). This patient exhibited progression toward severe cerebral acidosis and complete energy failure. The other patient to exhibit brain acidosis had marked pH heterogeneity ranging from 6.24 to 7.19. Heterogeneity of changes in energy status was also apparent, ranging from relatively normal spectra to total absence of high-energy phosphates with only a solitary P_i peak remaining, as in Figure 5.

In summary, in all patients with global ischemia and reperfusion there was heterogeneity with respect to cerebral pH and energy metabolism. These findings are preliminary and require further accrual of numbers before any strong conclusions can be drawn. However, as in focal ischemia, alkalotic pH shifts continue to be a feature of ischemic brain injury, the significance and mechanisms of which remain to be established.

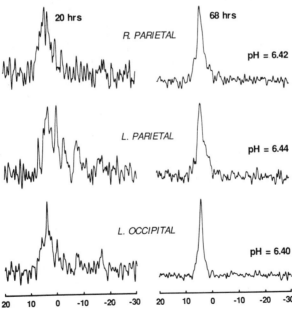

FIGURE 5. ^{31}P NMR spectra obtained from cortex of a patient with anoxic encephalopathy. Spectra serve to illustrate progression from some possibly discernible ^{31}P resonances to total obliteration of all peaks except P_i. At 68 hr the patient was clinically brain dead.

5. CONCLUSION

In summary, ischemic acidosis and subsequent acid-to-base pH "flip-flop," which have been documented previously in animal models of focal and complete ischemia, have now been seen in clinical stroke. The mechanisms and meaning of this acidosis and acid-to-base shift remain to be established in the clinical setting. The preliminary data obtained from our clinical studies suggest that the severity and duration of focal ischemic cerebral acidosis can predict the degree of energy metabolic damage, the extent of phospholipid breakdown, and the severity of neurological outcome. Furthermore, the data suggest that brain alkalosis represents a distinct stage in the evolution of ischemic infarction, with the timing of duration and degree of the acid-to-base pH "flip-flop" also possibly being dependent on the degree and duration of preceding brain acidosis. The probable multifactorial mechanisms of ischemic brain alkalosis appear related less to a combination of reparative cellular processes (including cell buffering) and more to reperfusion of ischemic brain, development of edema, and metabolic paralysis in view of alkalosis being related to a worse neurological outcome.

We have shown that systemic blood glucose levels influence brain intracellular pH in focal ischemia; hyperglycemia worsens and may prolong brain intracellular acidosis, resulting in further deterioration of energy phosphate and phospholipid metabolism. During ischemic alkalosis the influence of blood glucose is no longer seen. It remains to be seen whether the neurological outcome can be improved by control of systemic arterial blood glucose levels during the evolution of the stroke and whether the timing of the acid-to-base pH "flip-flop" provides a therapeutic window for judging the effectiveness of blood glucose control or cytoprotective pharmacotherapy in improvement of the neurological outcome.

ACKNOWLEDGMENTS

The work described in this report was support by Public Health Service grant NS23393 from the National Institutes of Health and by the American Heart Association of Michigan.

REFERENCES

Ackerman, J. J. H., Grove, T. H., Wong, G. G., Gadian, D. G., and Radda, G. K., 1980, Mapping of metabolites in whole animals by ^{31}P NMR using surface coils, *Nature* **283**:167–170.

Adams, H. P., Olinger, C., Marler, J. R., Biller, J., Brott, T. G., Barsan, W. G., and Banwalt, K., 1988, Comparison of admission serum glucose concentration with neurologic outcome in cerebral infarction, *Stroke* **19**:455–458.

Asplund, K., Hagg, E., and Helmers, C., 1980, The natural history of stroke in diabetic patients, *Acta Med. Scand.* **207**:417–424.

Atkinson, D. E., 1968, The energy change of the adenylate pool as a regulatory parameter, *Biochemistry* **7**:4030–4034.

Behar, K. L., den Hollander, J. A., Stromski, M. E., Ogino, T., Shulman, R. G., Petroff, O. A. C., and Prichard, J. W., 1983, High-resolution ¹H nuclear magnetic resonance study of cerebral hypoxia *in vivo*, *Proc. Natl. Acad. Sci. USA* **80**:4945–4948.

Berger, L., and Hakim, A. M., 1986, The association of hyperglycemia with cerebral edema in stroke, *Stroke* **17**:865–871.

Bottomley, P. A., Drayer, B. P., and Smith, L. S., 1986, Chronic adult cerebral infarction studied by phosphorous NMR spectroscopy, *Radiology* **160**:763–766.

Choi, M. U., and Abramson, M. B., 1978, Effects of pH changes and charge characteristics in the uptake of norepinephrine by synaptosomes of rat brain, *Biochim. Biophys. Acta* **540**:337–345.

Chopp, M., Frinak, S., Walton, D. R., Smith, M. B., and Welch, K. M. A., 1987, Intracellular acidosis during and after cerebral ischemia: In vivo nuclear magnetic resonance study of hyperglycemia in cats, *Stroke* **18**:919–923.

Chopp, M., Welch, K. M. A., Tidwell, C., and Helpern, J. A., 1988, Global cerebral ischemia and intracellular pH during hyperglycemia and hypoglycemia in the cat, *Stroke* **19**:1383–1387.

Cox, N. H., and Lorains, J. W., 1986, The prognostic value of blood glucose and glycosylated hemoglobin in patients with stroke, *Postgrad. Med. J.* **62**:7–10.

Degani, H., Laughlin, M., Campbell, S., and Shulman, R. G., 1984, Kinetics of creatine kinase in heart: A 31-P NMR saturation and inversion-transfer study, *Biochemistry* **24**:5510–5516.

Fishman, R. A., 1973, Brain edema, *N. Engl. J. Med.* **293**:706–711.

Gadian, D. B., 1982, "Nuclear Magnetic Resonance and its Application to Living Systems," Oxford University Press, Oxford, England.

Gadian, D. G., Radda, G. K., Richard, R. E., and Seeley, P. J., 1979, 31-P NMR in living tissue: The road from a promising to an important tool in biology, *in* "Biological Applications of Magnetic Resonance" (R. G. Shulman, ed.), pp. 463–535, Academic Press, New York.

Goldberg, N. D., Passonneau, J. V., and Lowry, O. H., 1986, Effects of changes in brain metabolism on the levels of critic acid cycle intermediates, *J. Biol. Chem.* **241**:3997–3402.

Gordon, R. E., Hanley, P. E., Shaw, D., Gadian, D. G., Radda, G. K., Stout, P., Bore, P. J., and Chan, L., 1980, Localization of metabolites in animals using 31-P topical magnetic resonance, *Nature* **287**:736–738.

Gordon, R. E., Hanley, P. E., and Shaw, D., 1982, Topical magnetic resonance, *Prog. NMR Spectrosc.* **15**:1–47.

Hakim, A. M., Pokrupa, R. P., Villanueva, J., Diksic, M., Evans, A. C., Thompson, C. J., Meyer, E., Yamamoto, Y. L., and Feindel, W. H., 1987, The effect of spontaneous reperfusion on metabolic function in early human cerebral infarcts, *Ann. Neurol.* **21**:279–289.

Hope, P. L., Costello, A. M., Cady, E. B., Delpy, D. T., Tofts, P. S., Chu, A., Hamilton, P. A., Reynolds, E. O. R., and Wilkie, D. R., 1984, Cerebral energy metabolism studied with phosphorous NMR spectroscopy in normal and birth-asphyxiated infants, *Lancet* **ii**:366–370.

Horikawa, Y., Naruse, S., Tanaka, C., Kimiyoshi, H., and Nishikawa, H., 1986, Proton NMR relaxation times in ischemic brain edema, *Stroke* **17**:1149–1151.

Jacobson, K., and Cohen, J. S., 1981, Improved technique for investigation of cell metabolism by 31-P NMR spectroscopy, *Biosci. Rep.* **1**:141–150.

Kempski, O., Staub, F., Jansen, M., Schodel, F., and Baethmann, A., 1988, Glial swelling during extracellular acidosis *in vitro*, *Stroke* **19**:386–392.

Kogure, K., Busto, R., Schwartzman, R. J., and Scheinberg, P., 1980, The dissociation of cerebral blood flow, metabolism, and function in the early stages of developing cerebral infarction, *Ann. Neurol.* **8**:278–290.

Kraig, R. P., 1989, Interrelation of glial pH to ischemic brain edema, *in* "Proceedings from the 16th Princeton-Williamsburg Conference," *Stroke.*

Kraig, R. P., Pulsinelli, W. A., and Plum, F., 1985, Behavior of brain bicarbonate ions during complete ischemia, *J. Cereb. Blood Flow Metab.* **5:**S227–S228.

Kraig, R. P., Pulsinelli, W. A., and Plum, F., 1986, Heterogeneous distribution of hydrogen and bicarbonate ions during complete brain ischemia, *Prog. Brain Res.* **63:**155–156.

Kuschinsky, W., and Wahl, M., 1978, Local chemical and neurogenic regulation of cerebral vascular resistance, *Physiol. Rev.* **58:**656–689.

Kwee, I. L., and Nakada, T., 1988, Phospholipid profile of the human brain: 31-P NMR spectroscopic study, *Magn. Res. Med.* **6:**296–299.

Levine, S. R., Welch, K. M. A., Bruce, R., and Smith, M. B., 1987, Brain intracellular pH "flip-flop" in human ischemic stroke identified by ^{31}P NMR, *Ann. Neurol.* **22:**137.

Levine, S. R., Welch, K. M. A., Dietrich, K., and Helpern, J. A., 1988a, Regional heterogeneity of brain pH and phosphate metabolism in early humans stroke, *Ann. Neurol.* **24:**128.

Levine, S. R., Welch, K. M. A., Helpern, J. A., Chopp, M., Bruce, R., Selwa, J., and Smith, M. B., 1988b, Prolonged deterioration of ischemic brain energy metabolism and acidosis association with hyperglycemia. Human cerebral infarction studied by serial 31-P NMR spectroscopy, *Ann. Neurol.* **23:**416–418.

Lowry, O. H., and Passonneau, J. V., 1964, The relationship between substrates and enzymes of glycolysis in brain, *J. Biol. Chem.* **239:**31–42.

Lund-Anderson, H., 1979, Transport of glucose from blood to brain, *Physiol. Rev.* **59:**305–352.

Mabe, H., Blomqvist, P., and Siesjö, B. K., 1983, Intracellular pH in the brain following transient ischemia, *J. Cereb. Blood Flow Metab.* **3:**109–114.

Mayevsky, A., Nioka, S., Subramanian, V. H., and Chance, B., 1988, Brain oxidative metabolism of the newborn dog—correlation between 31-P NMR spectroscopy and pyridine nucleotide redox state, *J. Cereb. Blood Flow Metab.* **8:**201–207.

McMillan, V., and Siesjö, B. K., 1983, The effect of phenobarbital anesthesia upon some organic phosphates, glycolytic metabolites and citric acid cycle-associated intermediates of the rat brain, *J. Neurochem.* **20:**1669–1681.

Melamed, E., 1976. Reactive hyperglycemia in patients with acute stroke, *J. Neurol. Sci.* **29:**267–275.

Michenfelder, J. D., and Theye, R. A., 1979, The effects of anesthesia and hypothermia on canine cerebral ATP and lactate during anoxia produced by decapitation, *Anesthesiology* **33:**430.

Mitchell, P., 1961, Coupling of phosphorylation to electron and hydrogen transfer by a chemi-osmotic type of mechanism, *Nature* **191:**144–148.

Mohr, J. P., Rubenstein, L. V., Tatemichi, T. K., Nichols, F. T., Caplan, L. R., Hier, D. B., Kase, C. S., Price, T. R., and Wolf, P. A., 1985, Blood sugar and acute stroke: the NINCDS pilot stroke data bank, *Stroke* **16:**143.

Moon, R. G., and Richards, J. H., 1973, Determination of intracellular pH by 31-P magnetic resonance, *J. Biol. Chem.* **248:**7276–7278.

Myers, R. E., and Yamaguchi, M., 1976, Tissue lactate accumulation as cause of cerebral edema, *Neurosci. Abstr.* **2:**1042.

Nedergaard, M., and Diemer, N. H., 1989, Hypoglycemia reduces infarct size in experimental focal cerebral ischemia, *in* "Proceedings from the 16th Princeton-Williamsburg Conference," *Stroke.*

Nencini, P., Kushner, M., Reivich, M., Chawluk, J. B., Zimmerman, M., Rango, M., Jamieson, D. G., and Alavi, A., 1988, Hyperglycemia and metabolism in cerebral infarction, *Neurology* **38:**368.

Nunnally, R. L., and Hollis, D. P., 1970, Adenosine triphosphate compartmentation in living hearts: A phosphorous NMR saturation transfer study, *Biochemistry* **18:**3642–3646.

Paschen, W., Sato, W., Pawlik, G., Umbach, C., and Heiss, W.-D., 1985, Neurologic deficit, blood flow and biochemical sequelae of reversible focal cerebral ischemia in cats, *J. Neurol. Sci.* **68:**119–134.

Pelligrino, D., and Siesjö, B. K., 1981, Regulation of extra- and intracellular pH in the brain in severe hypoglycemia, *J. Cereb. Blood Flow Metab.* **1:**85–96.

Petito, C. K., 1987, Post ischemic transformation of perineuronal glial cells, *in* "Cerebrovascular Diseases" (M. E. Raichle and W. J. Powers, eds.), pp. 103–106, Raven Press, New York.

Petroff, O. A. C., Prichard, J. W., Behar, K. L., Alger, J. R., den Hollender, J. A., and Shullman, R. G., 1985, Cerebral intracellular pH by 31-P NMR spectroscopy, *Neurology* **35:**781–788.

Pettegrew, J. W., Kopp, S. J., Dadok, J., Minshew, N. J., Feliksik, J. M., Glonek, T., and Cohen, M. M., 1986, Chemical characterization of a prominent phosphomonoester resonance from mammalian brain. 31-P and 1-H NMR analysis at 4.7 and 14.1 Tesla, *J. Magn. Reson.* **67:**443–450.

Pettegrew, J. W., Kopp, S. J., Minshew, N. J., Glonek, T., Feliksik, B. C., Tow, J. P., and Cohen, M. M., 1987, ^{31}P nuclear magnetic resonance studies of phosphoglyceride metabolism in developing and degenerating brain: Preliminary observations, *J. Neuropathol. Exp. Neurol.* **46:**419–430.

Plum, F., Cooper, A. J. L., Kraig, R. P., Petito, C. K., and Pulsinelli, W. A., 1985, Glial cells: The silent partners of the working brain, *J. Cereb. Blood Flow Metab.* **5:**S1–S4.

Prichard, J. W., Alger, J. R., Behar, K. L., Petroff, O. A. C., and Shulman, R. G., 1983, Cerebral metabolic studies in vivo by 31-P NMR, *Proc. Natl. Acad. Sci. USA* **80:**2748–2751.

Pulsinelli, W., Sigsbee, B., Waldman, S., Rawlinson, D., Scherer, P., and Plum, G., 1980, Experimental hyperglycemia and diabetes mellitus worsen stroke outcome, *Ann. Neurol.* **8:**91.

Radda, G. K., 1986, The use of NMR spectroscopy for the understanding of disease, *Science* **233:** 640–645.

Roberts, J. K. M., Wade-Jardetzky, N., and Jardetzky, O., 1981, Intracellular pH measurements by 31-P NMR. Influence of factors other than pH on 31-P chemical shifts, *Biochemistry* **20:**5389–5394.

Shoubridge, E. A., Briggs, R. W., and Radda, G. K., 1982, 31-P NMR saturation transfer measurements of the steady state rates of creatine kinase and ATP synthetase in the rat brain, *FEBS Lett.* **140:**288–292.

Siesjö, B. K., 1978, "Brain Energy and Metabolism," pp. 327–329, John Wiley & Sons, New York.

Siesjö, B. K., 1981, Cell damage in the brain: A speculative synthesis, *J. Cereb. Blood Flow Metab.* **1:** 155–185.

Siesjö, B. K., 1985a, Acidosis and brain damage: Possible molecular mechanisms, *J. Cereb. Blood Flow Metab.* **5:**S225–S226.

Siesjö, B. K., 1985b, Acid-base homeostasis in the brain: Physiology, chemistry, and neurochemical pathology, *Prog. Brain Res.* **63:**121–154.

Siesjö, B. K., Smith, M. L., and Warner, D. S., 1987, Acidosis and ischemic brain damage, *in* "Cerebrovascular Disease" (M. E. Raichle and W. J. Powers, eds.), pp. 83–95, Raven Press, New York.

Syrota, A., Samson, Y., Boullais, C., Wajnberg, P., Loc'h, C., Crouzel, C., Maziere, B., Soussaline, F., and Baron, J. C., 1985, Tomographic mapping of brain intracellular pH and extracellular water space in stroke patients, *J. Cereb. Blood Flow Metab.* **5:**358–368.

Wanke, E., Carbone, E., and Testa, P. L., 1979, K^+ conductance modified by a titratable group accessible to protons from the intracellular side of the squid axon membrane, *Biophys. J.* **26:** 319–324.

Welch, K. M. A., and Barkley, G. L., 1986, Biochemistry and pharmacology of cerebral ischemia, *in* "Stroke, Pathophysiology, Diagnosis and Management" (J. M. Barnett, J. P. Mohr, B. M. Stein, and F. M. Yatsu, eds.), pp. 75–90, Churchill-Livingstone, New York.

Welch, K. M. A., Helpern, J. A., Robertson, W. M., and Ewing, J. R., 1985, ^{31}P topical magnetic resonance measurement of high energy phosphates in normal and infarcted brain, *Stroke* **16:**151.

Welsh, F. A., Ginsberg, M. D., and Rieder, W., 1980, Deleterious effect of glucose pretreatment on recovery from diffuse cerebral ischemia in the cat, *Stroke* **11:**355–363.

Yoshida, S., Busto, R., Martinez, E., and Ginsberg, M. D., 1985, Regional energy metabolism after complete versus incomplete cerebral ischemia in the absence of severe lactic acidosis, *J. Cereb. Blood Flow Metab.* **5:**490–501.

INDEX

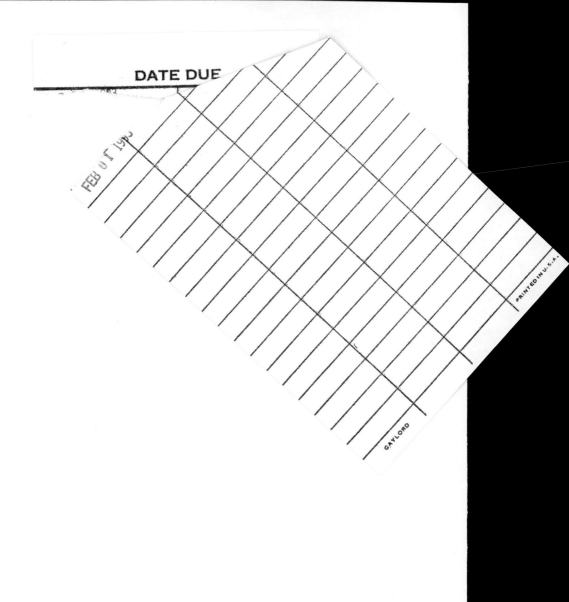

DATE DUE

FEB 07 1983

GAYLORD   PRINTED IN U.S.A.